NEW YORK SCHOOL OF REGIONAL ANESTHESIA

PERIPHERAL NERVE BLOCKS

PRINCIPLES AND PRACTICE

NEW YORK SCHOOL OF REGIONAL ANESTHESIA

PERIPHERAL NERVE BLOCKS

PRINCIPLES AND PRACTICE

ADMIR HADŽIĆ, MD, PHD

Associate Professor of Clinical Anesthesiology
College of Physicians and Surgeons
Columbia University
Director of Regional Anesthesia
Department of Anesthesiology
St. Luke's—Roosevelt Hospital Center
New York, New York

JERRY D. VLOKA, MD, PHD

Associate Professor of Anesthesiology
College of Physicians and Surgeons
Columbia University
Department of Anesthesiology
St. Luke's—Roosevelt Hospital Center
New York, New York

McGRAW-HILL

PROFESSIONAL

New York / Chicago / San Francisco / Lisbon / London / Madrid / Mexico City / Milan
New Delhi / San Juan / Seoul / Singapore / Sydney / Toronto

Copyright © 2004 by The McGraw-Hill Companies, Inc. All rights
reserved. Printed in China. Except as permitted under the United
States Copyright Act of 1976, no part of this publication may be
reproduced or distributed in any form or by any means, or stored
in a data base or retrieval system, without the prior written permission of the authors and publisher.

4567890 CTP CTP 09876

ISBN-13: 978-0-07-140918-6
ISBN-10: 0-07-140918-1

This book was set in New Aster by Parallelogram Graphics.
The editors were James Shanahan and Karen G. Edmonson.
The production supervisor was Catherine H. Saggese.
The text designer was Marsha Cohen.
The cover designer was Jeannet Leenderte.
The indexer was Pamela J. Edwards.
China Translation & Printing Services Ltd was printer and binder.

This book is printed on acid-free paper.

CIP information on file with publisher.

Dedication

We dedicate this book to our colleagues
and to the patients who have touched our personal and professional lives.
They have influenced our thoughts and enthusiasm for
regional anesthesia as articulated in this book.
JERRY D. VLOKA AND ADMIR HADŽIĆ

I dedicate this book to my wife, Margot,
and my children Caroline and Alexander.
Their love, support, and encouragement have made this book possible.
I extend my gratitude to my best friend, Admir Hadžić,
with whom years of academic pursuit seem like years of endless discovery.
JERRY D. VLOKA

To Gorica, Alen, Dennis,
my parents Junuz and Safeta, and my sister Admira,
with undying love.
ADMIR HADŽIĆ

CONTENTS

FOREWORD

All around the world, interest in regional anesthesia is growing rapidly. Many anesthesiologists recognize the numerous benefits of regional anesthesia for their patients and their practices. This textbook is the work of two remarkable individuals who have dedicated their professional lives to the practice, investigation, and teaching of regional anesthesia.

Jerry Vloka, MD, PhD, and Admir Hadžić MD, PhD, both acquired their medical education in Europe. After migrating to the United States, they completed their postgraduate education as residents in anesthesiology at the Department of Anesthesiology of St. Luke's–Roosevelt Hospital Center, New York. The two anesthesiologists rapidly recognized a common passion for regional anesthesia and began a successful professional association dedicated to its art. In addition to being superb clinicians, Jerry and Admir are recognized as accomplished creative investigators. This recognition stems from their exceptional dedication to the study of the relationship between the anatomy and physiology of peripheral nerves and regional anesthesia. In a number of cadaver models, they have elucidated the anatomy of the nerves of the upper and lower extremities, particularly as it concerns neuronal blockade. The relation between the functional regional anatomy and its clinical applications had been poorly defined, yet it is crucial in the clinical practice of peripheral neural blockade. Their anatomic findings have also allowed them to devise a number of modern, highly reliable approaches to neuronal blockade of the peripheral extremities. Many of their observations have been made available to the medical community through their publications in peer-reviewed journals and their popular, award-winning Web site www.nysora.com.

This book compiles the detailed knowledge and broad clinical experience of its two authors. The clarity and quality of this presentation reflects the authors' boundless energy and infectious enthusiasm for the teaching of peripheral nerve blocks. No reader will remain indifferent to the clear, systematic manner in which successful techniques for peripheral blockade are described. The neophyte as well as the experienced practitioner will find pearls that will facilitate their performance of peripheral nerve blocks and will be amazed by the quality of the book's illustrations.

The reader of this book will not remain indifferent to the message of its authors: An active regional anesthesia practice by well-trained practitioners benefits patients and enhances operating room efficiency. The learning of peripheral nerve blocks requires dedication, just like any other field of medicine. However, once the anatomic, pharmacologic, and technical principles of peripheral nerve blockade are well understood, nerve blocks can reliably and easily be applied with predictable success. Each step toward success is exquisitely described and illustrated in the book.

Many anesthesia residency programs lack the necessary training to successfully prepare their graduates for an active practice of peripheral nerve blocks. This textbook, however, will be of great aid and service to all such programs. For making the study of regional anesthesia accessible and fun, Jerry Vloka and Admir Hadžić deserve the gratitude and admiration of every anesthesiologist. They decidedly have earned mine.

Daniel M. Thys, MD

GOAL

The goal of this book is to provide the most accurate and practical instructional teaching text of peripheral nerve block procedures possible in a book format.

Many physicians believe that regional anesthesia is an "art". We have committed our professional lives, countless hours of research, and this book to prove the opposite, that regional anesthesia is an exact, objective science and not the privilege of a few "artistically inclined" clinicians. With proper training, equipment, and determination, every clinician can successfully and reproducibly implement peripheral nerve blocks in his or her practice.

Rationale

Many texts on nerve blocks are multiauthored and provide an encyclopedic review of a multitude of nerve block techniques and their modifications. In contrast, we wanted to create a highly didactic, consistent and detailed book that focused only on highly effective, reliable, and well-defined nerve block techniques. Although the primary focus of this book is on nerve blocks used for surgical anesthesia, the same techniques can be applied in pain management with the appropriate modification of local anesthetic agents, volumes, and concentrations.

New York School of Regional Anesthesia

The New York School of Regional Anesthesia (NYSORA) is an educational program in regional anesthesia founded by Drs. Jerry D. Vloka and Admir Hadžić in 1996 (www.nysora.com). One of the main goals of NYSORA, in its educational mission, is to transition regional anesthesia from an "art," as few clinicians view it, to a more objective, defined, exacting clinical discipline. The educational program content is the result of our clinical research and research on functional regional anesthesia anatomy in human cadaver models. The techniques taught by NYSORA feature precise, logical descriptions of regional anesthesia procedures. This approach is without a doubt the reason that NYSORA enjoys enormous popularity today. Since its creation, the NYSORA Web site has evolved into a standard teaching tool in many residency training programs throughout the world. With its current weekly readership of 6,000, it stands out as a leader in education in regional anesthesia.

Choice of Techniques

Readers with experience in regional anesthesia may quickly notice the omission of some common nerve block techniques. In particular, we omitted strictly "pain block" techniques and procedures that rely on subjective end points such as "feel," "pops," and paresthesia. In preparation for this book, we used our departmental computerized anesthesia record-keeping system to compile a database of all peripheral nerve blocks performed for surgical anesthesia at St. Luke's–Roosevelt Hospital Center over a 3-year period. After analyzing this large database, we selected only those nerve block procedures that were frequently and successfully performed during the specified period. Risking the possibility that such exclusion may result in some shortfalls, we felt that clinicians, instructors, and trainees in need of this book would be best served if we focused on techniques which are associated with a high success rate and reproducibility. Indeed, those who master the techniques described in this book will acquire an impressive set of skills necessary to practice a full scope of peripheral nerve blocks.

Authenticity

In our quest to present the most practical, real-life text possible, one of the principles guiding the development of this book was that all images and technique descriptions had to show real patients. Hence, almost all the photographs demonstrating block techniques and landmarks are of patients who successfully underwent the described procedures. To provide a real-life tutorial, wherever possible we have used anatomic descriptions, landmarks, technique details, and troubleshooting illustrations for the same patient. In addition, numerous original illustrations are included with specific block techniques to emphasize important anatomic and technical principles.

Organization of the Technique Descriptions

The New York School of Regional Anesthesia Peripheral Nerve Blocks Teaching Manual opens each block section with "Block at a Glance," which lists the most important, salient features of the block. This section is meant to serve as a "flash card" for quick memory refreshment before beginning the block procedure. An indication of the complexity level, based on the NYSORA classification of regional anesthesia procedures, is given as a general guide for teachers and students. The next section is a general description of the block technique that provides the reader with an idea of the philosophy and applicability of the technique.

The description of the anatomy focuses primarily on the specific anatomic aspects of relevance to performance of the technique rather than on a distracting, exhaustive listing of dry anatomic facts. To prepare for this part of the book, we searched our digital library, which houses more than 10,000 original anatomic and clinical videos and still images that we have compiled over the years. The video images were studied to demonstrate important technical aspects and highlight common mistakes of our trainees. This information was used to provide numerous technical pearls and "tips" to avoid common errors.

In addition to the anatomic landmarks for each block, we have also included surface landmarks. While this may at first seem superfluous, we felt that this feature would better orient students to the surface anatomy clues, thus leading to more accurate identification of landmarks. Although there are many surface landmarks that can be helpful, we limited the anatomic landmarks to *three* in order to simplify retention and performance of the blocks.

In the description of the techniques, we attempted to provide the most detailed, richly illustrated, methodical description of the block procedure possible. In particular, step-by-step, itemized instructions are provided for situations where the anticipated responses to nerve stimulation are not obtained. Most of these troubleshooting principles are also applicable to the continuous block technique. Some anatomic and technical points have necessarily been repeated due to the similarity between the single-injection and continuous block techniques; however, we feel that this was necessary in order to accurately and vividly emphasize the differences between the two.

A table of commonly used local anesthetics specific to the block is included in every chapter because block duration may vary among different block techniques even when the same local anesthetic is used. The information provided in these tables includes only the local anesthetics and concentrations that we use in our practice or those well-documented in peer-reviewed, published information. A considerable degree of variability may also be present as a result of interpatient variability and differences in block quality achieved. It should be kept in mind that the described block procedures and doses are for adult patients.

A section on block dynamics and perioperative management has been added to provide readers with some general expectations regarding block onset and distribution, as well as suggestions for successful perioperative management. Potential complications associated with each technique, information on their incidence, and clear, specific instructions on how to decrease the risks are also included.

For clarity, we refrained from using sterile drapes to better illustrate the anatomy and planes of needle insertion. In actual practice, clear drapes, sterile towels, and other principles of aseptic techniques should be strictly adhered to.

Where to Go From Here

Readers with less experience with peripheral nerve blocks should start at the beginning of the book and focus on the basic concepts of regional anesthesia anatomy, neuronal blockade, pharmacology of local anesthetics, and equipment. A certain level of basic training is a prerequisite for successful learning of all highly specialized anesthesia procedures (e.g., fiberoptic intubation, invasive monitoring, lung separation, and transesophageal echocardiography). Similarly, in our residency/fellowship program at St. Luke's–Roosevelt Hospital Center, the teaching of advanced nerve block procedures is reserved primarily for the more senior residents who are already experienced in basic regional anesthesia techniques.

Regardless of what method the reader uses to study peripheral nerve blocks, we are convinced that he or she will enjoy browsing through this book. We present a compendium of 20 years of combined clinical experience and countless hours of anatomic and clinical studies to bridge the gap between the "art" and science of the practice of nerve blocks in the most practical book format possible. As a result, we believe that we have created a uniquely practical, pertinent, anatomically logical text for generations of students of regional anesthesia.

ACKNOWLEDGMENTS

We extend our appreciation to all the staff anesthesiologists and surgeons, residents, regional anesthesia fellows, and research students at St. Luke's–Roosevelt Hospital Center, New York. We would like to acknowledge Nino and Lejla Hadžić as well as Richard Claudio for their contributions of time and artistic talent to the New York School of Regional Anesthesia (NYSORA) and to this book. Special thanks to Drs. Emine Karaca, Marina Yufa, Alex Visan, Alan Santos, Beklen Kerimoglu, Henri Shih, Aurimas Knepa, Jonathan Koenigsamen, Shruti Shah, Robert Mulcare, Kevin Sanborn and Paul Hobeika for their help in the preparation of this book. We also thank the Department Chairman, Dr. Daniel Thys. His support and encouragement, wisdom, and exemplary leadership allowed us to accomplish all that we have. Finally, we thank all our colleagues and visiting trainees at our Center of Excellence in Regional Anesthesia, whose many requests for the NYSORA book, inspired us to write this text. Finally, we would like to thank Lejla Hadžić for the outstanding work in creating the illustrations for this book.

Admir Hadžić
Jerry D. Vloka

1 TRAINING
IN PERIPHERAL NERVE BLOCKS

Peripheral nerve blocks are cost-effective anesthetic techniques used to provide superb anesthesia and analgesia while avoiding airway instrumentation and the hemodynamic consequences of general and neuraxial anesthesia. Patient satisfaction, a growing demand for cost-effective anesthesia, and a favorable postoperative recovery profile have resulted in an increasing demand for regional anesthesia. Although there are relatively few published reports of serious complications associated with the use of peripheral nerve blocks, the risk of complications is real and the consequences can be catastrophic. Therefore, just as with any other medical procedure, proper training is a prerequisite for the safe, successful implementation of nerve blocks. Indeed, the complications commonly associated with the use of regional anesthesia are often attributed to a lack of appropriate training and exposure to proper techniques during the residency training program. In this chapter, we outline the current training requirements in regional anesthesia in the United States, discuss their drawbacks, and suggest a model for a more structured, effective training.

Current Training Requirements in Regional Anesthesia

Anesthesiology education has seen several changes in the past decade. A third year of training in clinical anesthesia has been added, and significant emphasis is now placed on the development of and training in anesthesiology subspecialties such as cardiothoracic anesthesia, obstetric anesthesia, neuroanesthesia, ambulatory anesthesia, and pain management. Similarly, the subspecialty of regional anesthesia is undergoing a renaissance. The number of high-quality scientific publications on regional anesthesia has grown significantly over the past decade, and new techniques and procedures have been introduced. There has also been a remarkable increase in awareness of the advantages of regional anesthesia in a wide variety of clinical situations. However, although the ASA Residency Review Committee (RRC) clearly specifies the training requirements for spinal and epidural anesthesia (50 epidural anesthetic procedures, 50 spinal anesthetic procedures), the current recommendations for training in peripheral nerve blocks remain vague. These recommendations suggest that to achieve clinical competency, a trainee must perform 40 peripheral nerve blocks for surgical anesthesia and 25 for pain management. These suggestions do not specify which blocks should be included in a core curriculum of training in anesthesia, therefore, it is nearly impossible to ensure that residents graduating from different programs will have comparable degrees of expertise in all nerve block procedures. For instance, if a resident performed each of the approximately 34 block techniques listed in **Table 1.1** with equal frequency (2 blocks in each technique), he or she would actually surpass the RRC training recommendations but still would not have mastered any of the techniques specified.

Do All Residency Programs Provide Similar Exposure to Regional Anesthesia?

There is ample evidence that current training in regional anesthesia leaves residents unprepared to implement the full breadth of regional anesthesia techniques. Almost two decades ago, it was suggested that large discrepancies existed among training programs (2.8% to 55.7% of total delivered anesthetics) in the use of regional anesthesia and that some anesthesiology residency programs failed to teach regional anesthesia adequately. A report in 1993 claimed that the overall use of regional anesthesia had increased to almost 30%; however, the disparity among teaching programs persists. Several surveys of residents conducted nationally and internationally have established that the number of peripheral nerve blocks performed during a residency is limited and that residents lack confidence in their ability to perform such procedures. A survey of exposure to regional anesthesia techniques indicated that 51%, 62%, and 75% of graduating residents may not be confident in performing interscalene, femoral, and sciatic blocks, respectively. These results are not surprising, as the survey also indicated that the residents surveyed had performed 5 or fewer of each type of block by the end of their residency training. Currently, there are more than 40 widely accepted peripheral nerve block procedures. It is unlikely that the exposure of trainees during their residency training program is sufficient to achieve clinical competency in all regional anesthesia procedures, particularly in specific peripheral nerve blocks. Unfortunately, there is still little guidance for instructors on how to teach modern regional anesthesia techniques and insufficient research on the educational methods directly relevant to postgraduate training in anesthesia.

How Many Procedures Are Needed for Clinical Competency?

Completion of an approved residency training program is generally accepted to indicate that a graduate possesses the skills and knowledge required to deliver state-of-the art, high-quality anesthesia care. However, whereas the American Board of Anesthesiology examination assesses the theoretical knowledge of graduates, objective grading of their procedural skills is lacking. Such a grading system has been recommended for epidural anesthesia, and subjective criteria have been proposed to foster the cognitive and noncognitive maturation of residents. Two recent studies suggested that 60 to 90 procedures may be required before epidural anesthesia is mastered and a sufficiently high success rate is attained. A study by Kopacz et al claimed that for the attainment and maintenance of a 90% success rate, 45 and 60 attempts at spinal and epidural anesthesia are required, respectively. It seems unrealistic to suggest that trainees can acquire equal proficiency by performing fewer peripheral nerve block procedures, which are often much more complex than those of neuraxial anesthesia.

The learning curve and the number of procedures required before adequate technical skill is achieved have been the subject of studies in other medical disciplines. For example, Cass et al concluded that performance of an initial supervised 50 gastrointestinal endoscopies and of a subsequent 100 upper and lower gastrointestinal endoscopies is necessary to achieve clinical competence (defined as a 90% success rate). Family practice residents and untrained family practitioners have been shown to require 25 supervised attempts at performing flexible fiberoptic sigmoidoscopy to attain proficiency comparable with that of experienced practitioners. Duong and Havel concluded that 20 to 30 cases are required to achieve satisfactory skill in managing anesthesia in cardiac patients. Many experts agree that after performing only 30 endotracheal intubations by the conclusion of a residency program, few residents are adequately trained to perform intubations with an acceptable degree of safety and reliability. Therefore, it is quite clear that current training recommendations do not translate into a guarantee that anesthesiology graduates have acquired sufficient expertise in regional anesthesia procedures, particularly in peripheral nerve blocks.

Problems With Assessment of Attained Training

Defining the end points that qualify an anesthesiologist as competent in the performance of regional anesthesia techniques is difficult. An indication of the difficulty of learning these techniques is the finding of Kopacz et al that each trainee should be required to perform at least 45 spinal and 60 epidural anesthetic procedures to achieve competency (i.e. a 90% success rate). No existing methods can reliably predict eventual performance of the skills required in anesthesiology, and such assessments of technical performance are often unreliable at best. Whereas written in-training examinations are reliable in assessing a resident's fundamental knowledge of anesthesiology principles, they are obviously inadequate for assessing practical skills. The current American Board of Anesthesiology method of logging the number of procedures performed (in-training reports) ignores the assessment of quality. Simply performing a given procedure a certain number of times does not ensure that the procedure has been learned or performed well. Direct observation without established criteria, currently used in many training programs, clearly lacks reliability.

How Can We Improve Training in Regional Anesthesia?

The teaching of regional anesthesia should ideally consist of a multifaceted approach and, in addition to clinical mentoring, should include didactic lessons, training on mannequins, workshops on live models, and perhaps even theater-type simulations.

Selection of Nerve Block Techniques

One of the most confusing issues in the training of regional anesthesia is selection of the nerve block techniques to be included in the training curriculum. In recent years, there has been a plethora of publications introducing new techniques, approaches, and modifications of the classic techniques. Even abbreviated atlases of peripheral nerve block procedures describe more than 40 different techniques (excluding various modifications). In our teaching program, nerve block procedures are divided into three groups according to difficulty of performance, time required to master them, and potential for complications **(Tables 1.1 and 1.2).** To avoid the confusion that inevitably arises when introducing several advanced or alternative techniques, the residents in our program are first taught an essential core of peripheral nerve block techniques (basic nerve block techniques). The teaching of these procedures at our institution is facilitated by the fact that most faculty members have adopted "standard" nerve block techniques, as on the New York School of Regional Anesthesia (NYSORA) Web site (www.nysora.com). Thus, our trainees are repeatedly exposed to consistent techniques, which facilitates retention of knowledge of the landmarks, drugs, dosages, equipment, and other block procedures. On the basis of our experience, adherence to these principles ensures that all residents perform at least 10 to 20 procedures for each basic nerve block technique by the end of their residency, which translates into clinical competency in performing basic nerve blocks. Our residents perform between 150 and 300 nerve block procedures by the end of their residency training which makes them capable of performing peripheral nerve blocks for a wide spectrum of surgical indications.

Regional Anesthesia Rotation

In the regional anesthesia training model at St. Luke's–Roosevelt Hospital, New York, residents are required to master basic nerve block techniques during the first 2 years of clinical training **(Table 1.1).** Sizable orthopedic, hand, foot, and vascular surgery volumes, combined with the routine use of regional anesthesia for a majority of these procedures, allow a sufficient number of these procedures for residents to achieve adequate proficiency in basic regional anesthesia techniques during the CA-1 and CA-2 years. As the entire staff is competent in performing most basic and many intermediate block techniques by the time they reach their senior year of training, most trainees become proficient in the use of basic techniques, the pharmacology of local anesthetics, and the principles of nerve stimulation.

TABLE 1.1
New York School of Regional Anesthesia Classification of Regional Anesthesia Procedures

BASIC	INTERMEDIATE	ADVANCED
Superficial cervical plexus block	Deep cervical plexus block	Continuous interscalene brachial plexus block
Axillary brachial plexus block	Interscalene block	Continuous infraclavicular brachial plexus block
Intravenous regional block (Bier block)	Supraclavicular interscalene block	Thoracic paravertebral block: single-injection, continuous
Wrist block	Infraclavicular brachial plexus block	Thoracolumbar paravertebral block
Digital nerve block	Sciatic nerve block: posterior approach	Combined lumbar plexus/sciatic blocks
Genitofemoral block	Femoral nerve block	Lumbar plexus block
Saphenous block	Popliteal block: intertendinous, lateral, and lithotomy approaches	Continuous femoral nerve block
Ankle block		Sciatic nerve block: anterior approach
Spinal anesthesia		Anterior sciatic nerve block: parafemoral technique
Epidural anesthesia		Obturator block
Combined spinal/epidural anesthesia		Continuous sciatic block: posterior approach Continuous popliteal nerve block: intertendinous and lateral approaches

Senior residents in their last year of training are then assigned to a 2-month rotation in advanced regional anesthesia, during which time they are instructed primarily in intermediate and advanced regional anesthesia techniques (e.g. lumbar plexus blocks, continuous blocks). We find that concentrated training in regional anesthesia during a designated month is much more effective in our setting than the daily "designated block resident" model. The main disadvantage of "nerve block rotation" is the lack of the continuity of care which prevents the resident who performs the blocks from participating in administration of the regional anesthetic from beginning to end. However, it is the perioperative (especially intraoperative) management that largely determines the success of any regional anesthetic.

TABLE 1.2

New York School of Regional Anesthesia Classification of Regional Anesthesia Procedures: Definitions

Basic	• Technically easy to perform, have a low risk of complications, and have wide clinical applicability. Ample expertise is present in most residency programs to allow the adequate training of residents. These procedures should be part of the armamentarium of every practicing anesthesiologist.
Intermediate	• Complexity and potential for complications is greater than for basic block techniques. These procedures are best mastered by spending 1–2 mo in a well-structured, mentored elective peripheral nerve block rotation during residency training or with a fellowship in regional anesthesia.
Advanced	• Highly specialized procedures, most of which require significant expertise in basic and intermediate nerve block procedures for their implementation. Advanced nerve block techniques are either deeper nerve blocks or blocks that require more specialized equipment and/or the insertion of indwelling catheters for continuous infusion of local anesthetic. These procedures can be learned during 1–2 mo of instruction in a mentored nerve block rotation during the senior year of anesthesia residency training. Most trainees however, require a 6- to 12-mo fellowship to acquire sufficient expertise in these techniques.

During the 2 month period of concentrated training in the regional anesthesia rotation, residents typically perform and perioperatively manage an additional 20 to 30 advanced nerve block procedures. As these residents are already well trained in all the basic and in some intermediate nerve block procedures, as well as in the pharmacology of local anesthetics, before their regional anesthesia rotation, they are able to acquire new techniques at an accelerated pace.

Teaching Staff

All staff members provide training in basic regional anesthesia skills in our anesthesia residency training program. The ample opportunity to practice regional anesthesia and the mentoring available to our faculty members ensure that all attending staff are proficient in these basic techniques. However, training in advanced regional anesthesia procedures is conducted by a core team of regional anesthesiologists who have completed a fellowship or possess substantial expertise in practicing and teaching these techniques.

This organization is of crucial importance to ensure quality training of residents and fellows. To advance the subspecialty, it is also important that we as members of the profession ensure the adequate education of regional anesthesiologists through structured fellowship programs.

Equipment

In our training program, nearly all major conduction blocks are performed using insulated nerve block needles with the aid of a nerve stimulator. The elicitation of specific objective responses to nerve stimulation during block performance not only adds significant educational value for trainees, but also allows patient sedation, which makes teaching more acceptable to patients. In addition, in our practice the use of a remotely-controlled nerve stimulator allows instructors to teach residents during the block performance and to control the current output of the nerve stimulator without the need for additional personnel.

Teaching Material

In recent years, several excellent texts, multimedia instruction programs, and other tools for teaching regional anesthesia have been developed. There are several mannequins, CD-ROMs, and Web sites that can be used to aid in the learning of regional anesthesia techniques. Virtual reality simulators for training in regional anesthesia are also likely to become available in the future. In our residency program, all residents receive an institutional regional anesthesia rotation manual. They are also provided with access to the Internet at several locations in the department and can simply print out the description of a technique from the Regional Anesthesia Website (www.nysora.com) and read about the blocks they are about to perform.

In summary, most anesthesiologists perceive a need to employ more peripheral nerve blocks in their practice, it is certain that the use of these techniques will increase in the future. A similar trend has been seen in Europe, where, for example, French anesthesiologists utilize regional anesthesia in 23% of cases, a 14-fold increase in comparison with the amount of regional anesthesia practiced in 1980. However, it has been well established that current teaching methods and requirements for training in regional anesthesia are suboptimal. A structured regional anesthesia rotation, a well-defined curriculum, a dedicated team of mentors with training in regional anesthesia, and an ample clinical volume are all prerequisites for the adequate training of residents. A core group of widely applicable, relatively simple nerve blocks (basic and more common intermediate nerve blocks) should be mastered by all graduating residents to achieve more consistent proficiency in these techniques.

SUGGESTED READINGS

- American Board of Anesthesiology. A modification in the training requirements in anesthesiology: requirements for the third clinical anesthesia year. *Anesthesiology* 1985;62:175–177.

- Benumof JL. Permanent loss of cervical spinal cord function associated with interscalene block performed under general anesthesia. *Anesthesiology* 2000;93:1541–1544.

- Bouaziz H, Mercier FJ, Narchi P, et al. Survey of regional anesthesia practice among French residents at time of certification. *Reg Anesth* 1997;22:218–222.

- Bridenbaugh L. Are anesthesia resident programs failing regional anesthesia? *Reg Anesth* 1982;7:26–28.

- Brown DL. *Atlas of Regional Anesthesia*. Philadelphia, Pa: WB Saunders; 1992.

- Buist RJ. A survey of the practice of regional anesthesia. *J R Soc Med* 1990;83:709–712.

- Cass OW, Freeman ML, Peine CJ, et al. Objective evaluation of endoscopy skills during training. *Ann Intern Med* 1993;118:40–44.

- Chelly JE, ed. *Peripheral Nerve Blocks: A Color Atlas*. Philadelphia, Pa: Lippincott Williams & Wilkins; 1999.

- Chelly JE, Greger J, Gebhard R, Hagberg CA, Al-Samsam T, Khan A. Training of residents in peripheral nerve blocks during anesthesiology residency. J Clin Anesth. 2000 Dec;14(8):584-8.

- Clergue F, Auroy Y, Pequignot F, et al. French survey of anesthesia in 1996. *Anesthesiology* 1999;91:1509–1520.

- Delbos A, Eisenach JC, Narchi P, Brasseur L. Peripheral nerve blocks [book on CD ROM]. Philadelphia, Pa: Lippincott-Raven; 1993.

- D'Ercole F, Bergh A, Klein S, et al. A teaching model for resident training in regional anesthesia. *Reg Anesth Pain Med* 1998;23:112.

- Duong T, Havel R. Resident clinical competence in cardiac anesthesia: a case performance-based evaluation study. *J Cardiothorac Vasc Anesth* 1992;6:399–403.

- Gaba DM. Improving anesthesiologist's performance by simulating reality. *Anesthesiology* 1992;76:491–494.

- Gaba DM, DeAnda A. A comprehensive anesthesia simulation environment: recreating the operating room for research and training. *Anesthesiology* 1988;69:387–394.

- Hadžić A, Vloka JD, Koenigsamen J. Training requirements for peripheral nerve blocks. *Curr Opin Anesthesiol* 2002;15:669–673.

- Hadžić A, Vloka JD, Kuroda MM, et al. The practice of peripheral nerve blocks in the United States: a national survey. *Reg Anesth Pain Med* 1998;23:241–246.

- Hadžić A, Vloka JD. Peripheral nerve stimulator for unassisted nerve blockade. *Anesthesiology* 1996;84:1528–1529.
- Horlocker TT. Peripheral nerve blocks—regional anesthesia for the new millennium. *Reg Anesth Pain Med* 1998;23:237–240.
- http://www.nysora.com.regionalblock.com, arl.com, www.medicaltechnologysystems.com,http://uianesthesia.com/rasci/. http://www.alrf.asso.fr. http://www.regionablock.com
- Jankovic D, Wells C. *Regional Nerve Blocks: Textbook and Color Atlas.* Berlin, Germany: Blackwell Scientific Publications; 2001.
- Konrad C, Schupfer G, Wietlisbach M, Gerber H. Learning manual skills in anesthesiology: is there a recommended number of cases for anesthetic procedures? *Anesth Analg* 1998;86:635–639.
- Kopacz DJ, Bridenbaugh LD. Are anesthesia residency programs failing regional anesthesia? The past, present, and future. *Reg Anesth* 1993;18:84–87.
- Kopacz D, Neal J, Pollock J. The regional anesthesia "learning curve": what is the minimum number of epidural and spinal blocks to reach consistency? *Reg Anesth* 1996;21:182–190.
- Mulroy M. *Regional Anesthesia: An Illustrated Procedural Guide.* Boston, Mass: Little, Brown; 1996.
- Schertz RD, Baskin WN, Frakes JT. Flexible fiberoptic sigmoidoscopy training for primary care physicians: results of a 5-year experience. *Gastrointest Endosc* 1989;35:316–320.
- Shevde K, Panagopoulos. A survey of 800 patients' knowledge, attitudes and concerns regarding anesthesia. *Anesth Analg* 1991;73:109–198.
- Smith M, Sprung J, Zura A, et al. A survey of exposure to regional anesthesia techniques in American anesthesia residency training programs. *Reg Anesth Pain Med* 1999;24:11–16.
- Spence AA. The expanding role of simulators in risk management. *Br J Anesth* 1997;78:633–634.

2 ESSENTIAL
REGIONAL ANESTHESIA ANATOMY

A sound knowledge of anatomy is a prerequisite for the successful practice of regional anesthesia. It is not surprising then that many anesthesiologists consider regional anesthesia a practice of applied anatomy. However, it is important to realize that such knowledge must be in the context of regional anesthesia techniques rather than just a knowledge of "dry" anatomic facts. Therefore, just as practitioners of surgical disciplines rely on surgical anatomy, regional anesthesiologists must understand how various anatomic details influence their techniques and the choice of technique. In this chapter, the basics of regional anesthesia anatomy necessary for successful implementation of various procedures described later in this book are outlined. For better clarity and in-depth understanding, some of the material covered will also necessarily be repeated in descriptions of individual techniques throughout the book.

Anatomy of Peripheral Nerves

All peripheral nerves are similar in structure. The *neuron* is the basic functional unit responsible for the conduction of nerve impulses. Neurons are the longest cells in the body, many reaching a meter in length. Most neurons are incapable of dividing under normal circumstances, and they have very limited ability to repair themselves after injury. A typical neuron consists of a cell body (soma) that contains a large nucleus **(Fig. 2-1)**. The cell body is attached to several branching processes, called dendrites, and a single axon. Dendrites receive incoming messages; axons conduct outgoing messages. Axons vary in length, and there is one only per neuron. In peripheral nerves, axons are very long and slender. They are also called nerve fibers.

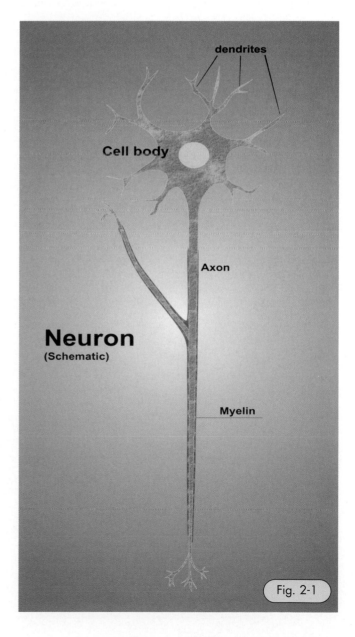

dendrites

Cell body

Axon

Neuron
(Schematic)

Myelin

Fig. 2-1

Connective Tissue

The individual nerve fibers that make up a nerve are bound together, somewhat like individual wires in an electrical cable. The connective tissue of a large nerve consists of three important envelopes: the epineurium, perineurium, and endoneurium **(Fig. 2-2)**. The *epineurium* surrounds the entire nerve and holds it loosely to the connective tissue through which it runs. This layer also sends septa into the nerve that divide the nerve fibers into bundles (fasciculi or funiculi) of varying sizes. The *perineurium* surrounds each fasciculus and splits with it at each branching point. The *endoneurium* is a delicate layer of connective tissue around each nerve that is embedded within the perineurium. The connective tissue of a nerve is tough compared to the nerve fibers themselves.

It permits a certain amount of stretch without damage to the nerve fibers. These fibers are somewhat "wavy," and when they are stretched, the connective tissue around them is also stretched—giving them some protection. This feature perhaps plays a "safety" role in nerve blockade by allowing nerves to be "pushed" rather than pierced by an advancing needle during nerve localization. For this reason, it is prudent to avoid stretching ("fixing") nerves and nerve plexuses during nerve blockade (such as in an axillary brachial plexus block and some approaches to a sciatic block).

Nerves receive blood from adjacent blood vessels running along their course. These feeding branches to larger nerves are macroscopic in size and irregularly arranged, forming anastomoses to

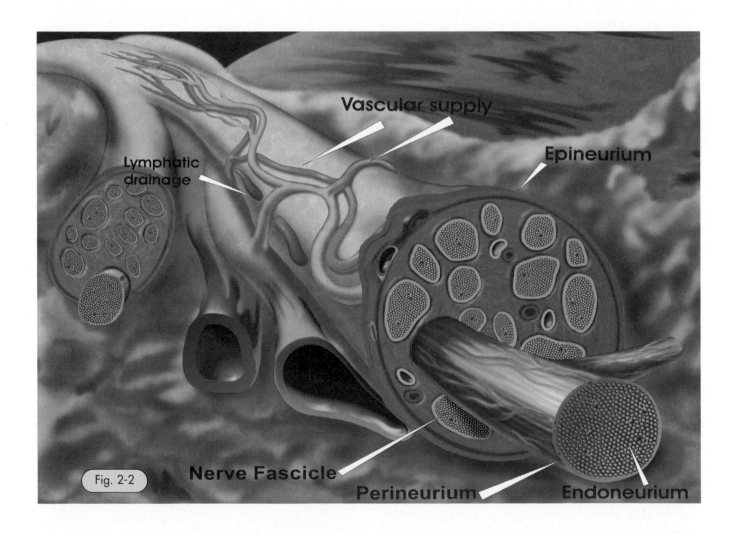

Fig. 2-2

become longitudinally running vessel(s) that supply the nerve and give off subsidiary branches. Although the connective tissue sheath enveloping nerves serves to protect them from stretching, it is possible that neuronal injury following nerve blockade may be at least partly due to the pressure or stretch within a poorly stretchable connective sheath and consequent interference with the vascular supply to the nerve.

Organization of Spinal Nerves

The neuronal system consists of central and peripheral parts. The central nervous system (CNS) includes the brain and spinal cord, and the peripheral nervous system consists of the spinal, cranial, and autonomic nerves and their associated ganglia. Nerves are bundles of nerve fibers that lie outside the CNS and serve to conduct electric impulses from one region of the body to another. The nerves that exit through the skull are known as cranial nerves, and there are 12 pairs of them. The nerves that exit below the skull and between the vertebrae are called spinal nerves, and there are 31 pairs of them **(Fig. 2-3)**. Each spinal nerve has a regional number and can be identified by its association with the adjacent vertebra. In the cervical region, the first pair of spinal nerves, C1, exits between the skull and the first cervical vertebra. For this reason, cervical nerves take their names from the vertebra immediately following them. In other words, cervical nerve C2 precedes vertebra C2, and the same system is used for the rest of the cervical series. The transition from this identification method occurs between the last cervical and first thoracic vertebrae. The spinal nerve lying between these two vertebrae has been designated C8. Thus, there are seven cervical vertebrae but eight cervical nerves. Spinal nerves caudal to the first thoracic vertebra take their names from the vertebra immediately preceding them. For instance, spinal nerve T1 emerges immediatcly caudal to vertebra T1, spinal nerve T2 following vertebra T2, and so on.

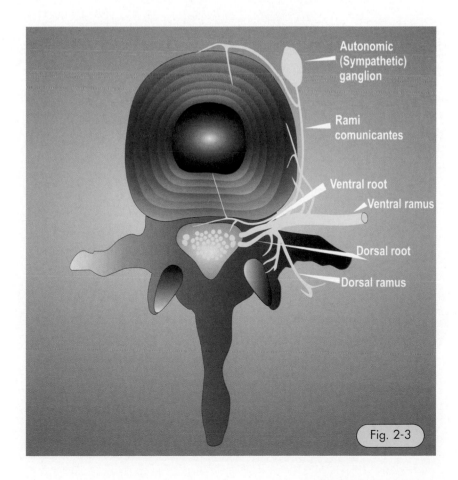

Autonomic (Sympathetic) ganglion

Rami comunicantes

Ventral root

Ventral ramus

Dorsal root

Dorsal ramus

Fig. 2-3

Origin and Peripheral Distribution of Spinal Nerves

Each spinal nerve forms through the fusion of dorsal and ventral nerve roots as these roots pass through the intervertebral foramen **(Fig. 2-3)**. At the thoracic and lumbar levels, the first branch of the spinal nerve carries visceral motor fibers to a nearby autonomic ganglion. Because preganglionic fibers are myelinated, they are light in color and are known as white rami. Two groups of unmyelinated postganglionic fibers leave the ganglion **(Fig. 2-4)**. Those fibers that innervate glands and smooth muscle in the body wall or limbs form the gray rami that rejoins the spinal nerve. The gray and white rami are collectively called the rami communicantes (communicating branches). Preganglionic or postgan-

glionic fibers that innervate internal organs do not rejoin the spinal nerves. Instead, they form a series of separate autonomic nerves and serve to regulate the activities of organs in the abdominal and pelvic cavities.

The dorsal ramus of each spinal nerve provides sensory innervation from, and motor innervation to, a specific segment of the skin and muscles of the back. The innervated region resembles a horizontal band that begins at the origin of the spinal nerve. The relatively large ventral ramus supplies the ventrolateral body surface, structures in the body wall, and the limbs. Each pair of spinal nerves innervates a specific region of the body surface, an area called a dermatome.

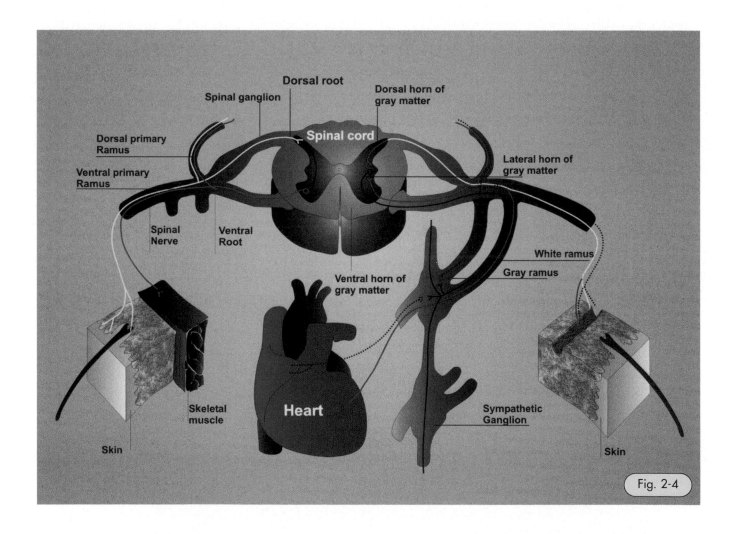

Fig. 2-4

Dermatomes

A dermatome is an area of the skin supplied by the dorsal (sensory) root of a spinal nerve **(Figs. 2-5, 2-6)**. In the head and trunk, each segment is horizontally disposed except C1, which does not have a sensory component. The dermatomes of the limbs from the fifth cervical to the first thoracic nerve and from the

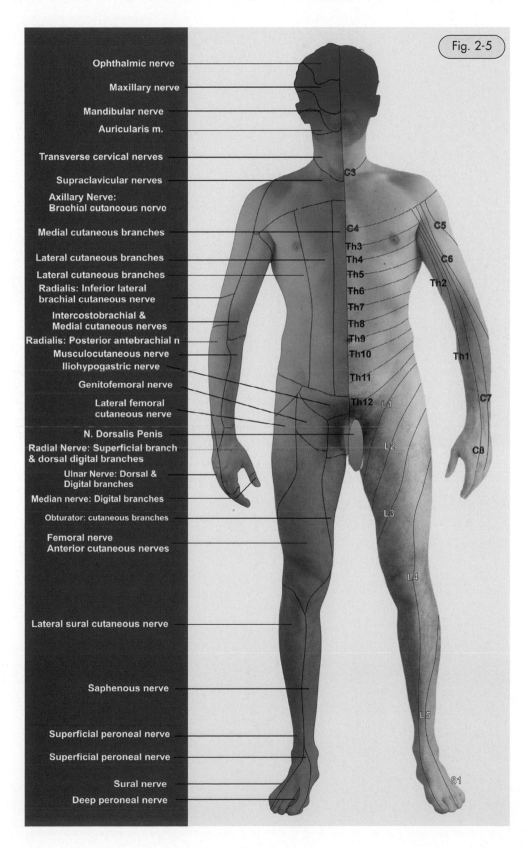

Fig. 2-5

Ophthalmic nerve
Maxillary nerve
Mandibular nerve
Auricularis m.
Transverse cervical nerves
Supraclavicular nerves
Axillary Nerve: Brachial cutaneous nerve
Medial cutaneous branches
Lateral cutaneous branches
Lateral cutaneous branches
Radialis: Inferior lateral brachial cutaneous nerve
Intercostobrachial & Medial cutaneous nerves
Radialis: Posterior antebrachial n
Musculocutaneous nerve
Iliohypogastric nerve
Genitofemoral nerve
Lateral femoral cutaneous nerve
N. Dorsalis Penis
Radial Nerve: Superficial branch & dorsal digital branches
Ulnar Nerve: Dorsal & Digital branches
Median nerve: Digital branches
Obturator: cutaneous branches
Femoral nerve Anterior cutaneous nerves
Lateral sural cutaneous nerve
Saphenous nerve
Superficial peroneal nerve
Superficial peroneal nerve
Sural nerve
Deep peroneal nerve

C3, C4, C5, Th3, Th4, Th5, Th6, Th7, Th8, Th9, Th10, Th11, Th12, L1, L2, L3, L4, L5, S1, C5, C6, Th2, Th1, C7, C8

third lumbar to the second sacral vertebra extend as a series of bands from the midline of the trunk posteriorly into the limbs. It should be noted that there is considerable overlapping of adjacent dermatomes; that is, each segmental nerve overlaps the territories of its neighbors.

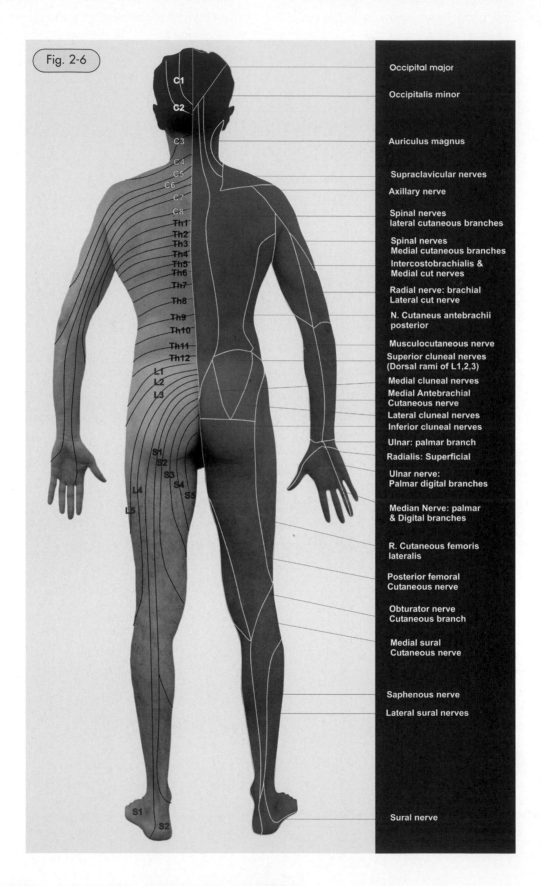

Fig. 2-6

Occipital major

Occipitalis minor

Auriculus magnus

Supraclavicular nerves

Axillary nerve

Spinal nerves
lateral cutaneous branches

Spinal nerves
Medial cutaneous branches

Intercostobrachialis &
Medial cut nerves

Radial nerve: brachial
Lateral cut nerve

N. Cutaneus antebrachii
posterior

Musculocutaneous nerve

Superior cluneal nerves
(Dorsal rami of L1,2,3)

Medial cluneal nerves

Medial Antebrachial
Cutaneous nerve

Lateral cluneal nerves

Inferior cluneal nerves

Ulnar: palmar branch

Radialis: Superficial

Ulnar nerve:
Palmar digital branches

Median Nerve: palmar
& Digital branches

R. Cutaneous femoris
lateralis

Posterior femoral
Cutaneous nerve

Obturator nerve
Cutaneous branch

Medial sural
Cutaneous nerve

Saphenous nerve

Lateral sural nerves

Sural nerve

Myotomes

A myotome is the segmental innervation of skeletal muscle by the ventral (motor) root(s) of a spinal nerve(s) **(Fig. 2-7)**.

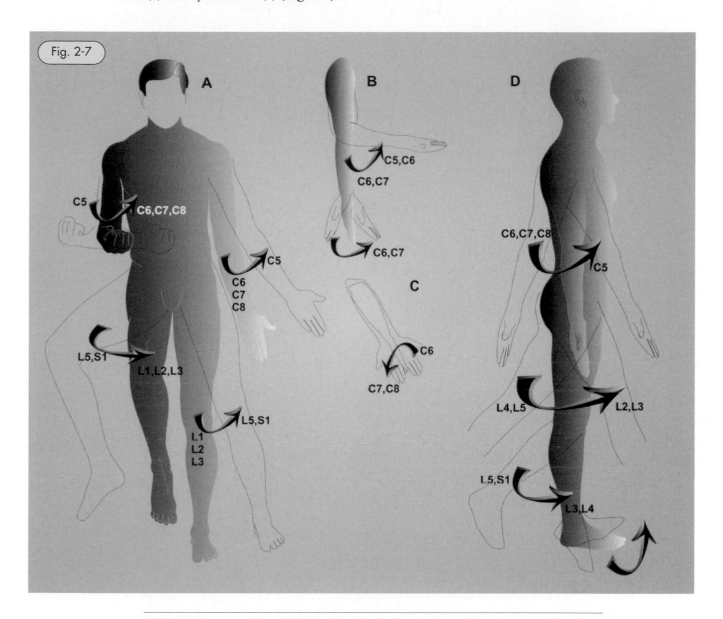

Fig. 2-7

A Medial and lateral rotation of shoulder and hip. Abduction and adduction of shoulder and hip.

B Flexion and extension of elbow and wrist.

C Pronation and supination of forearm.

D Flexion and extension of shoulder, hip, and knee. Dorsiflexion and plantar flexion of ankle, lateral views.

Osteotomes

The innervation of the bones often does not follow the same segmental pattern as the innervation of the muscles and other soft tissues **(Fig. 2-8)**.

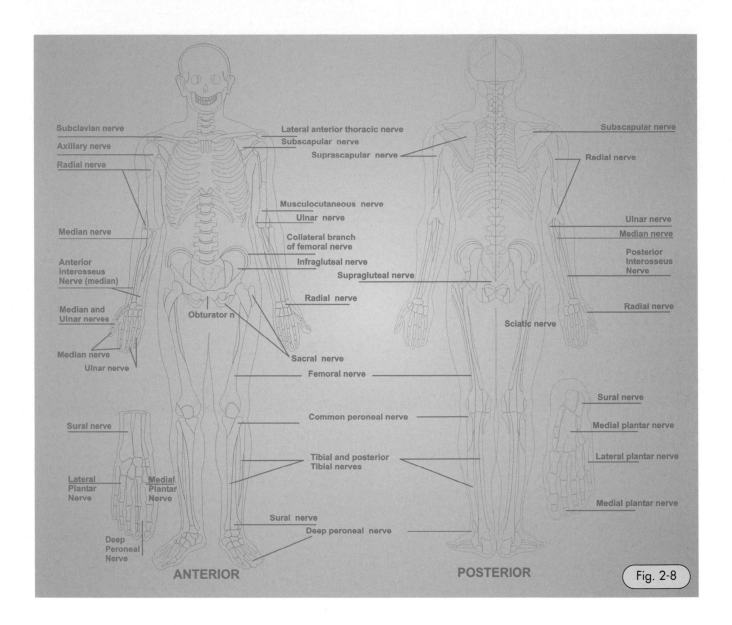

Subclavian nerve
Axillary nerve
Radial nerve
Median nerve
Anterior interosseus Nerve (median)
Median and Ulnar nerves
Median nerve
Ulnar nerve
Sural nerve
Lateral Plantar Nerve
Medial Plantar Nerve
Deep Peroneal Nerve

Lateral anterior thoracic nerve
Subscapular nerve
Suprascapular nerve
Musculocutaneous nerve
Ulnar nerve
Collateral branch of femoral nerve
Infragluteal nerve
Supragluteal nerve
Radial nerve
Obturator n
Sacral nerve
Femoral nerve
Common peroneal nerve
Tibial and posterior Tibial nerves
Sural nerve
Deep peroneal nerve

Subscapular nerve
Radial nerve
Ulnar nerve
Median nerve
Posterior Interosseus Nerve
Radial nerve
Sciatic nerve
Sural nerve
Medial plantar nerve
Lateral plantar nerve
Medial plantar nerve

ANTERIOR   POSTERIOR   Fig. 2-8

TIPS

► Although the differences among dermatomal, myotomal, and osteotomal innervation are often emphasized in anesthesiology texts as being important in the application of nerve blocks, it is impractical to think in these terms.

► Instead, it is more much practical to consider which block techniques provide adequate analgesia and anesthesia to various body areas (e.g., shoulder, hand, foot, etc.) rather than trying to match nerves and spinal segments to the desired dermatomes, myotomes, and osteotomes.

Nerve Plexuses

Although dermatomal innervation of the trunk is simple, the spinal segments controlling sensory and motor innervation of the upper and lower limbs are more complex. In these areas, the ventral rami from the contiguous spinal segments provide sensory and motor innervation. However, the ventral rami of adjacent spinal nerves blend their fibers to produce a series of compound nerve trunks, resulting in a complex, interwoven network of nerves called a nerve plexus. The four major nerve plexuses are the cervical, brachial, lumbar, and sacral.

Cervical Plexus

Branches from the cervical plexus innervate the muscles **(Table 2.1)** of the neck and extend into the thoracic cavity to control the diaphragmatic muscles. The cervical plexus consists of muscular and cutaneous branches in the ventral rami of spinal nerves (C1 through C4) and some nerve fibers from C5 **(Fig. 2-9)**. The phrenic nerve, the major nerve of this plexus, provides the nerve supply to the diaphragm. Branches are distributed to the skin of the neck, shoulder, and superior portion of the chest.

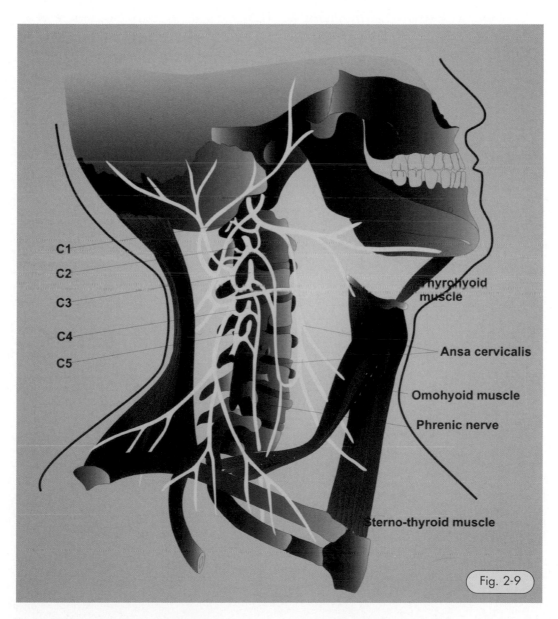

C1
C2
C3
C4
C5

Thyrohyoid muscle

Ansa cervicalis

Omohyoid muscle

Phrenic nerve

Sterno-thyroid muscle

Fig. 2-9

Organization of the cervical plexus

TABLE 2.1
Organization and Distribution of the Cervical Plexus

NERVES	SPINAL SEGMENTS	DISTRIBUTION
Ansa cervicalis (superior and inferior branches) nerve	C1 through C4	Five of the extrinsic laryngeal muscles (sternothyroid, sternohyoid, omohyoid, geniohyoid, and thyrohyoid) by way of N XII
Lesser occipital, transverse cervical, supraclavicular, and greater auricular nerves	C3	Skin of upper chest, shoulder, neck, and ear
Phrenic nerve	C3 through C5	Diaphragm
Cervical nerves	C2 through C5	Levator scapulae, scalene, sternocleidomastoid, and trapezius muscles (with N XI)

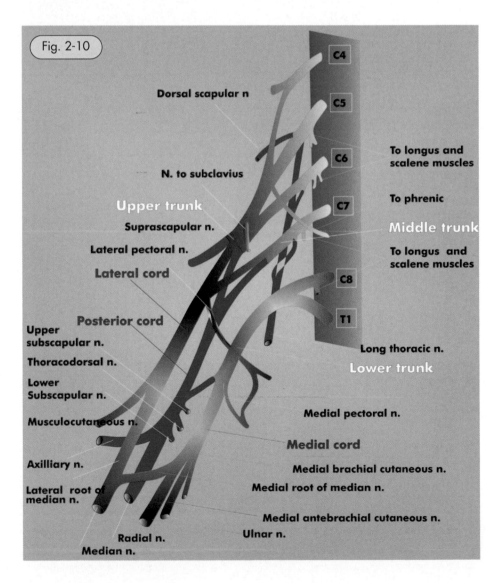

Fig. 2-10

Dorsal scapular n

N. to subclavius

Upper trunk

Suprascapular n.

Lateral pectoral n.

Lateral cord

Posterior cord

Upper subscapular n.

Thoracodorsal n.

Lower Subscapular n.

Musculocutaneous n.

Axilliary n.

Lateral root of median n.

Radial n.

Median n.

C4

C5

C6

C7

C8

T1

To longus and scalene muscles

To phrenic

Middle trunk

To longus and scalene muscles

Long thoracic n.

Lower trunk

Medial pectoral n.

Medial cord

Medial brachial cutaneous n.

Medial root of median n.

Medial antebrachial cutaneous n.

Ulnar n.

Organization of the brachial plexus

Brachial Plexus

The brachial plexus is both larger and more complex than the cervical plexus **(Fig. 2-10)**. It innervates the pectoral girdle and upper limb, with contributions from ventral rami of spinal nerves C5 through T1 **(Table 2.2)**. The spinal nerves converge to form the superior (C5 and C6), middle (C7), and inferior (C8 through T1) trunks. Divisions from these trunks then interconnect to form the lateral, medial, and posterior cords. The lateral cord forms the musculocutaneous nerve and contributes to the medial nerve together with the medial cord. The medial cord contributes to the medial nerve and forms the ulnar nerve. The posterior cord forms both the axillary and radial nerves.

TABLE 2.2
Organization and Distribution of the Brachial Plexus

NERVE(S)	SPINAL SEGMENTS	DISTRIBUTION
Nerves to subclavius	C4 through C6	Subclavius muscle
Dorsal scapular nerve	C5	Rhomboid muscles and levator scapulae muscle
Long thoracic nerve	C5 through C7	Serratus anterior muscle
Suprascapular nerve	C5 and C6	Supraspinatus and infraspinatus muscles
Pectoralis nerve (median and lateral)	C5 through T1	Pectoralis muscles
Subscapular nerves	C5 and C6	Subscapularis and teres major muscles
Thoracodorsal nerve	C6 through C8	Latissimus dorsi muscle
Axillary nerve	C5 and C6	Deltoid and teres minor muscles; skin of the shoulder
Radial nerve	C5 through T1	Extensor muscle of the arm and forearm (tricep brachii, extensor carpi radialis, extensor carpi ulnaris muscles) and brachioradialis muscle; digital extensors and abductor pollicis muscle; skin over posterolateral surface of the arm
Musculocutaneous nerve	C5 through C7	Flexor muscles of the arm (biceps brachii, brachialis, coracobrachialis muscles); skin over lateral surface of the forearm
Median nerve	C6 through T1	Flexor muscles of the forearm (flexor carpi radialis and palmaris longus muscles); pronator quadratus and pronator teres muscles; digital flexors (through the palmar interosseous nerve); skin over anterolateral surface of the hand
Ulnar nerve	C8 and T1	Flexor carpi ulnaris muscle, adductor pollicis muscle, and small digital muscles; skin over medial surface of the hand

Lumbar Plexus

The lumbar plexus arises from the lumbar segments of the spinal cord **(Fig. 2-11)**. The ventral rami of T12 through L4 supply the pelvic girdle and lower limb. Because the ventral rami of both the lumbar and sacral plexuses are distributed to the lower limb, they are often collectively referred to as the lumbosacral plexus.

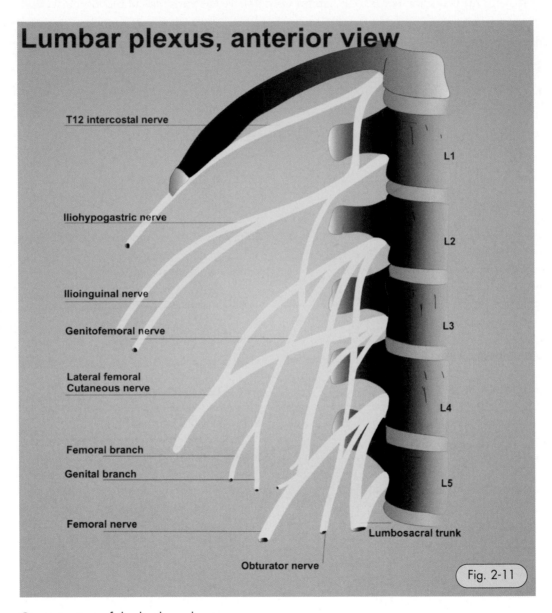

Lumbar plexus, anterior view

T12 intercostal nerve

Iliohypogastric nerve

Ilioinguinal nerve

Genitofemoral nerve

Lateral femoral
Cutaneous nerve

Femoral branch

Genital branch

Femoral nerve

Obturator nerve

L1

L2

L3

L4

L5

Lumbosacral trunk

Fig. 2-11

Organization of the lumbar plexus

The main nerves of the lumbar plexus are the genitofemoral, lateral femoral cutaneous, obturator, and femoral **(Table 2-3)**.

TABLE 2.3

Organization and Distribution of the Lumbar Plexus

NERVE(S)	SPINAL SEGMENTS	DISTRIBUTION
Iliohypogastric nerve	T12 through L1	Abdominal muscles (external and internal oblique muscles, transverse abdominis muscles); skin over inferior abdomen and buttocks
Ilioinguinal nerve	L1	Abdominal muscles (with iliohypogastric nerve); skin over superior medial thigh and portions of external genitalia
Genitofemoral nerve	L1 and L2	Skin over anteromedial surface of thigh and portions over genitalia
Lateral femoral cutaneous nerve	L2 and L3	Skin over anterior, lateral, and posterior surfaces of thigh
Femoral nerve	L2 through L4	Anterior muscles of thigh (sartorius muscle and quadriceps group); adductor of thigh (pectineus and iliopsoas muscles); skin over anteromedial surface of thigh, medial surface of leg, and foot
Obturator nerve	L2 through L4	Adductors of the thigh (magnus, brevis, and longus adductors); gracilis muscle; skin over medial surface of thigh
Saphenous nerve	L2 through L4	Skin over medial surface of leg

Sacral Plexus

The sacral plexus arises from the ventral rami of spinal nerves L4 through S4. The ventral rami of L4 and L5 form the lumbosacral trunk, which contributes to the sacral plexus along with the ventral rami of S1 through S4 **(Fig. 2-12)**. The major nerves of the sacral plexus are the sciatic and pudendal **(Table 2-4)**. The sciatic nerve passes posteriorly to the femur and deep into the long head of the biceps femoris muscle. As it approaches the popliteal fossa, it diverges into two nerves: the common peroneal (or the peroneal) and the tibial.

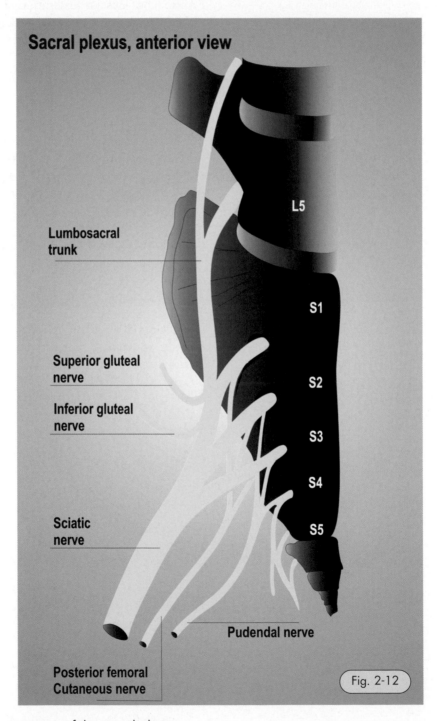

Sacral plexus, anterior view

L5

Lumbosacral trunk

S1

Superior gluteal nerve

S2

Inferior gluteal nerve

S3

S4

Sciatic nerve

S5

Pudendal nerve

Posterior femoral Cutaneous nerve

Fig. 2-12

Organization of the sacral plexus

TABLE 2.4

Organization and Distribution of the Sacral Plexus

NERVE(S)	SPINAL SEGMENTS	DISTRIBUTION
Gluteal nerves: superior, inferior	L4 through S2	Abductors of thigh (gluteus minimus, gluteus medius, tensor fasciae latae); extensor of thigh (gluteus maximus)
Posterior femoral cutaneous nerve	S1 through S3	Skin of perineum and posterior surface of thigh and leg
Sciatic nerve, tibial nerve	L4 through S3	Two of the hamstring muscles (semitendinosus and semimembranosus); adductor magnus (with obturator nerve)
Common peroneal nerve	L4 through S3	Flexor of knee and plantar flexors of ankle (popliteal, gastrocnemius, soleus, and tibialis posterior muscles and long head of biceps femoris muscle); flexors of toes; skin over posterior surface of leg and plantar surface of foot; biceps femoris muscle (short head); fibularis (brevis and longus) and tibialis anterior muscles; extensors of toes; skin over anterior surface of leg and dorsal surface of foot; skin over lateral portion of foot (through sural nerve)
Pudendal nerve	S2 through S4	Muscles of perineum, including urogenital diaphragm and external anal and urethral sphincter muscles; skin of external genitalia and related skeletal muscles (bulbospongiosus, ischiocavernosus muscles)

Thoracic and Abdominal Wall

Thoracic Wall

The intercostal nerves comprise the anterior rami of the upper 11 thoracic spinal nerves **(Fig. 2-13)**. Each intercostal nerve enters the neurovascular plane posteriorly and produces a collateral branch that supplies the intercostal muscles of the space. Except for the first, each intercostal nerve gives off a lateral cutaneous branch that pierces the overlying muscle near the midaxillary line. This cutaneous nerve divides into anterior and posterior branches, which supply the adjacent skin. The intercostal nerves of the second to the sixth spaces enter the superficial fascia near the lateral border of the sternum and divide into medial and lateral cutaneous branches. Most of the fibers of the anterior ramus of the first thoracic spinal nerve join the brachial plexus for distribution to the upper limb. The small first intercostal nerve is a collateral branch and supplies only the muscles of the intercostal space, not the overlying skin. The intercostal nerves of the lower five spaces continue in the neurovascular plane beyond the costal margin to supply the muscles and skin of the abdominal wall.

Anterior Abdominal Wall

The skin muscles and parietal peritoneum, or anterior abdominal wall, are innervated by the lower six thoracic nerves and the first lumbar nerve **(Fig. 2-13)**. At the costal margin, thoracic nerves T7 through T11 leave their intercostal spaces and enter the neurovascular plane of the abdominal wall between the transversus abdominis and internal oblique. The 7th and 8th nerves slope upward, the 9th runs horizontally, and the 10th and 11th incline downward. The nerves pierce the rectus abdominis and the anterior layer of the rectus sheath to emerge as anterior cutaneous branches supplying the overlying skin.

The subcostal nerve (T12) takes the line of the 12th rib across the posterior abdominal wall. It continues around the flank in the neurovascular plane and terminates similarly to the lower intercostal nerves. T7 through T12 give off lateral cutaneous nerves that further divide into anterior and posterior branches. The anterior branches supply the skin as far forward as the

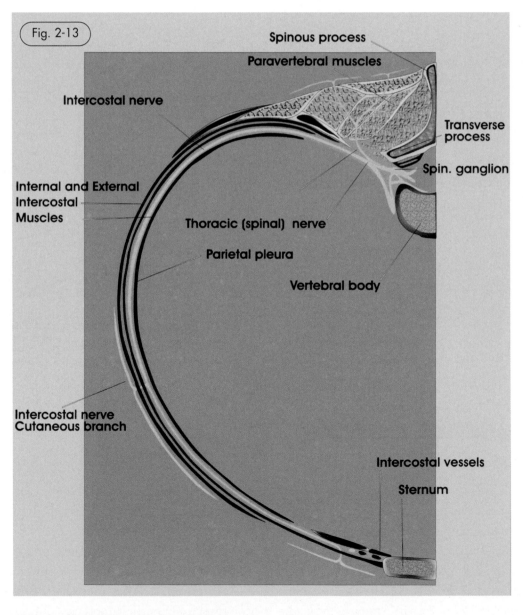

Fig. 2-13

Spinous process

Paravertebral muscles

Intercostal nerve

Transverse process

Spin. ganglion

Internal and External Intercostal Muscles

Thoracic (spinal) nerve

Parietal pleura

Vertebral body

Intercostal nerve Cutaneous branch

Intercostal vessels

Sternum

Organization of the intercostal nerve

lateral edge of the rectus abdominis. The posterior branches supply the skin overlying the latissimus dorsi. The lateral cutaneous branch of the subcostal nerve is distributed to the skin on the side of the buttock.

The first lumbar nerve divides into upper and lower branches, and the iliohypogastric and the ilioinguinal nerves. The iliohypogastric nerve divides just above the iliac crest into two terminal branches. The lateral cutaneous branch supplies the side of the buttock, and the anterior cutaneous branch supplies the suprapubic region.

The ilioinguinal nerve leaves the neurovascular plane by piercing the internal oblique muscle above the iliac crest. It continues between the two oblique muscles and accompanies the spermatic cord (or round ligament of the uterus) in the inguinal canal. Emerging from the superficial inguinal ring, it pro-vides cutaneous branches to the skin on the medial side of the root of the thigh, the proximal part of the penis, and the front of the scrotum (or the mons pubis and the anterior part of the labium majus).

Nerve Supply to the Peritoneum

The parietal peritoneum of the abdominal wall is innervated by the lower thoracic and first lumbar nerves. The lower thoracic nerves also innervate the peritoneum, which covers the periphery of the diaphragm. Inflammation of the peritoneum gives rise to pain in the lower thoracic wall and abdominal wall. By contrast, the peritoneum on the central part of the diaphragm receives sensory branches from the phrenic nerves (C3 through C5), and irritation in this area may produce pain referred to the region of the shoulder (the fourth cervical dermatome).

Innervation of the Major Joints

In this chapter, the discussion has dealt mostly with cutaneous innervation and myotomal and skeletal neuronal distribution. However, because much of the practice of peripheral nerve blocks involves orthopedic and other joint surgery, it is also important to review innervation of the major joints to better understand the neuronal components that need to be blocked to achieve anesthesia for joint surgery.

Shoulder Joint

Innervation to the shoulder joints stems mostly from the axillary and suprascapular nerves **(Fig. 2-14)**. The skin over most medial parts of the shoulder receives nerves from the cervical plexus. Such an arrangement explains why a brachial plexus block at the interscalene level is the most appropriate for achieving anesthesia of the shoulder.

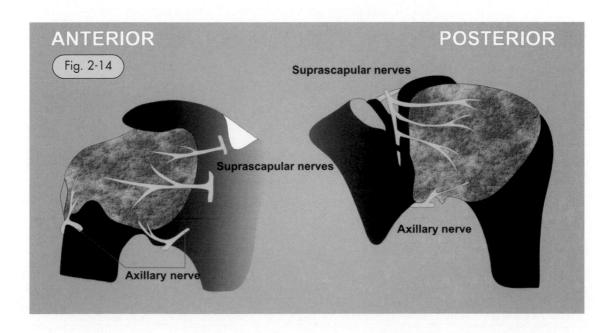

ANTERIOR   POSTERIOR

Fig. 2-14

Suprascapular nerves

Suprascapular nerves

Axillary nerve

Axillary nerve

Elbow Joint

The nerve supply to the elbow joint includes branches of all the major nerves of the brachial plexus: musculocutaneous, radial, medial, and ulnar **(Fig. 2-15)**.

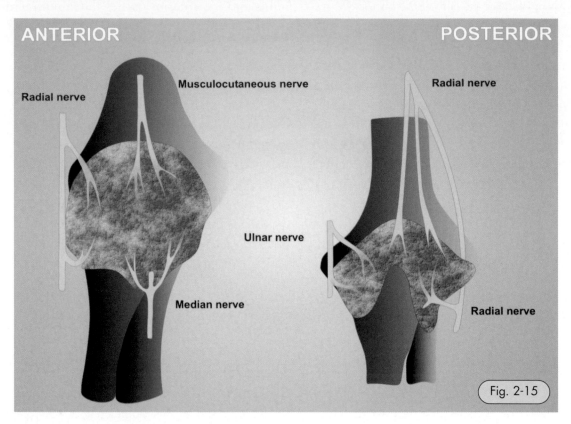

ANTERIOR

POSTERIOR

Radial nerve

Musculocutaneous nerve

Radial nerve

Ulnar nerve

Median nerve

Radial nerve

Fig. 2-15

Hip Joint

Nerves to the hip joint include the nerve to the rectus femoris from the femoral nerve, branches from the anterior division of the obturator nerve, and the nerve to the quadratus femoris from the sacral plexus **(Fig. 2-16)**.

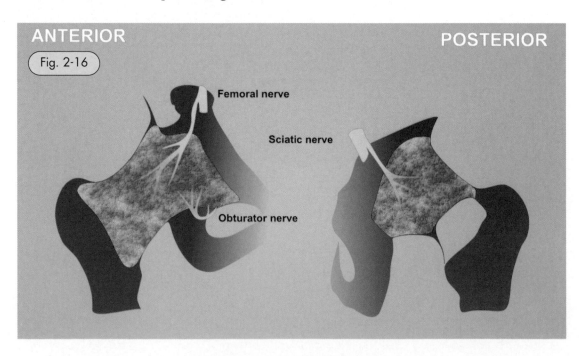

ANTERIOR

POSTERIOR

Fig. 2-16

Femoral nerve

Sciatic nerve

Obturator nerve

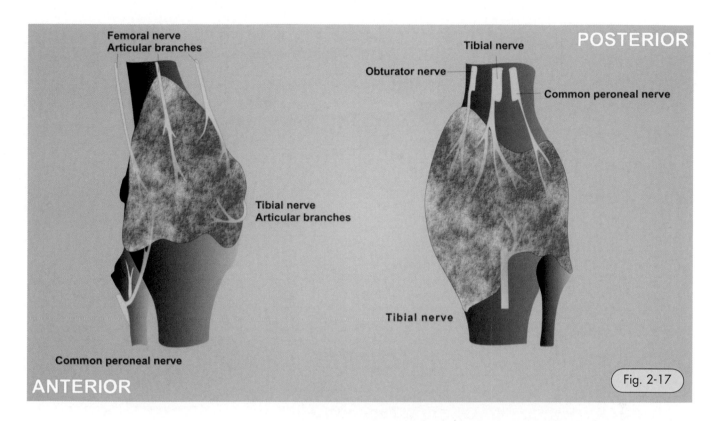

Fig. 2-17

Knee Joint

Knee innervation is obtained from branches from the femoral, obturator, and sciatic nerves **(Fig. 2-17)**. Articular branches from the tibial and common fibular divisions of the sciatic nerve, together with fibers from the posterior division of the obturator nerve, may also contribute to the innervation of the joint.

Ankle Joint

Innervation of the ankle joint is quite complex and involves the terminal branches of the peroneal nerves (deep and superficial peroneal), tibial nerves (posterior tibial), and femoral nerve (saphenous) **(Fig. 2-18)**. A more simplistic view is that the entire innervation of the ankle joint stems from the sciatic nerve, with the exception of the skin on the medial aspect around the medial malleolus (the saphenous nerve, a branch of the femoral nerve).

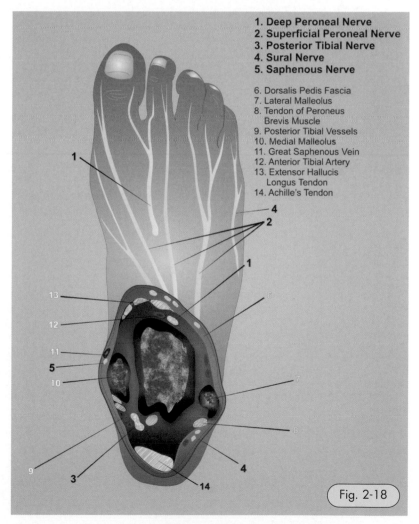

1. Deep Peroneal Nerve
2. Superficial Peroneal Nerve
3. Posterior Tibial Nerve
4. Sural Nerve
5. Saphenous Nerve

6. Dorsalis Pedis Fascia
7. Lateral Malleolus
8. Tendon of Peroneus Brevis Muscle
9. Posterior Tibial Vessels
10. Medial Malleolus
11. Great Saphenous Vein
12. Anterior Tibial Artery
13. Extensor Hallucis Longus Tendon
14. Achille's Tendon

Fig. 2-18

Wrist Joint

The wrist joint and hand are innervated by branches of almost the entire brachial plexus, including the radial, medial, and ulnar nerves **(Fig. 2-19)**.

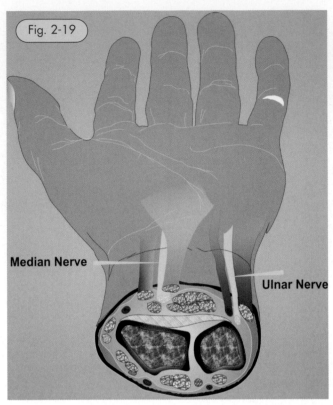

Fig. 2-19

Median Nerve

Ulnar Nerve

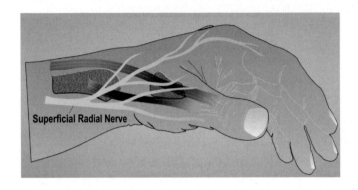

Superficial Radial Nerve

SUGGESTED READINGS

- Clemente CD. *Anatomy: A Regional Atlas of the Human Body.* 4th ed. Philadelphia, Pa: Lippincott; 1997.

- Dean D, Herbener TE. *Cross-sectional Human Anatomy.* Philadelphia, Pa: Lippincott; 2000.

- Gosling JA, Harris PF, Whitmore I, Willan PLT. *Human Anatomy: Color Atlas and Text.* 4th ed. London, England: Mosby International; 2002.

- Hahn MB, McQuillan PM, Sheplock GJ. *Regional Anesthesia: An Atlas of Anatomy and Techniques.* St. Louis, Mo: Mosby; 1996.

- Martini FH, Timmons MJ, Tallitsch RB. *Human Anatomy.* 4th ed. Upper Saddle River, NJ: Prentice Hall; 2003.

- Netter FH. *Atlas of Human Anatomy.* Summit, NJ: Ceiba Geigy; 1989.

- Pernkopf E. *Atlas of Topographical and Applied Human Anatomy. Vol I: Head and Neck.* 2nd ed. Munich, Germany: U&S Saunders; 1980.

- Pernkopf E. *Atlas of Topographical and Applied Human Anatomy.* Vol II: *Thorax, Abdomen and Extremities.* 2nd ed. Munich, Germany: U&S Saunders; 1980.

- Pick TP, Howden R, eds. *Gray's Anatomy: Descriptive and Surgical.* New York, NY: Portland House; 1977.

- Rohen JW, Yokochi C, Lütjen-Drecoll E. *Color Atlas of Anatomy.* 4th ed. Baltimore, Md: Williams & Wilkins; 1998.

- Rosse C, Gaddum-Rosse P. *Hillinshead's Textbook of Anatomy.* 5th ed. Philadelphia, Pa: Lippincott-Raven; 1997.

- Vloka JD, Hadžić A, April EW, Geatz H, Thys, DM. Division of the sciatic nerve in the popliteal fossa and its possible implications in the popliteal nerve blockade. *Anesth Analg* 2001;92:215–217.

- Vloka JD, Hadžić A, Kitain E, Lesser JB, Kuroda MM, April EW, Thys DM. Anatomic considerations for sciatic nerve block in the popliteal fossa through the lateral approach. *Reg Anesth* 1996;21:414–418.

- Vloka JD, Hadžić A, Lesser JB, Kitain E, Geatz H, April EW, Thys DM. A common epineural sheath for the nerves in the popliteal fossa and its possible implications for sciatic nerve block. *Anesth Analg* 1997; 84:387–390.

3 EQUIPMENT
AND PATIENT MONITORING
IN REGIONAL ANESTHESIA

Peripheral nerve blocks can be performed in a separate block-placement area or in the operating room **(Fig. 3-1)**. Regardless of where the actual procedure is performed, adequate space, equipment, and monitoring are imperative to ensure time-efficient care of the patient. One of the key requirements for successful implementation of nerve blocks is that all supplies, drugs, and other equipment for the block procedure be readily available in the room and prepared at the bedside. The physical size of the block room should allow enough room for proper monitoring, emergency access, and resuscitation of the patient. At the very minimum, proper lighting, oxygen administration, and emergency airway management with positive-pressure ventilation and suction must be available at all times.

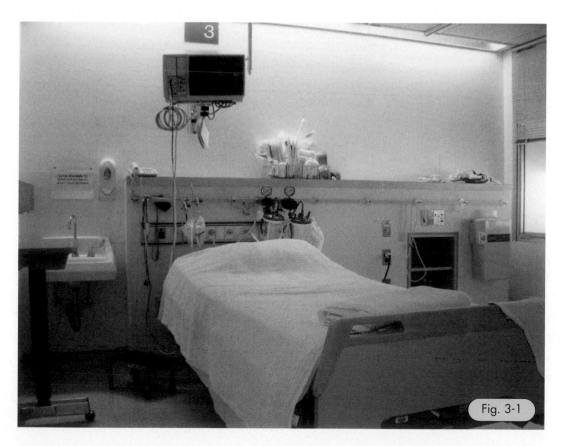

Fig. 3-1

An example of a block-placement room with basic monitoring equipment.

Emergency Drugs and Supplies

Adverse effects and difficulties associated with peripheral nerve blocks are relatively rare. However, when they occur, immediate and astute intervention is necessary to prevent severe complications. The block-placement area must be equipped with a source of oxygen, suction apparatus, and equipment for airway management and positive-pressure ventilation, as well as emergency drugs.

All drugs should be neatly organized in an immediately accessible drawer and checked on a daily basis for availability and expiration date. In our practice, emergency drugs are stored in a designated drawer in nerve block carts along with the rest of the nerve block equipment **(Table 3.1)**. Thus, they are immediately available throughout any nerve block procedure.

TABLE 3.1
Suggested Emergency Drugs Required During Nerve Block Procedures

DRUG	SUGGESTED DOSE FOR A 70-KG ADULT
Atropine	0.2–0.4 mg intravenous (IV) increments
Ephedrine	5–10 mg IV
Phenylephrine	50–200 µg IV
Epinephrine	10–100 µg IV
Midazolam	2.0–10 mg IV
Propofol*	30–200 mg IV
Muscle relaxant (succinylcholine or mivacurium)	mivacurium 0.1–0.2 mg/kg Succinylcholine 20–80 mg IV

* A short-acting barbiturate (e.g., thiopental, Brevital) can be used instead of propofol; however, this requires dilution of the drug at the time when its prompt administration is of utmost importance. In addition, the hypnotic and sedative effects of a barbiturate may be longer-lived than those of propofol.

Equipment for Emergency Airway Management

Toxicity of local anesthetics resulting in cessation of breathing and tonic-clonic seizure activity with resultant hypoxia, hypercarbia, and profound acidosis is an ever-present risk in the practice of peripheral nerve blocks. Proper, immediate treatment and airway management are necessary to avoid more severe complications of persistent hypoxia and acidosis. For this reason, emergency airway equipment must be immediately available at all times at all regional anesthesia placement and patient-monitoring locations. At the very least, this equipment should consist of laryngoscopic equipment with an assortment of commonly used blades, styletted endotracheal tubes of various sizes, airways of various sizes, and a mask-valve ventilation device (Ambu bag) with an oxygen source and a suction apparatus. These items ideally should be a part of the nerve block cart so that they are immediately available and accessible.

Needles and Needle–Catheter Systems

To perform successful nerve block anesthesia, appropriate equipment should be available, including needles, syringes, and the ancillary equipment necessary for the block. A needle of appropriate size should be chosen for each and every block technique to optimize precision and needle control and decrease the risk of complications. A needle that is too short will obviously not reach its targeted depth, whereas a needle of excessive length is much more difficult to control during advancement. In addition, excessively long needles tend to be inserted too deep and carry a higher risk of complications. The suggestions for needle length provided in this chapter are based on our practice and should be considered as general recommendations only **(Table 3.2)**.

Nerve injuries associated with peripheral nerve blocks occur for three main reasons. The first is direct injury of the nerve by the advancing needle. The second is injection of local anesthetic into the nerve or nerve sheath under high pressure (with resultant mechanical neural damage or ischemia of the nerve). Third, injury can be caused by a combination of these reasons, with possible contributing toxic effects of the local anesthetic or its preservative. To decrease the risk of needle-related injuries during nerve blockade, needles with short, blunt bevels are suggested by most expert anesthesiologists **(Fig. 3-2)**. Short-bevel needles are much less likely to penetrate nerves during needle advancement than long (cutting) bevel needles.

To avoid tissue trauma and unnecessary discomfort, it is important to use a needle with a relatively small diameter. Unfortunately, the limitations of small-diameter needle designs include difficulties in controlling the needle path due to bending of the needle during advancement and in the difficulty to inject local

TABLE 3.2
Suggested Needle Sizes For Some Common Nerve Block Procedures

Cervical plexus block	50 mm (2 in)
Interscalene brachial plexus block	25 mm (1 in) to 50 mm (2 in)
Infraclavicular brachial plexus block	100 mm (4 in)
Axillary brachial plexus block	25 mm (1 in) to 50 mm (2 in)
Thoracic paravertebral block	90 mm (3.5–4 in)
Lumbar paravertebral block	100 mm (4 in)
Lumbar plexus block	100 mm (4 in)
Sciatic block—posterior approach	100 mm (4 in)
Sciatic block—anterior approach	150 mm (6 in)
Femoral block	50 mm (2 in)
Popliteal block—posterior approach	50 mm (2 in)
Popliteal block—lateral approach	100 mm (4 in)

An example of common needle tip designs.

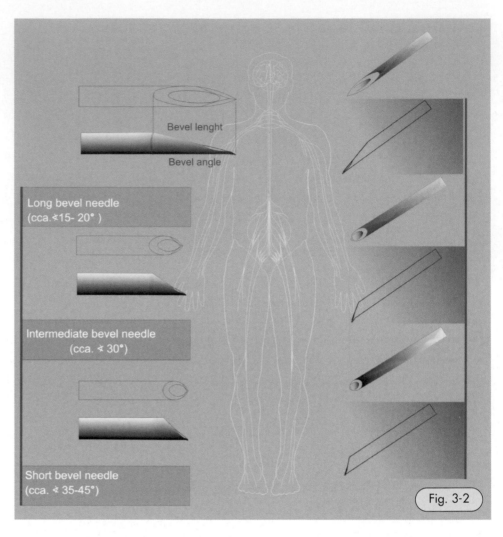

Bevel lenght

Bevel angle

Long bevel needle
(cca.∢15- 20°)

Intermediate bevel needle
(cca. ∢ 30°)

Short bevel needle
(cca. ∢ 35-45°)

Fig. 3-2

anesthetics and aspirate blood easily. In general, a 22-gauge needle is perhaps the smallest needle suitable for major conduction blocks. With longer needles, the needle diameter must be increased (e.g., 20- to 21-gauge) to prevent bending of the needle along its shaft and to retain control over the insertion path. On the other hand, needles of smaller internal diameter (e.g., 25- to 26-gauge) can be used for superficial and field blocks. It should be kept in mind that the high internal resistance of these needles during block injection makes it difficult to detect high pressures such as in the case of an intraneural injection. The future designs of nerve block needles may incorporate some means of pressure monitoring during injection to decrease the risk of inadvertent injection into the nerve.

Extension tubing attached to the needle is very useful in achieving proper needle stabilization. It is often included with the needle block kits currently marketed. Extension tubing also allows for an aspiration test to be performed, in case of inadvertent intravascular needle

placement as well as a syringe change, without moving the needle from its intended position.

When continuous infusion is planned, a wide variety of specially designed needles with larger diameters, catheters **(Fig. 3-3)**, and infusion pumps are also available **(Fig. 3-4)**. Some needle designs incorporate styletted catheters for increased ease and control of insertion or the ability to attach the nerve stimulator to a built-in lead to stimulate nerves before securing the catheter.

A more recent technical advance is a stimulating catheter for continuous nerve blocks. With this technology, a continuous catheter can be placed with a greater degree of precision. The infusion is initiated only after its successful placement is confirmed using nerve stimulation. Similarly, several different infusion pumps and systems have been recently introduced to allow continuous infusion for both inpatients and outpatients. These systems can be mechanically driven, spring-driven, balloon-driven, or of an electrical pump design **(Fig. 3-4)**.

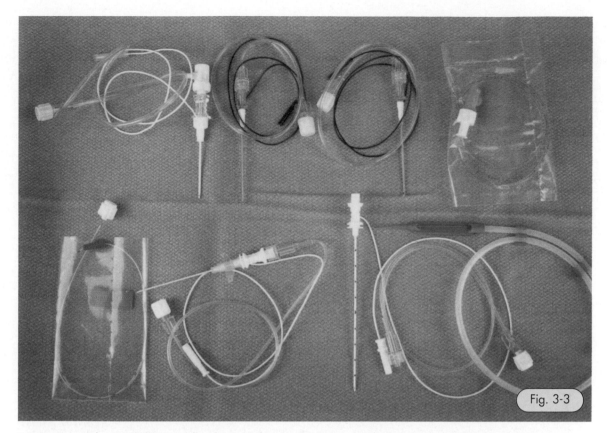

Fig. 3-3

Some currently available needle designs for continuous peripheral nerve blocks.

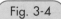

Fig. 3-4

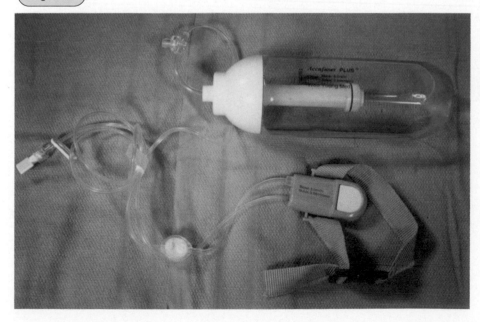

An example of continuous block infusion pumps.

Nerve Block Trays

A commercially or institutionally prepared nerve block tray is a prerequisite for time-efficient, successful performance of peripheral nerve block procedures. Such trays should be properly prepared to contain all necessary equipment to perform the intended regional anesthesia procedure without interruption. The basic items on each nerve block tray should include items for sterile skin preparation and draping, syringes with local anesthetic for skin infiltration, anesthesia, and performance of the block, a needle for skin infiltration and block performance, a skin surface electrode of good quality, and a marking pen with a ruler to outline the anatomy **(Fig. 3-5)**. A nerve stimulator or bottles of disinfectant are not sterile and should not be placed on the tray. With proper preparation, an anesthesiologist should be able to perform the entire procedure without distraction or without interrupting the process to look for additional or missing equipment.

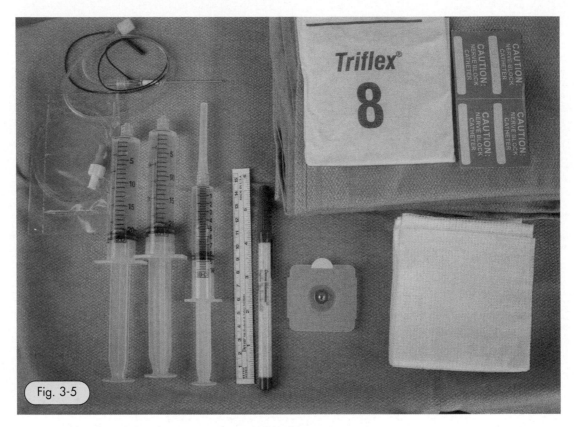

Fig. 3-5

An example of a properly prepared nerve block tray.

Organization of the Regional Anesthesia Cart

A designated, well-stocked, and well-maintained cart for regional anesthesia is extremely useful in a busy regional anesthesia practice **(Fig. 3-6)**. Such a cart should be organized logically to include all equipment and local anesthetics commonly used, draping and skin disinfecting supplies, nerve stimulators, and resuscitation drugs and equipment **(Figs. 3-6 to 3–12)**. The cart should be organized and stocked so that just about any regional block procedure can be performed time-efficiently and without interruption in the block area, on the ward, or in the operating room.

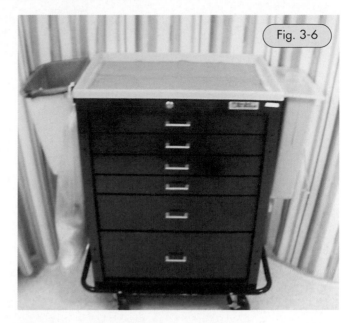

Fig. 3-6

Regional anesthesia cart.

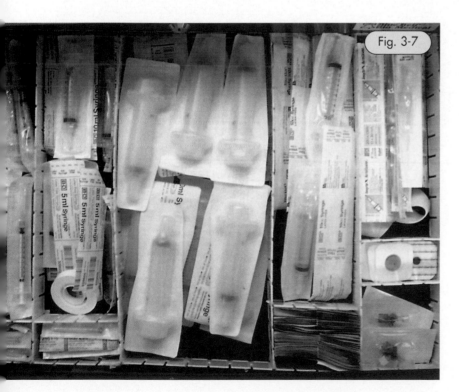

Fig. 3-7

The top drawer contains mostly various needles and syringes.

- 1- and 3-mL syringes
- 5- and 10-mL syringes and blank label tape
- 20-mL syringes
- 10-mL and control syringes
- Intravenous (IV) catheters and a tourniquet
- 18-gauge needles
- $1^1/_2$-in, 25-gauge needles
- Alcohol swabs
- Stopcocks
- Return electrodes (high-quality electrocardiogram [ECG] surface leads)

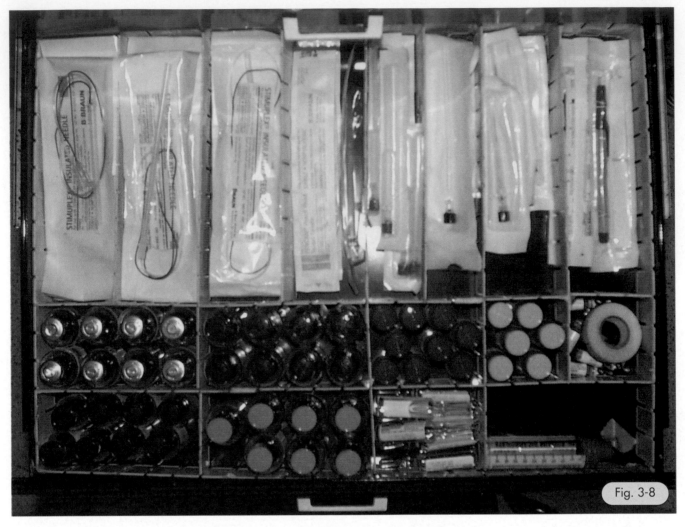

Fig. 3-8

The second drawer contains block needles, local anesthetics, and additives.

- 50-mm insulated needles
- 100-mm insulated needles
- 150-mm insulated needles
- 127-mm, 27-gauge pencil-point spinal needle
- 90-mm and 120-mm, 24-gauge Sprotte spinal needles
- 90-mm and 120-mm, 22-gauge Quincke-type spinal needles
- 80-mm, 22-gauge Tuohy epidural needle
- Skin markers

- 3% Chloroprocaine bottles
- 1% Ropivacaine
- Sterile water
- 0.9% Sodium chloride
- 1 mL 1:1000 epinephrine
- Label tape
- 1.5% Mepivacaine
- 0.5% Bupivacaine
- 2% Lidocaine
- Bicarbonate

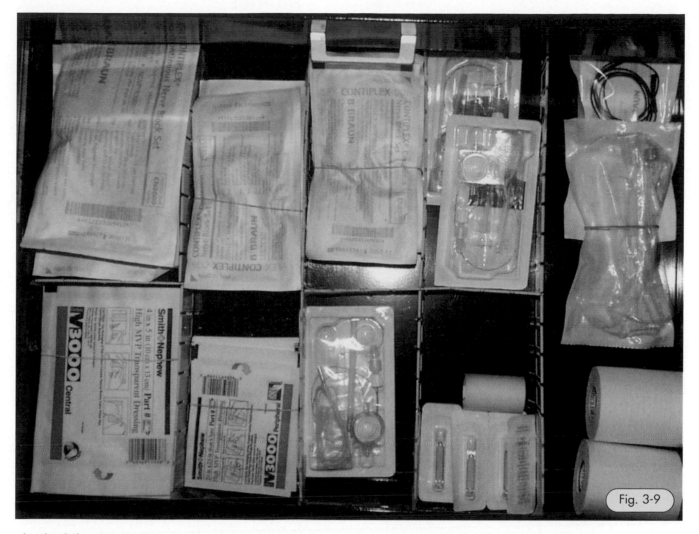

Fig. 3-9

The third drawer contains mostly continuous nerve block sets and various items for securing catheters.

- Continuous nerve block set with a 100-mm needle

- Continuous nerve block set with a 50-mm needle

- Various other continuous nerve block sets

- Various tubing and nerve stimulator electrode extension sets

- Clear dressing material

- Adhesive tape and other accessories for securing catheters

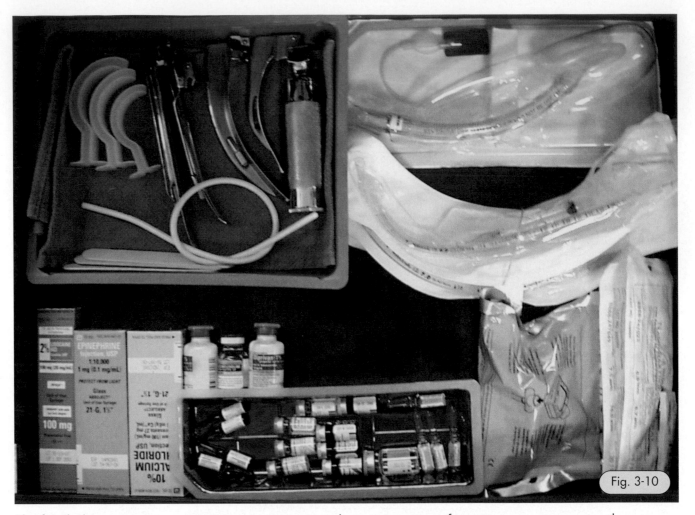

Fig. 3-10

The fourth drawer contains resuscitation equipment, such as various items for airway management and cardiovascular drugs.

- Laryngoscope handle and blades of various types and sizes

- Oral airways

- Intubating stylettes

- Tongue depressors

- Laryngeal mask airway (LMA)

- Several endotracheal tubes of various sizes

- Nasal airways

- End-tidal carbon dioxide detector

- Various emergency and IV induction medications: lidocaine, ephedrine, phenylephrine, epinephrine, atropine, calcium, propofol, succinylcholine, flumazenil, naloxone **(see Table 3.1)**

The organization of the cart suggested here can be further customized to accommodate the specifics of an individual practice.

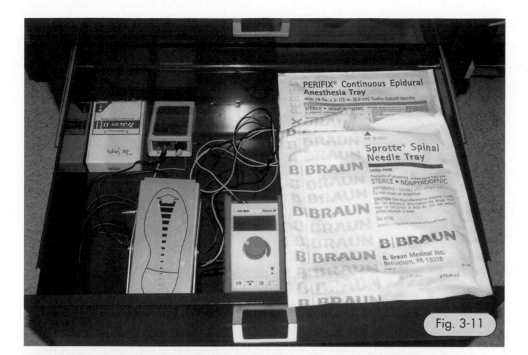

The fifth drawer contains various epidural and spinal trays and nerve stimulator(s).

Fig. 3-11

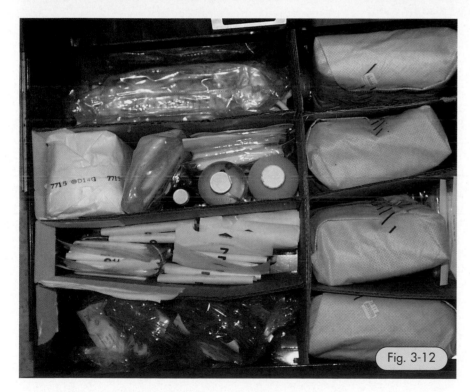

The bottom drawer contains various ancillary items.

Fig. 3-12

- Intravenous (IV) fluids

- IV sets for emergency vascular access

- Packs of sterile towels

- Oxygen masks

- 4-in × 4-in gauze packs

- Iodine and alcohol skin-disinfecting solutions

- Sterile plastic drape kits

- Sterile gloves and examining gloves of various sizes

Monitoring of Patients Receiving Regional Anesthetic

The majority of peripheral nerve block procedures proceed smoothly and without any complications. However, the risk of inadvertent intravascular injection or rapid absorption or channeling of local anesthetic into the systemic circulation with consequent toxic effects is always present. For this reason, every patient undergoing a major conduction nerve block should receive an intravenous infusion line and be adequately monitored to allow timely detection of any systemic toxicity produced by a local anesthetic and immediate vascular access for its treatment.

The monitoring of patients undergoing major conduction blocks should include recording a baseline level of consciousness, pulse oximetry, vital signs (blood pressure and heart rate), and an electrocardiogram (ECG). The respiratory rate must also be monitored throughout the block procedure. After completion of the procedure, all patients receiving large doses of local anesthetic for major conduction or plexus blocks are routinely monitored for signs of local anesthetic toxicity for 30 minutes following block placement. Although in almost all instances a toxic reaction occurs during or immediately on injection, the peak serum levels of local anesthetic are typically observed 20 minutes after the injection.

Intraoperative monitoring of patients undergoing surgery under regional anesthesia is identical to that of patients undergoing general anesthesia and consists of measuring arterial blood pressure, heart rate, respiratory rate and continuous ECG monitoring. For minimally sedated and conversing patients, temperature measurements are not necessary.

Documenting Nerve Block Procedures

Medical documentation pertaining to the induction and maintenance of general anesthesia has been standardized in most countries. Such documentation not only collects the physiologic data, such as arterial blood pressure, heart rate, and oxygenation, but also the details of various procedures such as endotracheal intubation, airway examination, laryngoscopy grades, and so on. Similarly, documentation of neuraxial anesthesia procedures routinely includes comments on level of blockade, sterility precautions, choice of equipment and technique, presence or absence of cerebrospinal fluid, blood, or paresthesia during needle placement, and injection of local anesthetic. However, it is puzzling that at present there are no standard documenting procedures for peripheral nerve blocks.

The lack of such standardized documentation for peripheral nerve blocks has several drawbacks because it makes retrospective analyses, whether for the purpose of research, quality assurance, or medicolegal issues, very difficult and sometimes impossible.

At St. Luke's-Roosevelt Hospital Center, we use a documentation procedure that allows an easy, reasonably accurate retrospective review of a peripheral nerve block procedure. This documentation is based on a computerized record-keeping system and consists of a description of the type of block, sterility procedures, equipment, and a number of other relevant details:

- Nerve block procedure
- Approach used
- Premedication
- Skin preparation
- Equipment used (needle and nerve stimulator)
- Number of attempts (needle insertions)
- Type of response obtained on nerve stimulation
- Minimal current (mA) accepted
- Local anesthetic (type, concentration, additives, volume)
- Abnormal pressure or pain during injection
- Signs of block onset
- Comments

Although not exhaustive, this information allows a reasonably accurate review of periblock events that may have led to a failure or any other problems. In addition, it helps trainees develop a consistent, organized approach to nerve blockade, which is necessary for a successful, objective, and more scientific approach to the practice of peripheral nerve blocks.

SUGGESTED READINGS

- Benumof JL. Permanent loss of cervical spinal cord function associated with interscalene block performed under general anesthesia. *Anesthesiology* 2000;93:1541.
- Birnbach DJ, Stein DJ, Murray O, Thys DM, Sordillo EM. Povidone iodine and skin disinfection before initiation of epidural anesthesia. *Anesthesiology* 1998;88:668.
- Benzon HT, Raja SN, Borsook D, Molloy RE, Strichartz G: *Essentials of Pain Medicine and Regional Anesthesia.* Philadelphia, Pa: Churchill Livingstone; 1999.
- Jankovic D, Wells C. *Regional Nerve Blocks.* 2nd ed. Wissenchafts-Verlag Berlin, Germany: Blackwell Scientific Publications, 2001.
- Hadžić A, Vloka JD. Peripheral nerve stimulator for unassisted nerve blockade. *Anesthesiology* 1996; 84:1528–1529.
- Mulroy MF: *Regional Anesthesia: An Illustrated Procedural Guide.* 3rd ed. Philadelphia, Pa: Lippincott, 2002.
- New York School of Regional Anesthesia Web site at www.nysora.com.
- Raj PP. *Textbook of Regional Anesthesia.* London, England: Churchill Livingstone, 2002.
- Steele SM, Klien SM, D'Ercole FJ, Greengrass RA, Gleason D. A new continuous catheter delivery system. *Anesth Analg* 1998;87:228.

PERIPHERAL
NERVE STIMULATORS AND
NERVE STIMULATION

Eliciting paresthesia or nerve stimulation is a commonly used method for localizing nerves prior to the injection of local anesthetic. Paresthesia is thought to result from mechanical stimulation of the nerve, causing a sensory feeling described as "an electric current" or "a shock" in the sensory distribution of the nerve being touched. Thus, paresthesia can indicate that the needle is in close proximity to the nerve and is a warning sign of impending mechanical contact should the needle be further advanced. In contrast, nerve stimulation techniques rely on the use of electric current to elicit motor stimulation of nerves and confirm the proximity of the needle to the nerve.

Nerve Localization: Paresthesia or Nerve Stimulation?

The debate over which technique, paresthesia or nerve stimulation, is safer and more efficacious is moot. The discussion must be limited only to brachial plexus blockade, as the use of paresthesia techniques in infraclavicular, lumbar plexus, femoral, sciatic, popliteal, and other "deep" blocks is both unreliable and unacceptable in modern practice. Consequently, modern regional anesthesia practice is nearly impossible without nerve stimulators. Most recently published reports in the field describe the use of nerve stimulators in their methods.

Regardless, the question of whether eliciting paresthesia or nerve stimulation is safer in brachial plexus blockade still continues to be debated by some researchers. Selander and Plevak suggest that the paresthesia technique increases the risk of postblock neuropathies. Indeed, the frequency of postanesthesia neuropathy was significantly greater when paresthesia techniques were utilized as compared with "nonparesthesia" techniques. On the other hand, careful use of the paresthesia technique to localize the brachial plexus is successfully used at many centers without a significant increase in the risk of nerve injury. The major drawback of the paresthesia technique is that it is associated with greater patient discomfort. Compared to the nerve stimulator technique, it is also much more difficult to teach.

Peripheral Nerve Stimulators

Peripheral nerve stimulators (PNSs) have become indispensable in the practice of modern regional anesthesia. A more in-depth understanding of how they function is required so that their full potential can be realized in a clinical setting. In this chapter, we review some basic engineering principles behind nerve stimulators and provide tips on how to choose a nerve stimulator for your practice and make the most out of it. Although the use of PNSs for regional anesthesia was first suggested by Von Perthes in 1912, it has gained wider acceptance concurrent only with the resurgence of interest in regional anesthesia during the last two decades. The manufacturing industry has met the demand for devices that are more accurate in determining nerve location prior to the injection of local anesthetic, and several makes and models are commercially available. Though the newer models are inherently more accurate, they often include a plethora of functions with controls that are not intuitive.

Nerve Stimulator Components

This is a standard block circuit of a modern PNS. The circuit has six main parts as seen in the block diagram **(Fig. 4-1)**.

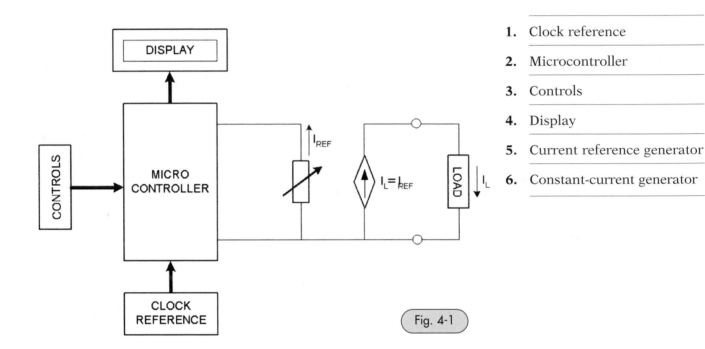

1. Clock reference
2. Microcontroller
3. Controls
4. Display
5. Current reference generator
6. Constant-current generator

Fig. 4-1

Clock Reference

The clock reference functions as a synchronizing mechanism for the PNS. Generally, it is a crystal oscillator that produces an accurate, high-frequency clock signal. This clock signal is then fed to the microcontroller as input and used to control all the functions. The specific frequency of the oscillator depends on the type of microcontroller used in the design.

Microcontroller

The microcontroller functions as the brain of the nerve stimulator. Most nerve stimulators run on battery power, and so choosing a low-power microcontroller is of the utmost importance. The microcontroller receives input from the controls and, according to the instructions received, changes the value of the current, frequency, or pulse width. In addition to changing the value, it also relays it to the display so that the user is aware of the new setting.

Constant-Current Generator

The constant-current generator can be modeled as a reference current. An ideal constant-current source could deliver the same current regardless of the value of the impedance (resistance) load connected to it. Because ideal constant-current source intensity does

Constant Current Output

volts

0.3 mA	■
0.5mA	◇
1 mA	▲
5mA	△

Impedance in kOhm

Fig. 4-2

not exist, a clinically acceptable compromise can be achieved using a current generator to provide a stable current over the clinically expected range of impedance loads. This is achieved by generating a progressively higher voltage output as the impedance between the electrodes is increased. For instance, when set to deliver a current of 1 mA and the tissue impedance between the two electrodes is 1 kΩ, the nerve stimulator delivers 1 V. If the impedance between the electrodes is 5 kΩ, the stimulator automatically increases the voltage output and delivers 5 V to maintain the same set current of 1 mA ($I = U/R$) **(Fig. 4-2)**.

Controls

There are usually three sets of controls on a typical PNS: frequency, pulse width, and current. The controls can be analog or digital, and each control increases or decreases the value of the controlled parameter. Once the user sets a value, the microcontroller changes the value of the desired parameter. A current controlled via a remote foot pedal facilitates quick current adjustment and allows a single operator to perform the nerve block procedure without the help of an assistant **(Fig. 4-3)**. More recently, hand-held remote controllers have also been introduced to allow unassisted nerve localization.

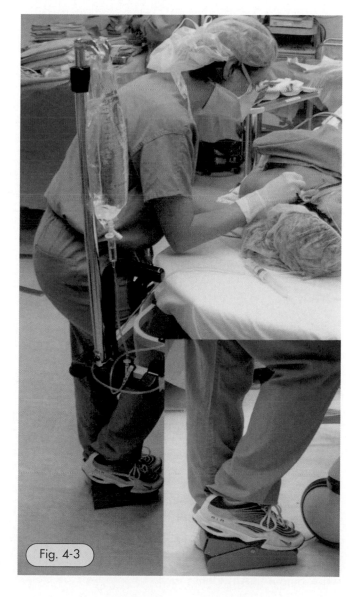

An example of a remote (foot-controlled) nerve stimulator.

Fig. 4-3

Current Reference Generator

The current reference generator is based on a precisely known voltage source and a low-tolerance digital potentiometer **(Fig. 4-1)**. A voltage regulator usually supplies the voltage source. A low-tolerance digital potentiometer is similar to a standard potentiometer in that it changes resistance over its entire range. It is controlled by the microcontroller using a series of command pulses that tell it to increase or decrease the value. Unlike analog potentiometers, digital potentiometers adjust values in discrete increments, and so it is important to choose one with enough steps. Generally, a 10-bit potentiometer, giving 1024 steps, is sufficient for the application.

Display

A typical PNS has a standard liquid crystal display (LCD) that uses less current and is more versatile than seven-segment, light-emitting diode displays. Most displays show the set value of current, frequency, and pulse width. Other indicators, such as low battery level and probe disconnect, can also be included.

| | | 2. | 0 | H | z | | | 1 | 0 | 0 | μ | s | |
| | | 0. | 5 | m | A | | | | | | | | |

An example of a typical PNS LCD display.

Electrophysiology of Nerve Stimulation

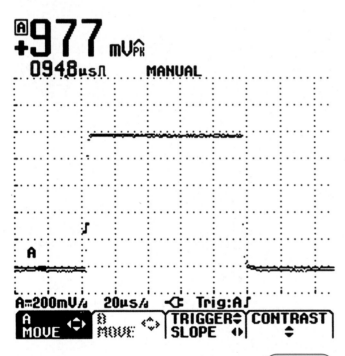

Fig. 4-4

A typical output of a nerve stimulator as analyzed by an oscilloscope. The nerve stimulator was set to deliver 1 mA into a 1-kΩ impedance load. The x-axis displays the duration of the stimulus (pulse width) (100 μs). The y-axis displays the amplitude of the voltage output (0.977 V). The actual current output by the stimulator is calculated as voltage output (voltage [V]/impedance [Ω] = output [mA]) (Ohm's law).

Of particular importance to nerve stimulation is the relationship between the strength and duration of the current and the polarity of the stimulus. To propagate a nerve impulse, a certain threshold level of stimulus must be applied to the nerve. Below this threshold, no impulse is propagated. Any increase in the stimulus above this threshold results in a corresponding increase in the intensity of the impulse. Assuming that a square pulse of current is used to stimulate the nerve **(Fig. 4-4)**, the total energy (charge) applied to the nerve is a product of current intensity and pulse duration.

The following two terms are of importance for nerve stimulation:

- Rheobase: the minimal current required to stimulate the nerve with a long pulse.
- Chronaxie: the duration of current required to achieve twice the stimulation that the rheobase produces.

The current intensity required to stimulate the nerve depends on the rheobase (Ir), chronaxie (C), and duration of the stimulus (t).

$$I = Ir(1 + C/t)$$

The chronaxie can be used to measure the stimulation threshold of any particular nerve and is useful when comparing different nerves or types of nerve fibers. The chronaxies of peripheral nerves are shown in **Table 4.1**.

TABLE 4.1
Chronaxies of Peripheral Nerves

TYPE OF FIBER	CHRONAXIE (μsec.)
α (alpha) fibers	50–100
Δ (delta) fibers	170
C fibers	400

The large α (or alpha) motor fibers are more readily stimulated than the smaller Δ (or delta) fibers or C fibers responsible for pain sensation. This makes it possible to achieve a motor response without significant patient discomfort. However, when a higher-intensity current is used (e.g., greater than 1.0 mA), preferential stimulation of the motor fibers may be lost, and uncomfortable paresthesia-like stimulation is often elicited. Significantly less current is required to elicit motor response with stimuli of longer duration (e.g. >0.5mA)

Orientation of the Electrodes

An important concept to keep in mind involving peripheral nerve stimulation is the principle of preferential cathodal stimulation, which states that when the cathode (negative electrode) is positioned closer to the nerve than the anode (positive electrode), significantly less current is needed to obtain a response to stimulation than if the positions are reversed. When the stimulating electrode is negative, the current flow alters the resting membrane potential adjacent to the needle, producing an area of depolarization which spreads across the nerve, initiating a motor response. When the electrode adjacent to the nerve is positive, the current causes hyperpolarization adjacent to the needle and a ring of depolarization distal to the needle tip. Such an arrangement of electrodes is less efficient in propagating the stimulus and has a clinical implication: significantly more current is required to stimulate the nerve. The site of placement of the positive (return) electrode is irrelevant with modern stimulators as long as quality electrodes are used and good electrical contact is achieved. The use of dry or poor-quality electrocardiograph electrodes for nerve localization should be avoided.

Relationship Between Needle-Nerve Distance and Current Intensity

One of the most common misconceptions about nerve stimulation is that nerve stimulators are considered "nerve finders." It is often claimed that a higher current can be used to identify the nerve first and that the needle can then be "guided" closer toward the nerve, by advancing it while progressively decreasing the stimulating current. However, the nature of the current-nerve distance is not that simplistic, as will be seen from the following discussion.

The relationship between the stimulus intensity and the distance from the nerve is governed by Coulomb's law:

$$I = K(Q/r^2)$$

where I is the current required to stimulate the nerve, K is a constant, Q is the minimal current needed for stimulation, and r is the distance from the stimulus to the nerve.

The presence of the inverse square means that a current of very high intensity is required as the needle moves away from the nerve. In addition, although stimulation with a current of high intensity (e.g., 4 to 8 mA) may result in nerve stimulation even though the needle is some distance away from the nerve, it does not offer information about the plane in which the needle must be advanced to get closer to the nerve. Besides, such high-current stimulation inevitably results in patient discomfort. Thus, nerve stimulators cannot be used as a substitute for a sound knowledge of regional anesthesia anatomy.

In contrast, when stimulation is accomplished using a current of low intensity, much more information can be obtained. For instance, a clear motor response achieved at 0.2 to 0.5 mA indicates an intimate needle–nerve relationship, which is associated with a higher success rate of achieving neuronal blockade. However, nerve stimulation using a stimulating current of less than 0.2 mA (0.1 – 0.3 msec) may be associated with intraneural placement of the needle and should be avoided. In our experience, stimulation at such a low-intensity current often results in pain and, occasionally, resistance on injection. In this case, the needle should be slightly withdrawn so that stimulation is achieved with a current between 0.20 and 0.50 mA and the injection carried out.

Important Features of Nerve Stimulators

In their pioneering work about two decades ago, Galindo and colleagues made recommendations about desirable features of PNSs. Although their suggestions are still valid today, current nerve stimulators have become much more specialized and advanced and incorporate rather complex, sophisticated electronics **(Fig. 4-1)**. Advances in technology have largely served the purpose of manufacturing more reliable, precise units. However, the plethora of functions and features on some models can make their use confusing. Based on our interactions with many anesthesiologists who attended our workshops on peripheral nerve blocks and participated in our recent survey on the use of nerve stimulators, it is clear that keeping pace with the technological advances in this field has become a challenge for many clinicians. For this and other practical reasons, we believe that nerve stimulators for regional anesthesia should be engineered specifically for the purpose of nerve stimulation, and be simple to operate, highly reliable, and ergonomic.

Important Features of Nerve Stimulators

- Constant-current output: The impedance of tissues, needles, connecting wires, and grounding electrodes may vary. A constant-current design incorporates automatic compensation in voltage output for changes in tissue or connection impedance during nerve stimulation, ensuring accurate delivery of the specified current within a clinically relevant range of impedance loads.
- Accurate current display: The ability to read the current being delivered is of utmost importance for both the success and safety of nerve blocks.
- Convenient means of current intensity control: Current can be controlled using either digital means or an analog dial. Alternatively, current intensity can be controlled using a remote controller, such as a foot pedal or hand-held controller, allowing a single operator to perform the procedure and control the current output. The stimulator design should allow for changes in the current intensity in increments of 0.01 mA in the range of 0.00 to 0.50 mA, and 0.1 mA thereafter.
- Pulse width: A short pulse width (e.g., 100 to 200 μs) corresponding to the chronaxies of A fibers appears to be the most suitable for nerve localization. Although some units allow the user to change the current duration, the clinical utility of such a feature is still not well defined.
- Stimulating frequency: A 2- to 2.5-Hz stimulating frequency appears optimal for nerve localization. When using older units with 1-Hz stimulation (one stimulus per second), the needle must be advanced very slowly to avoid missing the nerve between stimuli.
- Disconnect and malfunction indicator: This is an essential feature because the anesthesiologist should know when the stimulus is not being delivered due to a malfunction (e.g., disconnected, poor electrical connection, battery failure). The future needle designs may also incorporate an indicator of current intensity and disconnect on the hub of the needle.

SUGGESTED READINGS

- Bathram CN. Nerve stimulators for nerve localization—are they all the same? *Anaesthesia* 1997;52; 761–764.
- Choyce A, Chan VW, Middleton WJ, Knight PR, Peng P, McCartney CJ. What is the relationship between paresthesia and nerve stimulation for axillary brachial plexus block? *Reg Anesth Pain Med* 2001;26;100.
- Hadžić A, Vloka JD, Hadžić H, Thys DM, Santos AC. Nerve stimulators used for peripheral nerve blocks vary in their electrical characteristics. *Anesthesiology*, 2003;98:969–974.
- Hadžić A, Vloka JD, Koorn R. Effects of the auditory volume control knob on the stimulus amplitude display of the DualStim/Deluxe Model NS-2CA/DX peripheral nerve stimulator. *Anesthesiology* 1997;87: 714–715.
- Hadžić A, Vloka JD. Peripheral nerve stimulator for unassisted nerve blockade. *Anesthesiology* 1996;84: 1528–1529.

- Hadžić A, Vloka JD. Choice of local anesthetic. In: Chelly JE, ed. *Peripheral Nerve Blocks: A Color Atlas.* Philadelphia, Pa: Lippincott Williams & Wilkins, in press, 2003.
- Jankovic D, Wells C. *Regional Nerve Blocks.* 2nd ed. Wissenchafts-Verlag Berlin, Germany: Blackwell Scientific Publications, 2001.
- Pither CE, Raj PP, Ford DJ. The use of peripheral nerve stimulators for regional anesthesia: a review of experimental characteristics, technique, and clinical applications. *Reg Anesth* 1985;10:49–58.
- Tulchinsky A, Weller RS, Rosenblum M, Gross JB. Nerve stimulator polarity and brachial plexus block. *Anesth Analg* 1993; 77 (1):100–3.
- Vloka JD, Hadžić A, Kuroda MM, Koorn R, Birnbach DJ. Practice patterns in the use of peripheral nerve stimulators in peripheral nerve blockade: a national survey. *Reg Anesth* 1997; 22:61.
- Vloka JD, Hadžić A, Thys DM. Peripheral nerve stimulators for regional anesthesia can generate excessive voltage output with poor ground connection. *Anesth Analg* 2000; 91:1306–1313.

5 CLINICAL PHARMACOLOGY
OF LOCAL ANESTHETICS

Local anesthetics prevent or relieve pain by interrupting nerve conduction. They bind to specific receptor sites of the Na^+ channels in nerves and block the movement of ions through these pores. The action of local anesthetics is limited to the site of application and rapidly reverses on diffusion from the site of action. Both the chemical and pharmacologic properties of individual local anesthetic drugs determine their clinical properties. This chapter discusses the mechanism of action of local anesthetics and their physical properties, clinical use, and toxicity, and its prevention and treatment.

Nerve Conduction

Nerve conduction involves the propagation of an electrical signal generated by the rapid movement of small amounts of several ions (sodium and potassium) across a nerve cell membrane. The ionic gradient for sodium (high extracellularly and low intracellularly) and potassium (high intracellularly and low extracellularly) is maintained by a sodium-potassium pump mechanism within the nerve. In the resting state, the nerve membrane is more permeable to potassium ions than to sodium ions, resulting in the continuous leakage of potassium ions out of the interior of the nerve cell. This leakage of cations in turn creates a negatively charged interior relative to the exterior, resulting in an electric potential of -60 to -70 mV across the nerve membrane.

Receptors at the distal ends of sensory nerves serve as sensors and transducers of various mechanical, chemical, or thermal stimuli. Such stimuli are converted to miniscule electric currents. For example, chemical mediators released with a surgical incision react with these receptors and generate small electric currents. As a result, the electric potential across a nerve membrane near the receptor is altered, making it less negative. If the threshold potential is achieved, an action potential results, with a sudden increase in the permeability of the nerve membrane to sodium ions and a resultant rapid influx of positively charged sodium ions. This causes a transient reversal of charge, or depolarization. Repolarization occurs when sodium permeability decreases and potassium permeability increases, resulting in an efflux of potassium from within the cell and restoration of the electrical balance. Subsequently, both ions are restored to their initial intracellular and extracellular concentrations by the sodium-potassium adenosine triphosphatase-driven pump mechanism. Depolarization generates a current that sequentially depolarizes the adjacent segment of the nerve, thus "activating" the nerve.

The rapid influx of sodium ions that produces the initial upswing of the action potential occurs through specific sodium channels in the cell membrane. The sodium channel is a protein structure that penetrates the full depth of the membrane bilayer and is in communication with the extracellular surface of the nerve membrane and the axoplasm (interior) of the nerve. The physical properties of the sodium channel on the extracellular surface allow mainly sodium ions to move through it. Sodium channels can change the nerve from being nonconductive to conductive to an action potential and are commonly referred to as gated channels. If such a change in conductance is induced by electrical changes, the channel is said to be voltage-gated. The voltage-gated sodium channel in a nerve is generally considered to be the site of action of local anesthetics.

Local anesthetics prevent the generation and conduction of nerve impulses, and the primary site of action is the cell membrane. Local anesthetics block conduction by decreasing or preventing a large transient increase in the permeability of excitable membranes to Na^+. However, because the interaction of local anesthetic with K^+ channels requires higher drug concentrations, a blockade of conduction is not accompanied by any large or consistent change in resting membrane potential due to the blockade of K^+ channels.

Structure–Activity Relationship of Local Anesthetics

The typical structure of a local anesthetic consists of hydrophilic and hydrophobic domains separated by an intermediate ester or amide linkage. The hydrophilic group is usually a tertiary amine, and the hydrophobic domain is an aromatic moiety. The nature of the linking group determines the pharmacologic properties of local anesthetic agents. The physiochemical properties of these agents largely influence their potency and duration of action. For instance, hydrophobicity increases both the potency and duration of their action. This increase is due to an association of the drug at hydrophobic sites that enhances partitioning of the drug to its sites of action and decreases the rate of metabolism by plasma esterases as well as liver enzymes. In addition, the affinity of receptors in Na^+ channels for local anesthetic agents increases with hydrophobicity. Unfortunately, hydrophobicity also increases toxicity, decreasing the therapeutic index for more hydrophobic drugs.

An amino group present at the end of the molecule opposite the benzene ring determines the hydrophilic activity and ionization of a drug. The amino group usually has three organic groups attached (tertiary amine) and becomes charged (ionized) into a cationic form by the addition of a hydrogen ion. The pK_a of the local anesthetic determines the ratio of the ionized (cationic) and the uncharged (base) form of the drug. The pK_a for local anesthetic drugs falls within a narrow range.

By definition, the pK_a is the pH at which 50% of the drug is ionized and 50% is present as base. The relationship among pH, pK_a, and concentration of the cationic and base forms of a local anesthetic is described by the Henderson–Hasselbach equation:

$$pH = pK_a + \log ([base]/[cation])$$

The pK_a generally correlates with the speed of onset of action of most amide local anesthetic drugs; the closer the pK_a to the body pH, the faster the onset. The coexistence of the two forms of the drug—the charged cation and the uncharged base—is important because drug penetration of the nerve membrane by the local anesthetic requires the base (unionized) form to pass through the nerve lipid membrane; once in the axoplasm of the nerve, the base form can accept a hydrogen ion and equilibrate into the cationic form. The cationic form is predominant and produces a blockade of the sodium channel. The amount of base form that can be in solution is limited by its aqueous solubility.

An ester or an amide linkage is present between the lipophilic end (benzene ring) and the hydrophilic end (amino group) of the molecule. The type of linkage determines the site of metabolic degradation of the drug. Ester-linked local anesthetics are metabolized in plasma, whereas amide-linked drugs undergo metabolism in the liver.

Small structural modifications of local anesthetics can result in major changes in activity, such as significant differences in potency, onset, and duration of action of a local anesthetic.

Frequency and Voltage Dependence of Local Anesthetic Action

A resting nerve is much less sensitive to a local anesthetic than a nerve that is repeatedly stimulated. A higher frequency of stimulation and a more positive membrane potential cause a greater degree of anesthetic blockade. These frequency- and voltage-dependent effects of local anesthetics occur because in its charged form a molecule of local anesthetic gains access to its binding site within a pore only when the Na^+ channel is in an activated state and because the local anesthetic binds more tightly to and stabilizes the inactivated state of the channel. Local anesthetics exhibit these properties to different degrees depending on their pK_a, lipid solubility, and molecular size. In general, the frequency-dependence of local anesthetic action depends critically on the rate of dissociation from the receptor site in the pore of the Na^+ channel.

Differential Sensitivity of Nerve Fibers to Local Anesthetics

As a general rule, smaller nerve fibers are more susceptible to the action of local anesthetics than large fibers **(Fig. 5-1)**. Smaller fibers are preferentially blocked because the critical length over which an impulse can propagate passively is shorter. This length is related to the shorter space constant for the propagation of voltage changes along smaller unmyelinated nerves and to the shorter internodal distances. Smaller fibers, with their shorter critical lengths, are blocked more quickly by anesthetic solutions than larger fibers. The same reasoning accounts for the slower recovery of larger fibers when the process is reversed during washout of the local anesthetic. The sensitivity of a fiber to local anesthetics is not always determined by whether it is sensory or motor. Muscle proprioceptive afferent and motor efferent fibers are equally sensitive. These two types of fibers have the same diameter, which is larger than that of the alpha motor fibers

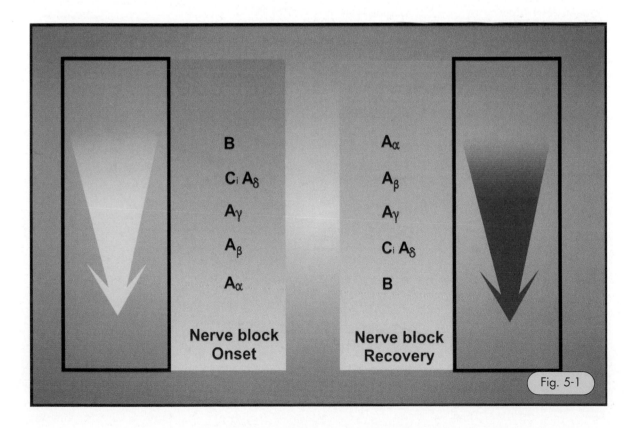

Nerve block Onset

B
$C_i\ A_\delta$
A_γ
A_β
A_α

Nerve block Recovery

A_α
A_β
A_γ
$C_i\ A_\delta$
B

Fig. 5-1

that supply the muscle spindles. It is the more rapid blockade of these smaller motor fibers, rather than of the sensory fibers, that leads to the preferential loss of muscle reflexes. Similarly, in large nerve trunks motor fibers are usually located in the outer portion of the bundle and are more accessible to local anesthetic. Thus, motor fibers may be blocked before sensory fibers in large mixed nerves.

The differential rate of blockade exhibited by fibers of varying sizes and firing rates is of considerable practical importance. Fortunately, the sensation of pain is usually the first modality to disappear; it is followed by the loss of sensations of cold, warmth, touch, deep pressure, and, finally, loss of motor function, although variation among patients and different nerves is considerable.

Local Anesthetics and pH

Local anesthetics are unprotonated amines and as such tend to be relatively insoluble (Fig. 5-2). For this reason, they are marketed as water-soluble salts, usually hydrochlorides. Although local anesthetics are weak bases (typical pK_a values range from 8 to 9), their hydrochloride salts are mildly acidic. This property increases the stability of local anesthetic esters and any accompanying vasoconstrictor substance. Local anesthetic drugs, as previously described, pass through the nerve membrane in a nonionized, lipid-soluble base form; when they are within the nerve axoplasm, they equilibrate into

an ionic form that is active within the sodium channel. The rate-limiting step in this cascade is penetration of the local anesthetic through the nerve membrane, and all the commercially available local anesthetic solutions contain very little drug in the nonionized, lipid-soluble base form that can penetrate the membrane.

The fraction of the nonionized form present, as well as that of the cationic form, is determined by the pK_a of the solution and the pH of the drug solution. Commercially available solutions are acidic, and the cationic form predominates in solution.

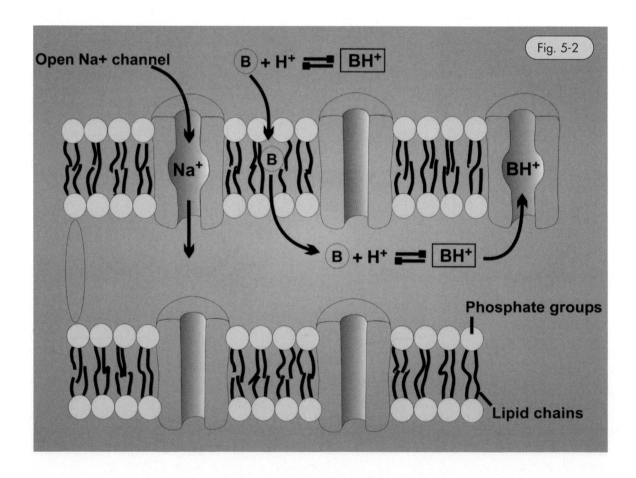

Fig. 5-2

Because this form does not cross biological membranes readily, sodium bicarbonate ($NaHCO_3$) is often added to local anesthetic. This increases the amount of drug in the base form, which shortens the onset time. Obviously, the limiting factor for pH adjustment is the solubility of the base form of the drug. Unfortunately, only small changes in pH can be achieved by the addition of bicarbonate because of the limited solubility of the base, only small decreases in onset time are realized. For instance, with the alkalinization of bupivacaine, an increase in the amount of base in solution is limited by the minimal solubility of free base in solution. For each local anesthetic, there is a pH at which the amount of base in solution is maximal (a saturated solution). Further increases in pH result in precipitation of the drug and do not produce an additional shortening of onset time.

Protein Binding

Local anesthetics are in large part bound to plasma and tissue proteins. However, they are pharmacologically active only in the free, unbound state. The most important binding proteins for local anesthetics in plasma are albumin and α-acid glycoprotein (AAG). The binding to AAG is characterized as high-affinity but low-capacity binding; hence, local anesthetics bind to AAG preferentially compared with albumin. However, binding to AAG is easily saturated with clinically achieved blood levels of local anesthetic. Once AAG saturation occurs, any additional binding is to albumin. Because the binding capacity of albumin for local anesthetic agents is very large, albumin can bind local anesthetic drugs in plasma in concentrations many times greater than those clinically achieved. Note that the fraction of drugs bound to protein in plasma correlates with the duration of local anesthetic activity: bupivacaine > etidocaine > ropivacaine > mepivacaine > lidocaine > procaine and 2-chloroprocaine. This suggests that the bond between the local anesthetic molecule and the sodium channel receptor protein may be similar to that in local anesthetic binding to plasma proteins.

The degree of protein binding of a particular local anesthetic is concentration-dependent and influenced by the pH of the plasma. The percentage of drug bound decreases as the pH decreases. This is important because with the development of acidosis, as may occur with local anesthetic-induced seizures or cardiac arrest, the amount of free drug increases. The magnitude of this phenomenon varies among local anesthetics, and it is much more pronounced with bupivacaine than with lidocaine. For instance, as the binding decreases from 95% to 70% with acidosis, the amount of free bupivacaine increases from 5% to 30% (a factor of 6) although the total drug concentration remains unchanged. Because of this increase in free drug, acidosis renders bupivacaine markedly more toxic.

Systemic Toxicity of Local Anesthetics

In addition to blocking conduction in nerve axons in the peripheral nervous system, local anesthetics interfere with the function of all organs in which the conduction or transmission of nerve impulses occurs. For instance, they have important effects on the central nervous system (CNS), the autonomic ganglia, the neuromuscular junction, and musculature. The risk of such adverse reactions is proportional to the concentration of local anesthetic achieved in the circulation. The toxic effects of local anesthetics on some important organs are reviewed later in this chapter.

Plasma Concentration of Local Anesthetics

The following factors determine the plasma concentration of local anesthetics:

- The dose of the drug administered
- The rate of absorption of the drug
  - (site injected, vasoactivity of the drug, use of vasoconstrictors)
- Biotransformation and elimination of the drug from the circulation.

It should be noted that although the peak level of a local anesthetic is directly related to the dose administered, administration of the same dose at different sites results in marked differences in peak blood levels. This explains why large doses of local anesthetic can be used with peripheral nerve blocks without the toxicity that would be seen with an intramuscular or intravenous (IV) injection. In the case of 2-chloroprocaine, peak blood levels achieved also are affected by the rate at which the local anesthetic drug undergoes biotransformation and elimination (plasma half-life of about 45 seconds to 1 minute). On the other hand, peak blood levels of amide-linked local anesthetic drugs are primarily the result of absorption.

Central Nervous System Toxicity

The symptoms of CNS toxicity associated with local anesthetics are a function of their plasma level **(Fig. 5-3)**.

Toxicity is typically first expressed as stimulation of the CNS, producing restlessness, disorientation, and tremor. As the plasma concentration of the local anesthetic increases, clonic-tonic convulsions occur; the more potent the anesthetic, the more readily convulsions may be produced. With even higher levels of local anesthetic, central stimulation is followed by depression and respiratory failure.

The apparent stimulation and subsequent depression produced by applying local anesthetics to the CNS presumably are due to depression of neuronal activity. Selective depression of inhibitory neurons is thought to account for the excitatory phase in vivo. However, rapid systemic administration of a local anesthetic may produce death with no, or only transient, signs of CNS stimulation. Under these conditions, the concentration of the drug probably rises so rapidly that all neurons are depressed simultaneously. Airway control and support of respiration constitute essential treatment. Benzo-

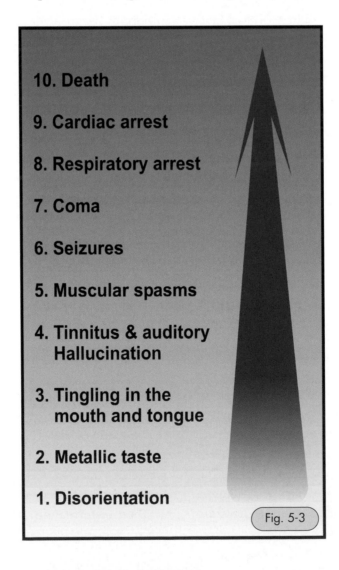

10. Death

9. Cardiac arrest

8. Respiratory arrest

7. Coma

6. Seizures

5. Muscular spasms

4. Tinnitus & auditory Hallucination

3. Tingling in the mouth and tongue

2. Metallic taste

1. Disorientation

Fig. 5-3

diazepines, barbiturates, or propofol administered IV in small doses are the drugs of choice for aborting convulsions. The use of benzodiazepines as premedication is often recommended; however, they must be used with caution as respiratory depression with excessive sedation may produce respiratory acidosis with a consequent higher level of free drug in the serum.

Cardiovascular Toxicity

The primary site of action of local anesthetics is the myocardium, where they decrease electrical excitability, conduction rate, and the force of myocardial contraction. Most local anesthetics also cause arteriolar dilatation, contributing to hypotension. Cardiovascular effects typically occur at higher systemic concentrations than those at which effects on the CNS are produced. However, it should be noted that it is possible for car-

diovascular collapse and death to occur even in an absence of the warning signs and symptoms of CNS toxicity. It is believed that this is probably the result of action on the pacemaker cells or the sudden onset of ventricular fibrillation. In animal studies on local anesthetic cardiotoxicity, all caused dose-dependent depression of the contractility of cardiac muscle. This depressant effect on cardiac contractility parallels the anesthetic potency of the local anesthetic in blocking nerves. Therefore, bupivacaine, which is four times more potent than lidocaine in blocking nerves, is also four times more potent in depressing cardiac contractility. Deaths caused by a bupivacaine overdose have been associated with progressive prolongation of ventricular conduction and widening of the QRS complex, followed by the sudden onset of arrhythmia such as ventricular fibrillation.

Pregnancy and Local Anesthetic Toxicity

Plasma concentrations of AAG are also decreased in pregnant women and in newborns. This lowered concentration effectively increases the free fraction of bupivacaine in plasma, and it may have been an important contributing factor to the bupivacaine toxicity in pregnant patients and to the number of cardiac arrests that took place with inadvertent overdoses of bupivacaine in pregnant women. However, with intermediate-duration local anesthetics (e.g., lidocaine and mepivacaine), smaller changes in protein binding occur during pregnancy, and the use of these local anesthetics is not associated with an increased risk of cardiac toxicity during pregnancy.

Pharmacodynamics and Treatment of Local Anesthetic Toxicity

Blood levels of lidocaine associated with the onset of seizures appear to be in the range of 10 to 12 μg/mL. At these concentrations, inhibitory pathways in the brain are selectively disabled, and facilitatory neurons can function unopposed. Prodromal symptoms appear before the onset of seizures and usually include slowed speech, jerky movements, tremors, and hallucinations. It should be noted that the prodromal symptoms are not consistent among different patients and local anes-

thetics. As the blood levels of lidocaine are increased further, respiratory depression becomes significant and at much higher levels (20 to 25 μg/mL), cardiotoxicity is manifested. In contrast, for bupivacaine, blood levels of approximately 4 μg/mL result in seizures, and blood levels of approximately 4 to 6 μg/mL are associated with cardiac toxicity. This is reflective of a much lower therapeutic index for bupivacaine compared with lidocaine in terms of cardiac toxicity. When cardiotoxicity has not developed, high levels of local anesthetics in the brain rapidly dissipate and are redistributed to other tissue compartments. However, when drug levels result in significant cardiotoxicity, cardiac output diminishes, resulting in impairment in redistribution. The cardiotoxicity of long-acting local anesthetics, such as bupivacaine and etidocaine, carries a risk of cardiac arrest and difficult resuscitation. It should be noted that such complications typically occur during or immediately on injection of a local anesthetic. Most of these toxic effects occur in pregnant patients, who apparently have high blood levels of local anesthetic resulting from inadvertent intravascular injection of large amounts of drugs (Albright, 1978). Most frequently, this occurs while an epidural anesthetic is being administered or results from tourniquet failure during IV administration of a regional anesthetic.

In patients with toxicity, treatment consists of administering a benzodiazepine (midazolam 0.05 to 0.1 mg) or a moderate dose of propofol (1 to 1.5 mg/kg) and preventing the detrimental effects of hypoxia and hypercarbia using hyperventilation with 100% oxygen. This can be accomplished using mask ventilation or hyperventilation through a laryngeal mask airway. With severe toxicity, rapid tracheal intubation is performed after mask hyperventilation with 100% oxygen and administration of a muscle relaxant. In addition to facilitating endotracheal intubation, an additional benefit of a mus-cle relaxant is cessation of tonic-clonic seizure activity and prevention of severe acidosis. Failure to stop seizure activity can lead to progressive acidosis, which further potentiates the toxicity of the circulating and intracellular local anesthetic by increasing the active free fraction of the local anesthetic and myocardial contractility. Additional therapy may include fluid resuscitation, vasopressor therapy, antiarrhythmic therapy (e.g., bretylium or magnesium), and inotropic support. In cases of severe toxicity with large doses of long-acting local anesthetics, aggressive resuscitation with chest compression and timely institution of cardiopulmonary bypass may prove lifesaving.

Types of Local Anesthetics

As previously mentioned, local anesthetic drugs are classified as esters or amides **(Fig. 5-4)**. A short overview of various local anesthetics with comments regarding their clinical applicability in peripheral blockade is provided in this section.

Ester-linked Local Anesthetics

Ester-linked local anesthetics are hydrolyzed at the ester linkage in plasma by the plasma pseudocholinesterase. This plasma enzyme also hydrolyzes natural choline esters and succinylcholine. The rate of hydrolysis of ester-linked local anesthetics depends on the type and location of the substitution in the aromatic ring. For example, 2-chloroprocaine is hydrolyzed about four times faster than procaine, which in turn is hydrolyzed about four times faster than tetracaine. With 2-chloroprocaine, this hydrolysis is extremely rapid, resulting in a half-life of less than a minute, making plasma determination of 2-chloroprocaine a challenge. However, the rate of hydrolysis of all ester-linked local anesthetics is markedly decreased in patients with atypical plasma pseudo-cholinesterase, and a prolonged half-life of these drugs may occur. Another hallmark of metabolism of ester-linked local anesthetics is that their hydrolysis leads to the formation of p-aminobenzoic acid (PABA). PABA and its derivatives carry a small risk potential for allergic reactions. A his-tory of an allergic reaction to a local anesthetic should immediately suggest that a current reaction is due to the presence of PABA derived from an ester-linked local anesthetic. However, although exceedingly rare, allergic reactions can also develop from the use of multiple-dose vials of amide-linked local anesthetics that contain PABA as a preservative.

Cocaine

Cocaine occurs naturally in the leaves of the coca shrub and is an ester of benzoic acid. The clinically desired actions of cocaine are blockade of nerve impulses and local vasoconstriction secondary to inhibition of local norepinephrine reuptake. However, its toxicity and the potential for abuse have precluded wider clinical use of cocaine in modern practice. Its high toxicity is primarily due to the blockade of catecholamine uptake in both the CNS and peripheral nervous system. Its euphoric properties are due primarily to inhibition of catecholamine uptake, particularly dopamine, at CNS synapses. Other local anesthetics do not block the uptake of norepinephrine and do not produce the sensitization to catecholamines, vasoconstriction, or mydriasis characteristics of cocaine. Currently, cocaine is used primarily to provide topical anesthesia of the upper respiratory tract, where its combined vasoconstrictor and local anesthetic properties provide anesthesia and shrinking of the mucosa with a single agent.

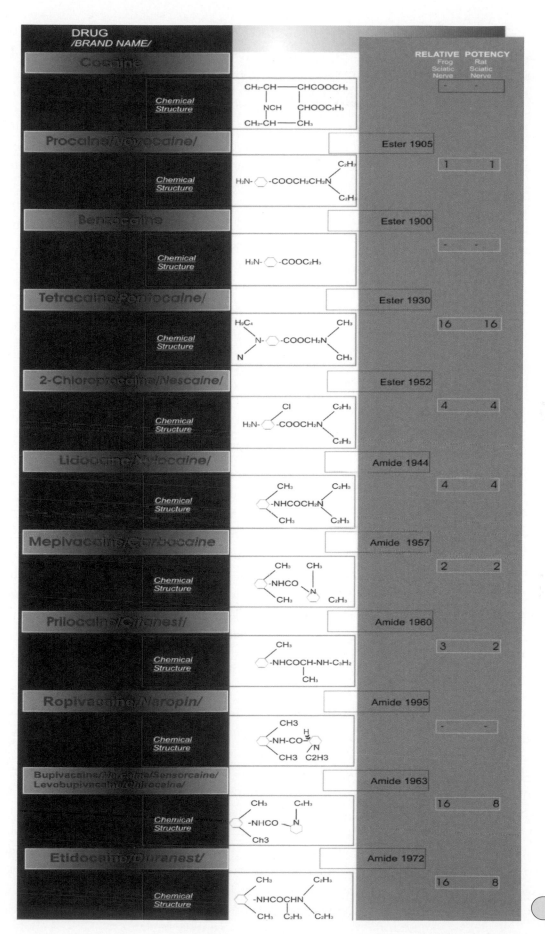

Fig. 5-4

Procaine

Procaine, an amino ester, was the first synthetic local anesthetic. Procaine is characterized by low potency, slow onset, and short duration of action. Consequently, although once widely used, its use now is largely confined to infiltration anesthesia and, perhaps, diagnostic nerve blocks.

2-Chloroprocaine

2-Chloroprocaine, an ester local anesthetic introduced in 1952, is a chlorinated derivative of procaine. Chloroprocaine is the most rapidly metabolized local anesthetic currently used. Because of its extremely rapid breakdown in plasma (less than 1 minute), it has a very low potential for systemic toxicity. Enthusiasm for its use in regional anesthesia has been tempered by reports of prolonged sensory and motor blockade after epidural or subarachnoid administration of large doses. Such toxicity appeared to have been a consequence of low pH and the use of sodium meta-bisulfite as a preservative in earlier formulations. However, there are no reports of neurotoxicity with newer preparations of chloroprocaine, which contain calcium ethylenediaminetetraacetic acid (EDTA) as the preservative, although these preparations also are not recommended for intrathecal administration. Muscular back pain after epidural anesthesia with 2-chloroprocaine has been reported and is thought to be due to tetany in the paraspinal muscles, which may be a consequence of Ca^{2+} binding by the EDTA included as a preservative. The incidence of back pain appears to be related to the volume of drug injected and its use for skin infiltration. A newer 2-chloroprocaine commercial preparation from which all preservatives have been removed has been released, and the initial studies appear to be promising.

However, while 2-chloroprocaine is not recommended for either spinal or IV regional anesthesia, we commonly use it for peripheral nerve blockade. In fact, 3% 2-chloroprocaine is our local anesthetic of choice for surgical anesthesia of short duration that result in relatively minor tissue trauma and postoperative pain (e.g., carpal tunnel syndrome, knee arthroscopy, muscle biopsy). Its characteristics in peripheral nerve blockade include fast onset and short duration of action (1.5–2 hours). The duration of blockade can be extended (up to 2 hours) by the addition of epinephrine (1:300,000).

Tetracaine

Tetracaine is the butylamino derivative of procaine. Tetracaine was introduced in 1932, and it is a long-acting amino ester. It is significantly more potent and has a longer duration of action than procaine or 2-chloroprocaine. Tetracaine is more slowly metabolized than the other commonly used ester local anesthetics, and it is considerably more toxic. Currently, it is used in spinal anesthesia when a drug of long duration is needed, as well as in various topical anesthetic preparations. Because of its slow onset and high toxicity, tetracaine is rarely used in peripheral nerve blocks.

Amide-linked Local Anesthetics

As opposed to ester-linked drugs, amide-linked local anesthetics are metabolized in the liver. The hepatic blood flow and liver function determine the clearance of these anesthetics by the liver. Consequently, factors that decrease hepatic blood flow or hepatic drug extraction both result in an increased elimination half-life. It should be noted that renal clearance of unchanged local anesthetics is a minor route of elimination, accounting for only 3% to 5% of the total drug administered. The primary biotransformation step for amide-type local anesthetics is a dealkylization reaction in which an ethyl group is cleaved from the tertiary amine.

Lidocaine

Lidocaine was introduced in 1948 and remains one of the most widely used local anesthetics. It is an aminoethylamide and is the prototype of the amide class of local anesthetics. Lidocaine is absorbed rapidly after parenteral administration and from the gastrointestinal and respiratory tracts. It is dealkylated in the liver by oxidases to monoethylglycine xylidide and glycine xylidide, which can be metabolized further to monoethylglycine and xylidide. Lidocaine can be used in almost any peripheral nerve block in which a local anesthetic of intermediate duration is needed. A concentration of 1.5% or 2% with or without the addition of epinephrine is most commonly used for surgical anesthesia. More diluted concentrations are suitable in pain management, particularly for diagnostic blocks.

Mepivacaine

Mepivacaine, introduced in 1957, is an intermediate-duration amino amide local anesthetic. Its pharmacologic properties are similar to those of lidocaine. Although mepivacaine has been suggested to be more toxic to neonates (and thus it is not used in obstetric anesthesia), it appears to have a slightly higher therapeutic index in adults than lidocaine. Its onset of action is similar to that of lidocaine, however, its duration is slightly longer than that of lidocaine. It is interesting that 1.5% mepivacaine is by and large the most commonly used local anesthetic in peripheral nerve blockade by institutions with substantial expertise in this area. It is our first choice in any peripheral nerve block technique when an intermediate-duration blockade is desired (3 to 6 hours, depending on the type of nerve block and addition of a vasoconstrictor).

Prilocaine

Prilocaine is an intermediate-duration amino amide local anesthetic with a pharmacologic profile similar to that of lidocaine. The primary differences are a lack of vasodilatation and an increased volume of distribution, which reduces its CNS toxicity. However, it is unique among local anesthetics for its propensity to cause methemoglobinemia, an effect of metabolism of the aromatic ring to o-toluidine. The development of methemoglobinemia is dependent on the total dose administered (8 mg/kg) and does not have significant consequences in healthy patients. If necessary, it can be treated by IV administration of methylene blue (1 to 2 mg/kg). Prilocaine is infrequently used in peripheral nerve blockade.

Etidocaine

Etidocaine is a long-acting amino amide introduced in 1972. Its neuronal blocking properties are characterized by an onset of action similar to that of lidocaine and a duration of action comparable to that of bupivacaine. Compared with bupivacaine, etidocaine produces pref-

erential motor blockade. Etidocaine is structurally similar to lidocaine, with alkyl substitution on the aliphatic connecting group between the hydrophilic amine and the amide linkage. This feature increases the lipid solubility of the drug and results in a drug more potent than lidocaine that has a very rapid onset of action and a prolonged duration of anesthesia. A major disadvantage of etidocaine is its profound motor blockade over a wide range of clinical concentrations, which often outlasts sensory blockade. For these reasons, etidocaine is not used for peripheral nerve blockade.

Bupivacaine

Since its introduction in 1963, bupivacaine has been one of the most commonly used local anesthetics in regional and infiltration anesthesia. Its structure is similar to that of lidocaine, except that the amine-containing group is a butylpiperidine. Bupivacaine is a long-acting agent capable of producing prolonged anesthesia and analgesia that can be even further prolonged by the addition of epinephrine. It is substantially more cardiotoxic than lidocaine. This toxicity is manifested by severe ventricular arrhythmias and myocardial depression after inadvertent intravascular administration of large doses of the drug. The cardiotoxicity of bupivacaine is cumulative and substantially greater than would be predicted by its local anesthetic potency. At least part of the cardiotoxicity of bupivacaine may be mediated centrally because direct injection of small quantities of bupivacaine into the medulla can produce malignant ventricular arrhythmias. Bupivacaine-induced cardiotoxicity can be difficult to treat. Acidosis, hypercarbia, and hypoxemia enhance the severity of the toxicity.

Bupivacaine is widely used both in neuraxial and peripheral nerve blockade. The blocking property is characterized by a slower onset and a long, somewhat unpredictable duration of blockade. Because of its toxicity profile, large doses of bupivacaine should be avoided.

Ropivacaine

The cardiotoxicity of bupivacaine stimulated interest in developing a less toxic, long-lasting local anesthetic. The development of ropivacaine, an enantiomer of

1-propyl-2′, 6′-pipecolocylidide, is the result of that search. The enantiomer, like most local anesthetics with a chiral center, was chosen because it has a lower toxicity than the R isomer. This is presumably because of slower uptake, resulting in lower blood levels for a given dose (5 to 7 hours, respectively). Ropivacaine undergoes extensive hepatic metabolism after IV administration, with only 1% of the drug eliminated unchanged in the urine. Ropivacaine is slightly less potent than bupivacaine in producing anesthesia when used in lower concentrations. However, in concentrations of 0.5% and higher, it produces dense blockade with slightly shorter duration than that of bupivacaine. In concentrations of 0.75%, the onset of blockade is almost as fast as that of 1.5% mepivacaine or 3% 2-chloroprocaine, with reduced CNS toxicity and cardiotoxic potential and a lower propensity for motor blockade than bupivacaine. For these reasons, ropivacaine has become one of the most commonly used long-acting local anesthetics in peripheral nerve blockade.

Levobupivacaine

Levobupivacaine contains a single enantiomer of bupivacaine hydrochloride, and it is related chemically and pharmacologically to the amino amide class of local anesthetics. Levobupivacaine is less cardiotoxic than bupivaicane. It is extensively metabolized with no unchanged levobupivacaine detected in the urine or feces. The blocking properties of levobupivacaine in peripheral nerve blockade are studied less than those of ropivacaine, however, research results suggest that they seem to parallel those of bupivacaine. Therefore, levobupivacaine is an excellent, less toxic alternative to bupivacaine.

Mixing of Local Anesthetics

Mixing of local anesthetics (e.g., lidocaine and bupivacaine) is often done in clinical practice with the intent of obtaining a faster onset and lower toxicity with shorter-acting local anesthetics and a longer duration of blockade with longer-acting local anesthetic. Unfortunately, when local anesthetics are mixed, their onset, duration, and potency become much less predictable and the end result is far from expected. For instance, mixing 3% 2-chloroprocaine with 0.5% bupivacaine results in a slower onset of blockade and only a slightly longer duration. In addition, mixing local anesthetics also carries a risk of a drug error. For this reason, we rarely mix local anesthetics; instead, we choose drugs and concentrations of single agents to achieve the desired effects.

Additives to Local Anesthetics

Vasoconstrictors

The addition of a vasoconstrictor to a local anesthetic delays its vascular absorption, increasing the duration of drug contact with nerve tissues. The net effect is prolongation of the blockade by as much as 50% and a decrease in the systemic absorption of local anesthetic. These effects vary significantly among different types of local anesthetics and individual nerve blocks. Epinephrine is the most commonly used vasoconstrictor in peripheral nerve blockade. Because the injection of a large volume of local anesthetic into nerve sheaths, the use of a tourniquet and the use of epinephrine may combine to produce a decrease in nerve blood supply, it is wise to limit the concentration of epinephrine to 1:300,000.

Opiates

The injection of opioids into the epidural or subarachnoid space to manage acute or chronic pain is based on the knowledge that opioid receptors are present in the substantia gelatinosa of the spinal cord. Thus, combinations of a local anesthetic and an opiate are often successfully used in neuroaxial blockade to both enhance the blockade and prolong analgesia. However, in peripheral nerves similar receptors are absent or the effects of opiates are negligibly weak. For this reason, it is our opinion that opiates do not have a significant clinical role in peripheral nerve blockade.

Clonidine

Clonidine is a centrally acting selective partial α_2-adrenergic agonist. Because of its ability to reduce sympathetic nervous system output from the CNS, clonidine acts as an antihypertensive drug. Preservative-free clonidine, administered into the epidural or subarachnoid space (150 to 450 μg), produces dose-dependent analgesia and, unlike opioids, does not produce depression of ventilation, pruritus, nausea, or vomiting. Clonidine produces analgesia by activating postsynaptic α2 receptors in the gelatinous substance of the spinal cord. Much less research has been done on the effects of clonidine in peripheral nerve blockade. However, it is quite clear that it can significantly prolong analgesia when combined in doses of 50 to 100 μg with short- and intermediate-acting local anesthetics. Its benefits, however, appear to be overshadowed by the analgesia achieved with long-acting local anesthetics. It should be noted that clonidine cannot produce surgical anesthesia and is not administered alone. These potentially useful effects of clonidine should be weighed against its side effects, including dose-dependent sedation and hypotension. Although life-threatening hypotension or bradycardia has not been reported when clonidine is used with peripheral nerve blocks, its circulatory effects may complicate resuscitation in a setting of local anesthetic toxicity.

The Onset and Duration of Blockade

Local Anesthetic Diffusion

A mixed peripheral nerve or nerve trunk consists of individual nerves surrounded by an investing epineurium (see Ch. 2 "Regional Anesthesia Anatomy"). When a local anesthetic is deposited in proximity to a peripheral nerve, it diffuses from the outer surface toward the core along a concentration gradient. Consequently, nerves located in the outer mantle of the mixed nerve are blocked first. These fibers are usually distributed to more proximal anatomic structures than those situated near the core of the mixed nerve and are often motor fibers. When the volume and concentration of local anesthetic solution deposited about the nerve are adequate, the local anesthetic eventually diffuses inward to block the more centrally located fibers. Lesser amounts and concentrations of a drug block only the nerves in the mantle and smaller and more sensitive central fibers.

Onset of Blockade

In general, local anesthetics are deposited as close to the nerve as possible, and preferably into the tissue sheaths (e.g., brachial plexus, lumbar plexus) or epineurial sheaths of the nerves (e.g., femoral, sciatic). The local anesthetic must diffuse from the site of injection into the nerve, where it acts. The rate of diffusion is determined by the concentration of the drug, its degree of ionization (ionized local anesthetic diffuses more slowly), its hydrophobicity, and the physical characteristics of the tissue surrounding the nerve. Higher concentrations of local anesthetic result in a more rapid onset of peripheral nerve blockade. Local anesthetics with lower pK_a values tend to have a more rapid onset of action for a given concentration, because more drug is ionized at neutral pH.

Duration of Blockade

The duration of nerve block anesthesia depends on the physical characteristics of the local anesthetic and the presence or absence of vasoconstrictors. Especially important physical characteristics are lipid solubility and protein binding. In general, local anesthetics can be divided into three categories: short-acting (e.g., 2-chloroprocaine, 45 to 90 minutes), intermediate duration (e.g., lidocaine, mepivacaine, 90 to 180 minutes), and long-acting (e.g., bupivacaine, levobupivacaine, ropivacaine, 4 to 18 hours). The degree of block prolongation with the addition of a vasoconstrictor appears to be related to the intrinsic vasodilatory properties of the local anesthetic; the more intrinsic vasodilatory action, the more prolongation (e.g., lidocaine, bupivacaine).

Although this discussion is in line with current clinical teaching, it is really more theoretical than of significant clinical relevance. For instance, a dense block of the brachial plexus with 2-chloroprocaine will likely outlast a weak, poor-quality block with bupivacaine. In addition, classical teaching does not take into account the type of block. As an example, a sciatic nerve block with bupivacaine lasts almost twice as long as an interscalene or lumbar plexus block with the same drug dose and concentration. These differences must be kept in mind to properly time and predict the resolution of blockade. The approximate duration of blockade with local anesthetics is detailed with the individual block techniques.

SUGGESTED READINGS

- Albright GA. Cardiac arrest following regional anesthesia with etidocaine or bupivacaine. *Anesthesiology* 1978;51:285–287.

- Auroy Y, Narchi P, Messiah A, et al. Serious complications related to regional anesthesia: results of a prospective survey in France. *Anesthesiology* 1997;87:479–486.

- Avery P, Redon D, Schaenzer G, et al. The influence of serum potassium on the cerebral and cardiac toxicity of bupivacaine and lidocaine. *Anesthesiology* 1985;61:134–138.

- Braid BP, Scott DB. The systemic absorption of local analgesic drugs. *Br J Anaesth* 1965;37:394.

- Burney RG, DiFazio CA, Foster JA. Effects of pH on protein binding of lidocaine. *Anesth Analg* 1978;57:478–480.

- Butterworth JF, Strichartz GR. The molecular mechanisms by which local anesthetics produce impulse blockade: a review. *Anesthesiology* 1990:72:711–734.

- Carpenter RI, Mackey DC. Local anesthetics. In: Barash PG, Cullen BF, Stoelting RK, eds. *Clinical Anesthesia.* 2nd ed. Philadelphia, Pa: Lippincott, 1992;509–541.

- Casati A, Magistris L, Fanelli G, Beccaria P, Cappellirri G, Aldegheri G, Torri G. Small-dose clonidine prolongs postoperative analgesia after sciatic-femoral nerve block with 0.75% ropivacaine for foot surgery. *Anesth Analg* 2000;91:388.

- Catterall WA. Cellular and molecular biology of voltage-gated sodium channels. *Physiol Rev* 1992;72:S15–S48.

- Clarkson CW, Hondeghem LM. Mechanism for bupivacaine depression of cardiac conduction: fast block of sodium channels during the action potential with slow recovery from block during diastole. *Anesthesiology* 1985; 62:396–405.

- Courtney KR, Strichartz GR. Structural elements which determine local anesthetic activity. In: Strichartz GR, ed. *Handbook of Experimental Pharmacology.* Vol 81. Berlin, Germany: Springer-Verlag, 1987;53–94.

- Cousins MJ, Bridenbaugh PO, eds. *Neural Blockade in Clinical Anesthesia and Management of Pain.* 3rd ed. Philadelphia, Pa: Lippincott; 1995.

- Cousins MJ, Mather LE. Intrathecal and epidural administration of opioids. *Anesthesiology* 1984;61:276–310.

- Covino BG. Toxicity and systemic effects of local anesthetic agents. In: Strichartz GR, ed. *Handbook of Experimental Pharmacology.* Vol 81. Berlin, Germany: Springer-Verlag, 1987;187–212.

- Covino BG, Vassallo HG. *Local Anesthetics: Mechanisms of Action and Clinical Use.* New York, NY: Grune & Stratton; 1976.

- De Negri P, Visconti C, DeVivo P, et al. Does clonidine added to epidural infusion of 0.2% ropivacaine enhance postoperative analgesia in adults? *Reg Anesth Pain Med* 2000;25:39.

- DiFazio CA, Rowlingson JC. Additives to local anesthetic solutions. In: Brown DL, ed. *Regional Anesthesia and Analgesia.* Philadelphia, Pa: WB Saunders, 1996;232–239.

- Gormley WP, Murray JM, Fee JPH, and Bower S. Effect of the addition of alfentanil to lignocaine during axillary brachial plexus anaesthesia. *Br J Anaesth* 1996;76:802–805.

- Fibuch EE, Opper SE. Back pain following epidurally administered Nesacaine MPF. *Anesth Analg* 69:1989; 113–115.

- Garfield JM, Gugino L. Central effects of local anesthetics. In: Strichartz GR, ed. *Handbook of Experimental Pharmacology.* Vol 81. Berlin, Germany: Springer-Verlag, 1987;187–212.

- Gissen AJ, Datta S, Lambert D. The chloroprocaine controversy. II. Is chloroprocaine neurotoxic? *Reg Anesth* 1984;9:135–145.

- Graf BM, Martin E, Bosnjak ZJ, et al. Stereospecific effect of bupivacaine isomers on atrioventricular conduction in the isolated perfused guinea pig heart. *Anesthesiology* 1997;86:410–419.

- Harwood TN, Butterworth JF, Colonna DM, et al. Plasma bupivacaine concentrations and effects of epinephrine after superficial cervical plexus blockade in patients undergoing carotid endarterectomy. *J Cardiothorac Vasc Anesth* 1999;3:703–706.

- Hilgier M. Alkalinization of bupivacaine for brachial plexus block. *Reg Anesth* 1985;10:59–61.
- Huang YF, Pryor ME, Mather LE, et al. Cardiovascular and central nervous system effects of intravenous levobupivacaine and bupivacaine in sheep. *Anesth Analg* 1998;86:797–804.
- Kasten GW, Martin ST. Bupivacaine cardiovascular toxicity: comparison of treatment with bretylium and lidocaine. *Anesth Analg* 1985;64:911–916.
- Moore DC. Administer oxygen first in the treatment of local anesthetic-induced convulsions. *Anesthesiology* 1980;53:346–347.
- Nath S, Haggmark S, Johansson G, et al. Differential depressant and electrophysiologic cardiotoxicity of local anesthetics: an experimental study with special reference to lidocaine and bupivacaine. *Anesth Analg* 1986; 65:1263–1270.
- Ragsdale DR, McPhee JC, Scheuer T, et al. Molecular determinants of state-dependent block of Na$^+$ channels by local anesthetics. *Science* 1994;265:1724–1728.
- Raymond SA, Gissen AJ. Mechanism of differential nerve block. In: Strichartz GR, ed. *Handbook of Experimental Pharmacology*. Vol 81. Berlin, Germany: Springer-Verlag, 1987;95–164.
- Reiz S, Haggmark S, Johansson G, et al. Cardiotoxicity of ropivacaine—a new amide local anesthetic agent. *Acta Anaesthesiol Scand* 1989;33:93–98.
- Ritchie JM, Greengard P. On the mode of action of local anesthetics. *Annu Rev Pharmacol* 1966;6:405–430.
- Rowlingson JC. Toxicity of local anesthetic additives. *Reg Anesth* 1993;18:453–460.
- Sage DJ, Feldman HS, Arthur GR, et al. Influence of bupivacaine and lidocaine on isolated guinea pig atria in the presence of acidosis and hypoxia. *Anesth Analg* 1984;63:1–7.
- Santos AC, Arthur GR, Lehning EJ, et al. Comparative pharmacokinetics of ropivacaine and bupivacaine in nonpregnant and pregnant ewes. *Anesth Analg* 1997;85: 87–93.
- Santos AC, Arthur GR, Padderson H, et al. Systemic toxicity of ropivacaine during bovine pregnancy. *Anesthesiology* 1994;75:137–141.
- Singelyn FJ, Gouvernuer JM, Robert A. A minimum dose of clonidine added to mepivacaine prolongs the duration of anesthesia and analgesia after axillary brachial plexus block. *Anesth Analg* 1996;83:1046.
- Stevens RA, Urmey WF, Urquhart BL, et al. Back pain after epidural anesthesia with chloroprocaine. *Anesthesiology* 1993;78:492–497.
- Strichartz GR, Ritchie JM. The action of local anesthetics on ion channels of excitable tissues. In: Strichartz GR, ed. *Handbook of Experimental Pharmacology*. Vol 81. Berlin, Germany: Springer-Verlag, 1987;21–53.
- Tucker GT, Mather LE. Pharmacokinetics of local anesthetic agents. *Br J Anaesth* 1975;47:213–224.
- Wagman IH, Dejong RH, Prince DA. Effect of lidocaine on the central nervous system. *Anesthesiology* 1967;28: 155–172.
- Wang BC, Hillman DE, Spiedholz NI, et al. Chronic neurologic deficits and Nesacaine-CE. An effect of the anesthetic, 2-chloro-procaine, or the antioxidant, sodium bisulfite. *Anesth Analg* 1984;63:445–447.
- Winnie AP, Tay CH, Patel KP, et al. Pharmacokinetics of local anesthetics during plexus blocks. *Anesth Analg* 1977;56:852–861.

6 NEUROLOGIC COMPLICATIONS OF PERIPHERAL NERVE BLOCKS

There are relatively few published reports of complications associated with the use of peripheral nerve blocks. Because there is a relative paucity of published information on the mechanisms of neuronal injury following nerve blockade and methods to prevent such injuries, some of the discussion will necessarily be theoretical. However, we believe that following the recommendations made in this chapter should substantially reduce the risks of complications following peripheral nerve blocks.

Complications After Nerve Blockade: How Common Are They?

The reported incidence of complications associated with peripheral nerve blocks is generally low and varies from 0% to 5%. Complications related to brachial plexus blocks are perhaps most commonly reported, whereas there are few reports of injuries to the lower-extremity nerves. Such a discrepancy is most likely related to the fact that a brachial plexus block is one of the most prevalent techniques in clinical practice. However, the disproportionately higher number of reported cases of neuropathies in the upper extremity (particularly axillary block) may also be a function of some anatomic features of the axillary brachial plexus. For instance, in a survey of hand surgeons, 171 (21%) of the 800 surgeons responding had seen a total of 249 major complications (those lasting a year or more) and 521 (65%) had seen patients with minor neurologic complications. The survey further suggested that about 1 in 5 hand surgeons had seen a major neurologic complication that might have been related to an axillary brachial plexus block.

It should be noted that the etiology of neurologic complications is often multifactorial. A relatively small proportion of postoperative neurologic sequelae are caused by the regional anesthetic alone; they can also be caused or compounded by underlying disease or surgery. For instance, the incidence of neurologic injury following hand surgery under an axillary block was 3.4% in a series of 533 patients. However, the nerve block itself was implicated in only 1.9% of these cases. Likewise, an increase in shoulder arthroscopic procedures in the past decade has been accompanied by a growing awareness of the potential for surgery-related neurologic injury. The occurrence of transient neuropraxia of the brachial plexus can be as high as 30% after shoulder arthroscopy, with the musculocutaneus nerve being the most vulnerable component of the brachial plexus. This has been attributed to a number of surgical factors, such as joint distention, excessive traction, and extravasation of fluid during surgery, and not to nerve block procedure.

Postoperative Neurologic Deficit: Regional Versus General Anesthesia

Although nerve injuries are commonly voiced concerns with the use of peripheral nerve blocks, postoperative neurologic complications may actually be more common after general and neuraxial anesthesia than after peripheral nerve blocks. In a closed-claims review of nerve injuries associated with anesthesia, 61% of the claims were related to the use of general anesthesia and 36% to the use of regional anesthesia. Such injuries were thought to be caused mostly by compression or stretching of the nerve(s) or plexuses during patient positioning. Peripheral nerve injuries associated with general anesthesia most commonly involve injuries to the ulnar nerve and brachial plexus, whereas injuries to the lumbosacral plexus primarily occur after central neuraxial blockade.

Symptoms of Nerve Injury

The symptoms of a nerve lesion following a peripheral nerve block manifest after the block has receded, usually within 48 hours. The perception of symptoms is influenced by the origin of the nerve lesion and other confounding factors such as postoperative pain, immobility, effects of surgery, position, application of casts, dressing, bandaging, and so forth. The intensity and duration of symptoms may also vary with the severity of the injury, from a light, intermittent tingling and numbness lasting a few weeks to persistent, painful paresthesia, neuropathic pain, sensory loss, and/or motor weakness lasting for several months or years. Some nerve injuries can even evolve into severe causalgia or reflex sympathetic dystrophy. It should be kept in mind that although dermatomes can provide clues to the location of injuries, the loss of sensation at the skin does not provide precise information concerning the site of injury because the boundaries of dermatomes are not precise, clearly defined lines. More useful information on the extent and level of nerve injury can be obtained from the loss of motor function on the basis of the origin and assessment of motor performance.

Peripheral Nerves: Functional Anatomy

The functional anatomy of the peripheral nerve is crucially important in understanding the mechanisms of peripheral nerve injury. A peripheral nerve is a complex structure consisting of fascicles held together by the epineurium, an enveloping external connective sheath **(Fig. 6-1)**. Each fascicle contains many nerve fibers and capillary blood vessels embedded in a loose connective tissue, the endoneurium. The perineurium is a multilayered epithelial sheath that surrounds individual fascicles. Nerve fibers depend on a specific endoneurial environment for their function. This differs from the regular extraneural interstitium. Peripheral nerves are richly supplied by an extensive vascular network in which the endoneurial capillaries have endothelial "tight junctions," a peripheral analogy to the blood-brain barrier. The entire vascular bed is regulated by the sympathetic nervous system, and its blood flow can be as high as 30 to 40 mL/100g per minute. In addition to conducting nerve impulses, nerve fibers also maintain axonal transport of various functionally important substances such as proteins and precursors of receptors and transmitters. This process is highly dependent on oxidative metabolism. Any of these structures and functions can be deranged during a traumatic nerve block and possibly result in temporary or permanent impairment or loss of neural function.

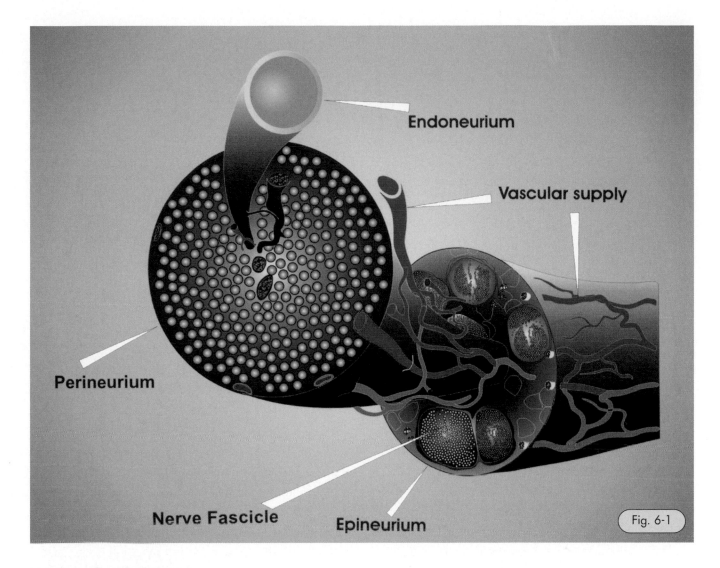

Pathophysiology

Complications following a peripheral nerve block fall into one of 6 major categories:

1. Mechanical trauma to the nerve
   a. Needle trauma
   b. Intraneuronal (fascicular) injection
2. Neuronal ischemia
3. Inadvertent needle placement at unwanted locations
4. Neurotoxicity of local anesthetics
5. Drug error (injection of the wrong drug)
6. Infection

In many instances, the insult may be caused by a combination of these factors.

Mechanical Trauma

Injuries to peripheral nerves after intrafascicular injection of therapeutic and other agents are well documented. Nerve injury following intraneural injection varies from minimal damage to severe axonal and myelin degeneration, depending upon the agent injected and dose of the drug used. Several studies have documented that regardless of the agent used, intrafascicular injection is the main determinant of nerve injury.

At present, there is no consensus on what constitutes proper monitoring and documentation of nerve block procedures. Much of the debate on how to prevent intraneural injection and nerve injury associated with PNB has focused on methods of nerve localization (e.g.,

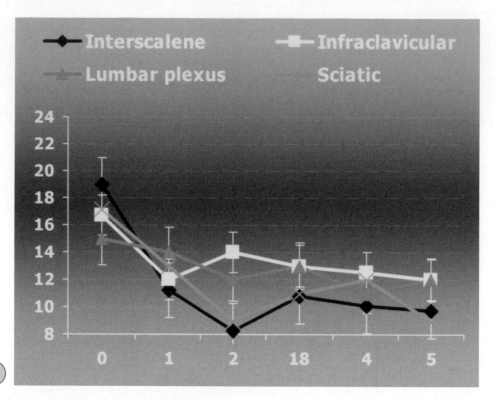

Intrafascicular injection of 1% lidocaine in a dog model of sciatic nerve block resulted in significantly higher injection pressures then during normal, perineural injection. The combination of intraneural needle placement and high pressure during injection was associated with nerve injury.

Fig. 6-2

paresthesia versus nerve stimulation). Still, there is no evidence that one method is safer than another, and nerve injury can occur even with experienced practitioners. Although there is a paucity of clinical data, educational material in regional anesthesia, including major textbooks, suggests that lancinating pain reported by the patient and high injection pressure may portend intraneural injection of local anesthetic and perhaps increase the potential for nerve injury. Consequently, many clinicians advise against performing PNBs in patients under excessive sedation or anesthesia. However, multiple case reports suggest that pain may be absent as a warning factor of pending nerve injury. Besides, administration of sedatives and analgesics is often necessary for performing nerve blocks and makes patient acceptance easier. The combination of premedication with sedatives and analgesics, along with the neuronal blocking properties of local anesthetics, may render pain on injection as a sole indicator of intraneural injection unreliable.

Experimental evidence suggests that such injections may be associated with a resistance to needle advancement and an increased pressure on injection of local anesthetic. For instance, in a model of nerve injury by Selander et al., generally higher pressures (e.g., ≥ 11 psi) were required to inject solution into a nerve fascicle of a rabbit sciatic nerve. Injection into a nerve fascicle using such a pressure results in rupture of the fascicle and its connective tissues sheath—the perineurium with a consequent histologic evidence of disruption of the neuronal anatomy. Similarly, in our large animal model, most intrafascicular injections were associated with high injection pressures (≥ 20 psi), **(Fig. 6-2)**. More importantly, the combination of insertion of the needle intrafascicularly and high resistance to injection (as indicated by injection pressures ≥ 20 psi) were associated with neurologic deficit in dogs and histologic evidence of severe fascicular injury with demyelination. These data suggest that high injection pressures during nerve block injection may indicate intrafascicular injection and as such, carry a risk of nerve injury.

Neurologic injuries resulting from an intraneuronal injection are probably due to a combination of factors. Examples include direct needle trauma with perforation of the perineurium and other nerve sheaths, physical disruption of the nerve fibers, and disruption of the neuronal microvasculature, with the consequent intraepineural or intrafascicular hematoma and nerve ischemia. Because the perineurium is a tough and resistant tissue layer, an injection into this compartment or a fascicle can cause a prolonged increase in endoneurial pressure, exceeding the capillary perfusion pressure. This pressure in turn may result in endoneural ischemia. The addition of a

▶ Based on our current understanding of mechanism of complications after neuronal blockade, it seems prudent to avoid high pressures and forceful, fast injections during administration of nerve blocks.

▶ Avoiding high injection pressures and controlling the speed of injection are perhaps the two single most important measures to avoid neurologic injury, inadvertent neuraxial spread of local anesthetic (centroneurally), as well as massive channeling of local anesthetic into the systemic circulation (via cut venules, lymphatic channels etc.).

vasoconstrictor and the application of a tourniquet over the site of nerve blockade will inevitably result in an additional decrease in blood supply to the nerve. The combination of all these factors contributes to neuronal ischemia and increases the risk of neurologic injury.

Another important complication of an intraneuronal injection is the potential for an intrafascicular spread of the local anesthetic proximally toward the spinal cord, resulting in central neuronal blockade. This is particularly a concern with block techniques that involve needle placement at the level of the nerve roots or spinal nerves, such as interscalene, paravertebral, and lumbar plexus block. Such injections within the dural cuffs or perineurium may result in inadvertent spinal or epidural anesthesia.

In an attempt to standardize pressures and speed of injection during nerve block procedures, we instruct our trainees to always use the same needle types, syringe sizes (20 mL) and one-hand injection technique to develop a more consistent "feel" for pressure during injection. Unfortunately, the perceptions of a "normal" and "abnormal" pressure during nerve block injections greatly vary among clinicians (*Reg Anesth Pain Med* 2004, in press). Even when an experienced anesthesiologist with a "developed feel" performs a nerve block procedure, it is usually another (helper) person who helps with the actual injection of local anesthetic. Besides, internal resistance of needles of various lengths, diameters and manufacturers all significantly vary, making it more difficult to reliably estimate the pressure during injection using a "feel" technique. Therefore, some means of objective measurements of pressures during nerve block injection may be beneficial to decrease a risk of neurologic complications after nerve blockade. Perhaps in the near future, nerve block kits will include a small, disposable, pressure measuring device to objectively monitor pressures during nerve block injections. Additionally, implementation of such monitoring would undoubtedly help to standardize injection practices and allow for objective documentation and meaningful retrospective analyses. The futuristic look into such design is shown in the figure below, where a small, calibrated manometer continuously displays the injection pressures during injection, **(Fig. 6-3)**.

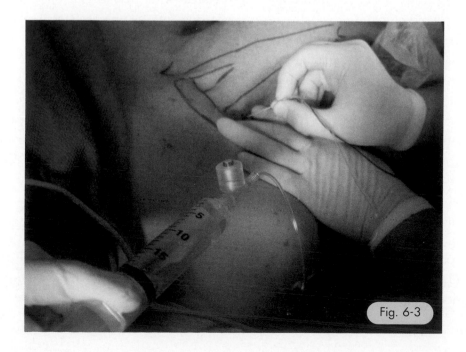

Fig. 6-3

Nerves may also be injured by other factors that may not be related to the nerve block procedure, such as compression, stretching during patient positioning, and the application of surgical retractors.

Needle Bevels

Most experts agree that short-bevel needles (i.e., with angles of 30° to 45°) carry less risk of causing nerve injuries during peripheral nerve blockade than sharp needles with longer-bevel tips **(Fig. 3-2)**. Recommendations on needle design are based largely on the work of Selander and colleagues, who clearly showed that the risk of perforating a nerve fascicle was significantly lower when a short-bevel (45°) needle was used as compared with a standard long-bevel (12° to 15°) needle. The results of their work certainly make clinical sense, and nowadays short-bevel needles are most commonly used for nerve blocks (excluding cutaneous blocks and local infiltration). In contrast, the work of Rice and McMahon suggested that shorter-bevel needles may cause more mechanical damage than long-bevel needles. In their experiment involving deliberate penetration of the largest fascicle of rat sciatic nerves with 12°- to 27° bevel injection needles, when the needle was actually inserted into the nerves, the degree of neuronal trauma was greater with short-bevel needles. On microscopic images, the sharp needles naturally produced clean cuts and the blunt needles produced messy cuts. The debate that ensued neglected the fact that blunt-tip needles are much less likely to be inserted into nonfixed nerves in the clinical setting. Thus, while their findings may hold true when the fascicle is indeed penetrated, short-bevel needles are much less likely to penetrate the nerves, thus reducing the risk of nerve penetration altogether.

Nerve Stimulators

Nerve stimulators have become indispensable tools in modern regional anesthesia practice. An important advantage of the nerve stimulator technique is that nerve response is an objective method of confirming the needle–nerve relationship, as opposed to the elicitation of paresthesia, which is invariably subjective. In addition, avoiding painful paresthesia and the ability to premedicate patients prior to block placement result in significantly greater patient satisfaction with the nerve stimulator technique. Thus, it is not surprising that most recent publications on major peripheral nerve blocks describe procedures that use nerve stimulation. Also, most experts today suggest obtaining nerve stimulation with a much lower current intensity (0.2–0.5 mA) than was the case with older recommendations. Nerve stimulation with a consequent motor response using a low-intensity current results in accurate needle placement with minimal discomfort to the patient.

However, it should be kept in mind that the use of nerve stimulators does not exclude the possibility of nerve damage, as a recent study by Auroy and colleagues points out. In particular, caution should be exercised when stimulation is obtained with currents of less than 0.2 mA. In our own clinical experience, stimulation with such a low current intensity is often associated with paresthesia on injection, perhaps suggesting intraneural placement of the needle. In this situation, we routinely withdraw the needle until the motor response is obtained at a current of 0.2 to 0.5 mA (with a pulse duration of 0.1 – 0.3 msec).

It should be noted that nerve stimulators used for peripheral nerve blockade can vary greatly in stimulating frequency, maximum voltage output, stimulus duration, and accuracy. Although most modern units studied in our laboratory performed adequately within a clinically relevant range of currents and impedance loads, some older models may be grossly inaccurate in the lower range settings (i.e., <0.5 mA). For that reason, the recommendations on current intensity in older books may not be applicable with all nerve stimulators.

To get the most out of a nerve stimulator, it should be tested for accuracy by the biomedical department. This is particularly important for older units. Unfortunately, most manufacturers suggest testing nerve stimulators with a current of 1.0 mA. Consequently, a routine test by biomedical engineers would involve testing stimulators at a current output of 1.0 mA and an impedance load of 1 kΩ, and, indeed, nearly all the stimulators we tested performed well in this current range. However, in peripheral nerve blockade it is much more important that these tests be done in the most relevant clinical current range (0.1 to 0.5 mA). At the very least, for both accuracy and safety, the type of nerve stimulators and their electrical characteristics (current accuracy and duration, stimulating frequency) should be taken into consideration when comparing results of clinical studies or when trying to implement published techniques in clinical practice.

Toxicity of Local Anesthetics

Local anesthetics are used in concentrations that, under normal clinical conditions, do not cause irreversible nerve damage. However, the combination of a relatively high concentration of local anesthetic, intraneural injection, and epinephrine, can result in neurotoxicity. The potential for neurotoxicity associated with a local anesthetic is a function of its potency, concentration, and the length of time the neuronal tissue is exposed to the agent. Exposure of the endoneurium to a very high concentration of local anesthetic may contribute to a neurologic deficit. Fortunately, under normal circumstances, the concentration of local anesthetic at the injection site decreases quickly because of dilution by the interstitial fluids and absorption into the blood. For this reason, as long as the local anesthetic is not injected intraneurally, there is no convincing evidence that the concentrations used clinically present an independent risk factor for neurologic dysfunction.

Neuronal Ischemia

A good neurologic outcome despite the widespread use of tourniquets during extremity surgery demonstrates that peripheral nerves are relatively resistant to ischemia of limited duration and magnitude. However, laboratory data unequivocally suggest that the combination of nerve compression and ischemia can indeed cause irreversible damage to the sciatic nerve in less than 4 hours. A combination of several factors, such as increased pressure due to inadvertent intraneural injection and reduced blood flow due to epinephrine, can result in severe neuronal demise. The endoneurial pressure under these circumstances can exceed the capillary perfusion pressure and result in ischemia of the nerve fascicles on top of the tissue toxicity of the local anesthetic. The addition of epinephrine can further enhance ischemia because it has a vasoconstrictive effect and reduces blood flow. Thus, the key to avoiding neuronal ischemia is avoidance of the combination of intraneural injection, epinephrine, and prolonged application of the tourniquet, particularly over the area of nerve block injection.

Methods and Techniques to Decrease the Risk of Nerve Injury After Peripheral Nerve Blocks*

Based on the aforementioned evidence, we routinely adhere to the following recommendations to decrease the risk of complications with peripheral nerve blockade.

- Aseptic technique
  Most nerve block techniques are merely percutaneous injections. However, infections are known

*Adapted with permission from www.NYSORA.com (New York School of Regional Anesthesia) to occur and can result in significant disability. Since this complication is almost entirely preventable, every effort should be made to adhere to a strictly aseptic technique.

- **Short bevel insulated needles**
  The short bevel design helps to prevent nerve penetration. Insulated needles are now widely available and result in much more precise needle placement when a nerve stimulator is used.

- **Needles of appropriate length for each and every block procedure**
  Excessively long needles should not be used for nerve blockade. For instance, NEVER insert needles longer than 50 mm in interscalene blockade. In addition, needles of appropriate length can be advanced with far greater precision than excessively long needles.

- **Needle advancement**
  During needle localization, advance and withdraw the needle slowly. Keep in mind that nerve stimulators deliver current of very short duration once (1 Hz) or twice (2 Hz) a second and that no current is delivered between the pulses. Fast insertion and withdrawal of the needle may result in failure to stimulate the nerve because the needle may pass near by, or even through, the nerve between the stimuli without eliciting nerve stimulation.

- **Fractionated injections**
  Inject smaller doses and volumes of local anesthetics (3–5 mL) with intermittent aspiration to avoid inadvertent intravascular injection. Always observe the patient during the injection of local anesthetic because negative aspiration of blood is not always present with an intravenous injection. This approach may allow detection of the signs of local anesthetic toxicity before the entire dose is injected.

- **Accuracy of the nerve stimulator**
  Always make sure that the nerve stimulator is operational, delivering the specified current, and that the leads are properly connected to the patient and the needle.

- **Avoidance of forceful, fast injections**
  Forceful, fast injections are more likely to result in channeling of local anesthetic to the unwanted tissue layers, lymphatic vessels, or small veins that may have been cut during needle advancement. Such injections may result in massive channeling of the local anesthetic in the systemic circulation, with consequent risk of severe CNS and cardiac toxicity. Forceful, fast injections under excessive pressure also may carry more risk of intrafascicular injection. Limit the injection speed to 15–20 mL/minute.

- **Avoidance of injection under high pressure**
  Intrafascicular needle placement results in higher resistance (pressure) to injection due to the compact nature of the neuronal tissue and its connective tissue sheaths. Always use the same syringe and needle size to develop a "feel" during the injection. As a rule, when injection of the first 1 mL of local anesthetic proves difficult, the injection should be abandoned and the needle completely withdrawn and checked for patency before reinserting.

- **Avoidance of paresthesia on injection**
  Severe pain or discomfort on injection may signify intraneuronal placement of the needle and should be avoided. This should not be confused with a normal mild "paresthesia-like" symptom, commonly reported by patients when the needle is placed in the immediate vicinity to the nerve. Keep in mind that published case reports suggest that absence of pain on injection alone does not guarantee that the needle is not placed intraneurally. Absence of pain and abnormal resistance on injection should be documented in the anesthetic record after each block procedure.

- **Choose your local anesthetic solution wisely**
  Always choose a shorter acting (and less toxic) local anesthetic for short procedures where long-lasting postoperative analgesia is not required.

Local anesthetic toxicity is the most common complication with neuronal blockade and it is much safer when this occurs with chloroprocaine or lidocaine than with bupivacaine.

- **Blocks in anesthetized patients**

  Blocks in anesthetized patients should be avoided or at least an uncommon practice. When it is necessary to place blocks in anesthetized patients, this should be done only by practitioners with substantial experience with the planned technique. Such cases should NEVER be considered "teaching."

- **Repeating blocks after a failed block**

  Repeating a block after a failed block should be avoided whenever possible. When indicated, it should be done only by those with substantial experience in the planned technique.

SUGGESTED READINGS

- Auroy Y, Benhamou D, Bargues L, Ecoffey C, Falissard B, Mercier F, Buaziz H, Samii K. Major complication of regional anesthesia in France. *Anesthesiology* 2002;97: 1274–1280.
- Auroy Y, Narchi P, Messiah A, Litt L, Rouvier B, Sami K. Serious complications related to regional anesthesia: Results of a prospective survey in France. *Anesthesiology* 1997;87:479.
- Bainton CR, Strichartz GR. Concentration dependence of lidocaine-induced irreversible conduction loss in frog nerve. *Anesthesiology* 1994;81:657.
- Bashein G, Robertson HT, Kennedy WF Jr. Persistent phrenic nerve paresis following interscalene brachial plexus block. *Anesthesiology* 1985;63:102–104.
- Benumoff JL. Permanent loss of cervical spinal cord function associated with interscalene block performed under general anesthesia. *Anesthesiology* 2000;93: 1541–1544.
- Bonica JJ, Moore DC, Orlov M. Brachial plexus block anesthesia. *Am J Surg* 1949;78:65.
- Bonica JJ. The Management of Pain, 2nd edition. Philadelphia: Lea & Febiger, 1954:227.
- Bonner SM, Pridie AK. Sciatic nerve palsy following uneventful sciatic nerve block. *Anaesthesia* 1997;52: 1205–1211.
- Borgeat A, Ekatodramis G, Kalberer F, Benz C. Acute and nonacute complications associated with interscalene block and shoulder surgery: A prospective study. *Anesthesiology* 2001;95:875.
- Brand L, Papper EM. A comparison of supraclavicular and axillary techniques for brachial plexus blocks *Anesthesiology* 1961;22:226.
- Brown DL, Ransom DH, Hall JA, Leicht CH, Schoeder DR, Offord KP. Regional anesthesia and local-induced systemic toxicity: Seizure frequency and accompanying cardiovascular changes. *Anesth Analg* 1995;81:321.
- Chang PC, Lang SA, Yip RW. Reevaluation of the sciatic nerve block. *Reg Anesth* 1993;18:18.
- Choyce A, Chan VWS, Middleton WJ, Knight PR, Peng P, McCartney CJL. What is the relationship between paresthesia and nerve stimulation for axillary brachial plexus block? *Ref Anesth Pain Med* 2001;26:100–104.
- Curtis PH, Tucker HJ. Sciatic palsy in premature infants: a report and follow up study of ten cases. *JAMA* 1960;174:1586.
- Davis WJ, Lennon RL, Wedel DJ. Brachial plexus anesthesia for outpatient surgical procedures on an upper extremity. *Mayo Clin Proc* 1991;66:470.
- de Jong RH. Axillary block of the brachial plexus. *Anesthesiology* 1961;22:215.
- de Jong RH. Physiology and Pharmacology of Local Anesthesia, 2nd ed. Springfield: Charles C. Thomas, 1970:122.
- Fink BR, Kennedy RD, Hendrickson AE, Middaugh ME. Lidocaine inhibition of rapid axonal transport. *Anesthesiology* 1972;5:422.
- Frederick HA, Carter PR, Littler JW. Injection injuries at the median and ulnar nerves at the wrist. *J Hand Surg* 1972;17:465–467.
- Fremling MA, Mackinnon SE. Injection injury to the median nerve. *Ann Plast Surg* 1996;37:561–567.
- Gentili F, Hudson A, Kline D, Hunter D. Early changes following injection injury of peripheral nerves. *Can J Surg* 1980;23:177.

- Gentili F, Hudson A, Hunter D, Kline DG. Nerve injury with local anesthetic agents: a light and electron microscopic, fluorescent microscopic, and horseradish peroxidase study. *Neurosurgery* 1980;6:263.
- Gilles FH, French JH. Postinjection sciatic nerve palsies in infants and children. *J Pediatr* 1961;58: 195–204.
- Gillespie JH, Menk EJ, Middaugh RE: Reflex sympathetic dystrophy: A complication of interscalene block. *Anesth Analg* 1987;66:1316–1317.
- Hadžić A, Vloka J, Hadžić N, Thys DM, Santos AC. Nerve Stimulators Used for Peripheral Nerve Blocks Vary in Their Electrical Characteristics. *Anesthesiology*, In Press, 2004.
- Hadžić A, Vloka JD, Koorn R. Effects of the auditory volume control knob on the stimulus amplitude display of the DualStim/Deluxe™ model NS-2CA/DX peripheral nerve stimulator. *Anesthesiology* 1997;87: 714–715.
- Hadžić A, Vloka JD, Kuroda MM, Koorn R, Birnbach DJ. The practice of peripheral nerve blocks in the United States. A national survey. *Reg Anesth Pain Med* 1998;23:241–246.
- Hamelberg W, Dysart R, Bosomworth P. Perivascular axillary versus supraclavicular brachial plexus block and general anesthesia. *Anesth Analg* 1962;41:85.
- Jankovic D, Wells C. Brachial plexus, Regional nerve blocks, 2nd Edition. Edited by Jankovic D, Wells C. Edinburgh, Blackwell Science Berlin, 2001:76–77.
- Kalichman MW, Powel HC, Myers RR. Quantitative histologic analysis of local anesthetic-induced injury to rat sciatic nerve. *The Journal of Pharmacology; and Experimental Therapeutics* 1989;250:406–413.
- Kalichman MW, Powel HC, Myers RR. Pathology of local anesthetic-induced nerve injury. *Acta Neuropathol* 1988;75:583–589.
- Kalichman MW, Moorhouse DF, Powell HC, Myers RR. Relative neural toxicity of local anesthetics. *Journal of Neuropathology and Experimental Neurology* 1993;52: 234–240.
- Kroll DA, Caplan RA, Posner K, et al. Nerve injury associated with anesthesia. *Anesthesiology* 1990;73:202.
- Lavoie P-A, Khazen T, Filion PR. Mechanisms of the inhibition of fast axonal transport by local anesthetics. *Neuropharmacology* 1989;2:175.
- Lim EK, Pereira R. Brachial plexus injury following brachial plexus block. *Anaesthesia* 1984;39:691–694.
- Lofstrom B, Wennberg A, Widen L. Late disturbances in nerve function after block with local anesthetic agents. *Acta Anesth Scand* 1966;10:111.
- Lundborg G. Ischemic nerve injury. *Scand J Plast Reconstr Surg* 1970;6:79.
- Lundborg G. Structure and function of the intraneural microvessels as related to trauma, edema formation and nerve function. *J Bone Joint Surg* 1975;57A:938.
- Mackinnon SE, Hudson AR, Gentili F, Kline DG, Hunter RT. Peripheral nerve injury with steroid agents. *Plastic and Reconstructive Surgery*, 1982;69: 482–489.
- Mackinnon SE, Hudson AR, Llamas F, Dellon AL, Kline DG, Dan A, Hunter RT. Peripheral nerve injury by chymopapain injection. *J Neurosurg* 1984;61:1–8.
- McFarland EG, O'Neill OR, Hsu CY. Complications of shoulder arthroscopy. *J South Orthop Assoc* 1997;6: 190–196.
- Moberg E, Dhuner K-G. Brachial plexus block analgesia with xylocaine. *J Bone Joint Surg* 1951;33A:884.
- Mogensen BA, Mattsson HS. Posttraumatic instability of the metacarpophalangeal joint of the thumb. *Hand* 1980;12:85.
- Moore DC, Bridenbaugh LD, Thompson GE, et al. Bupivacaine: A review of 11,080 cases. *Anesth Analg* 1978;57:42.
- Moore DC, Mulroy Bonica JJ. The Management of Pain, 2nd edition. Philadelphia: Lea & Febiger, 1954:227.
- Moore DC, Mulroy MF, Thompson GE. Peripheral nerve damage and regional anesthesia (editorial). *Br J Anaesth* 1994;73:435.
- Myers RR, Kalichman MW, Reisner LS, Powell HC. Neurotoxicity of local anesthetics: Altered perineurial permeability, edema, and nerve fiber injury. *Anesthesiology* 1986;64:29–35.
- Myers RR, Powell HC. Endoneurial fluid pressure in peripheral neuropathies. In: Hargens A. Tissue fluid pressure and composition. Baltimore: Williams and Wilkins, 1980:193–207.
- Neal JM. How close is close enough? Defining the "Paresthesia Chad". *Regional Anesthesia and Pain Medicine* 2001;26:97–99.

- Pither CE, Raj PP, Ford DJ. The use of peripheral nerve stimulators for regional anesthesia: A review of experimental characteristics. *Regional Anesthesia* 1985;10: 49–58.

- Pitman MI, Nainzadeh N, Ergas E, Springer S. The use of somatosensory evoked potentials for detection of neuropraxia during shoulder arthroscopy. *Arthroscopy* 1988;4:250–255.

- Plevak DJ, Linstromberg JW, Danielsson DR. Paresthesia vs. non paresthesia—the axillary block. *Anesthesiology* 1983;59:A216.

- Rice ASM, McMahon SB. Peripheral nerve injury caused by injection needles used in regional anesthesia: Influence of bevel configuration, studied in a rat model. *Br J Anaesth* 1992;69:433.

- Rodeo SA, Forster RA, Weiland AJ. Neurological complications due to arthroscopy. *J Bone Joint Surg Am* 1993;75:917–926.

- Selander D. Neurotoxicity of local anesthetics: animal data. *Reg Anesth* 1993;18:461–468.

- Selander D, Brattsand R, Lundborg G, et al. Local anesthetics: Importance of mode of application, concentration and adrenaline for the appearance of nerve lesions. *Acta Anaesth Scand* 1979;23:127–136.

- Selander D, Dhuner KG, Lundborg. Peripheral nerve injury due to injection needles used for regional anesthesia. *Acta Anaesthsiol Scand* 1977;21:182.

- Selander D, Edshage S, Wolff T. Parasthesiae or no parasthesiae? Nerve lesions after axillary blocks. *Acta Anaesth Scand* 1979;23:27.

- Selander D, Mansson LG, Karlsson L, Svanvik J. Adrenergic vasoconstriction in peripheral nerves of the rabbit. *Anesthesiology* 1985;62:6.

- Selander D, Sjostrand J. Longitudal spread of intraneurally injected local anesthetics. *Acta Anesth Scand* 1978;22:622.

- Selander D. Peripheral Nerve Injury After Regional Anesthesia. In: Finucane BT. Complications of Regional Anesthesia, Philadelphia: Churchill Livingstone, 1999:105–115.

- Selander D. Nerve toxicity of local anesthetics. In: Lofstrom JB, Sjostrand U (eds): Local Anesthesia and Regional Blockade. Amsterdam. Elsevier Science Publisher B. V., 1988:77.

- Selander D. Neurotoxicity of local anesthetics: Animal data. *Reg Anesth* 1993;18:461.

- Selander D. Peripheral nerve damage and regional anesthesia (letter). *Br J Anesth* 1995;75:116.

- Smith DR, Kabine AJ, Rizzoli HV. Blood flow in peripheral nerves: Normal and postseverance flow rates. *J Neurol Sci* 1977;33:341.

- Stan TC, Krantz MA, Solomon DL, et al. The incidence of neurovascular complications following axillary brachial plexus block using a transarterial approach. *Reg Anesth* 1995;20:486.

- Stanish WD, Peterson DC. Shoulder arthroscopy and nerve injury: pitfalls and prevention. *Arthroscopy* 1995;11:458–466.

- Stark RH. Neurologic injury from axillary block anesthesia. *J Hand Surg* 21A:391,1996.

- Strasberg JE, Atchabahian A, Strasberg SR, Watanabe O, Hunter DA, Mackinnon SE. Peripheral nerve injection injury with antiemetic agents. *Journal of Neurotrauma* 1999;16:99–107.

- Tourtier Y, Rebillion M, Delort J, et al. Complications of axillary block using two techniques: Experience with 1400 cases. *Anesthesiology* 1989;71:726.

- Urmey WF, Stanton J. Inability to consistently elicit a motor response following sensory paresthesia during interscalene block administration. *Anesthesiology* 2002;96:552–554.

- Vloka JD, Hadžić A, Thys DM. Peripheral nerve stimulators for regional anesthesia can generate excessive voltage output with poor ground connection. *Anesth Analg* 2000;91:1306–1313.

- Wall JJ. Axillary nerve blocks. *Ann Surg* 1959;149:53.

- Weaver MA, Tandatnick CA, Hahn MB. Peripheral Nerve Blockade. In: Raj PP. Textbook of Regional Anesthesia. Philadelphia: Churchill Livingstone, 2002;857–887.

- Winchell SW, Wolfe R: The incidence of neuropathy following upper extremity nerve blocks. *Reg Anesth* 1985;10:12.

- Wolley EJ, Vandam LD. Neurological sequelae of brachial plexus nerve block. *Ann Surg* 1959;149:53.

- Zeh DW, Katz RL. A new nerve stimulator for monitoring neuromuscular blockade and performing nerve blocks. *Anesth Analg* 1973;57:13–17.

Peripheral nerve block anesthesia offers many clinical advantages that contribute to both improved patient outcome and lower overall health care costs. Nerve blocks provide excellent anesthesia and postoperative pain relief and fewer side effects than general anesthesia and permit early physical activity. The use of nerve blocks is also associated with reduced use of opioids for postoperative pain, fewer postoperative complications, and earlier discharges. Regional anesthesia is particularly desirable and effective in elderly and high-risk patients undergoing a wide variety of surgical procedures, particularly on the extremities. However, the success achieved with peripheral nerve blocks is multifactorial **(Fig. 7-1)** and undoubtedly more anesthesiologist-dependent than in the case of neuraxial and general anesthesia. The main determining factor for success is the anesthesiologist's technical skills and determination, which are required for successful practice of peripheral nerve blocks. To establish a regional anesthesia and peripheral nerve block program, a dedicated team of well-trained anesthesiologists is necessary to ensure consistent peripheral nerve block service.

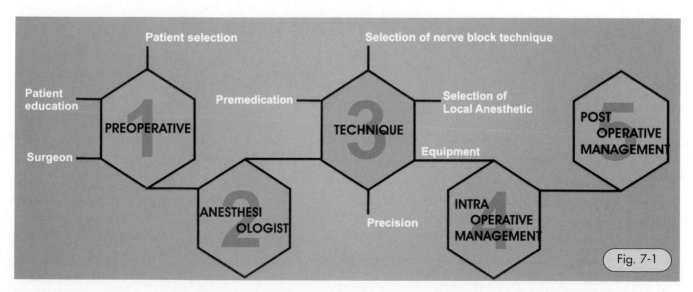

Five key elements for success with nerve blocks.

Patient

Patient Selection

To determine if a patient is a candidate for regional anesthesia, factors such as the primary indication for surgery, the presence of coexisting diseases, potential contraindications, and the patient's psychological state should all be considered. Regional anesthesia, alone or in combination with general anesthesia, is feasible and desirable in most surgical patients for almost any operative site. There are only a few absolute contraindications to regional anesthesia: patient refusal, the presence of an active infection at the site of puncture, and, perhaps, a true allergy to amide local anesthetics. In our practice the contraindications for the use of regional anesthesia are so rare that we do not emphasize them in the description of the block techniques to the patients. Regional anesthesia is particularly advantageous in high-risk surgical patients undergoing orthopedic, thoracic, abdominal, or vascular surgery. Patients with concomitant respiratory disease also benefit in that endotracheal intubation and mechanical ventilation are avoided.

Patient Education

Among the general public, there is a common lack of awareness regarding the potential uses and benefits of regional anesthesia. Patients are commonly asked to choose between two overly simplistic descriptions of anesthesia options: "a needle in the neck" or "go to sleep." However, neither of these accurately describes the nature of the anesthetic care. Many patients therefore have a tendency to choose general ("asleep") anesthesia because they lack an understanding of what regional anesthesia comprises and because of the anxiety related to needle insertion during block performance. In fact, in our practice most patients are appropriately sedated both during block performance and during the actual surgery. Resultantly, very few of our patients have an unpleasant recollection of their regional anesthesia experience. Another common misconception is that nerve blocks are associated with an increased risk of nerve injury. In fact, closed-claims studies by the American Society of Anesthesiologists suggest that the majority of reported neurologic complications are actually associated with general anesthesia because of problems with patient positioning.

During the preoperative visit, the anesthesiologist should help the patient understand the basics of anesthetic management and establish realistic expectations. Patients should be educated about the principal benefits of regional anesthesia—avoidance of general anesthesia and airway management, improved pain control, and reduced incidence of nausea and vomiting—all of which are evident immediately in the postoperative period. Patients should be instructed on what to expect during the postoperative period. In particular, they should be informed about the duration of the blockade, the need for analgesic therapy as the block wears off, and the care of the insensate extremity.

Surgeon

An insightful, educated surgeon is often the greatest advocate of regional anesthesia. At our institution, nearly all patients undergoing various orthopedic, vascular, hand, and podiatric surgical procedures are anesthetized using regional anesthesia. While some new surgeons joining the staff have reservations about regional anesthesia, their views are quickly changed once they realize that increased operating room efficiency and favorable outcomes are associated with expertly performed regional anesthesia procedures. However, the entire department of anesthesiology must be adequately trained in peripheral nerve blocks to provide consistent service and continuity of care. In such an environment, most of our surgeons routinely request regional anesthesia, and many patients coming in for procedures already have some basic information and expectations regarding the anesthetic plan. A discussion with the surgeon prior to choosing a regional anesthetic technique is crucially important.

The discussion must include considerations regarding the site, nature, extent, and duration of the planned surgical procedure. Discussion of the use of a tourniquet is always necessary to make sure that the intended technique will be adequate for the planned surgery.

Anesthesiologist

A confident, well-trained anesthesiologist is perhaps the single most important factor for the success of regional anesthetic. For acceptance by the patient and successful initiation and conductance of a regional anesthetic plan, it is primarily the anesthesiologist's confidence and ability to establish a rapport with the patient that determines the success. In our practice, we do not present the patient with a plethora of anesthetic options for a particular procedure, which many patients find confusing. Instead, we propose to the patient a regional anesthesia plan that is deemed optional based on the patient's physical status, the planned procedure, the surgical technique, and the experience of the anesthesia team. As the number and complexity of regional anesthesia techniques keep increasing, it is clear that regional anesthesia is a highly specialized subspecialty of anesthesiology. Thorough training during residency is necessary to obtain consistent results and decrease the risk of complications. A well-structured regional anesthesia fellowship is by far the best path toward success for those who chose to become regional anesthesiologists and acquire the skills necessary to practice the full scope of regional anesthesia and become effective instructors.

Technique

Technique Selection

Technique selection is of vital importance for the success of nerve block anesthesia. Choosing, initiating, and carrying out a regional anesthetic plan often require more thought than administering a general anesthetic. With general anesthesia, regardless of the technique, drugs, or ventilation modes chosen, adequate anesthesia is almost assured because patients typically are unconscious following administration of the anesthetic. In contrast, otherwise successful regional blocks may fail to provide adequate operating conditions because the site and duration of the surgery, the need for tourniquet application, or appropriate perioperative sedation was not considered. General guidelines on selecting nerve block techniques for some specific surgical procedures are provided in the appendix at the end of this chapter (**Table 7.2**).

Premedication

Most patients are apprehensive about pending anesthesia and surgery. Therefore, prior to placement of a peripheral nerve block for surgery, premedication is essential to alleviate anxiety and prevent unnecessary discomfort. Inadequately premedicated patients move during the block placement, making it difficult to interpret responses to nerve stimulation and possibly causing dislodgment of the needle from its intended position. In our practice, we prefer using a combination of benzodiazepine and a short acting narcotic (alfentanil). It should be noted that different block procedures are associated with varying degrees of discomfort. Premedication is adjusted for individual patients and for the procedure. A narcotic analgesic is introduced only at the time of needle placement. Alfentanil provides intense analgesia of short duration and in our practice is the narcotic most commonly used for this purpose.

All peripheral nerve blocks can be divided into two major groups—blocks associated with minor patient discomfort (*superficial blocks*) and blocks associated with more patient discomfort (*deep blocks*). A sedation protocol should be chosen according to the regional anesthesia technique planned and individual patient characteristics. For instance, an interscalene brachial plexus block can be administered to a minimally sedated, fully alert patient. On the other hand, an infraclavicular, sciatic, or lumbar plexus block necessitates, for most patients, a greater degree of sedation and analgesia

TABLE 7.1

Suggested Premedication For Common Nerve Block Procedures

BLOCK PLACEMENT	SEDATION
Blocks resulting in mild patient discomfort	Midazolam 2–4 mg ± alfentanil 50–100 µg
• Cervical blocks	
• Interscalene block	
• Supraclavicular block	
• Axillary block	
• Posterior popliteal block	
Blocks resulting in more patient discomfort	Midazolam 4–8 mg ± alfentanil 500–1000 µg
• Infraclavicular block	
• Wrist blocks	
• Paravertebral blocks	
• Lumbar plexus block	
• Lateral popliteal block	
• Saphenous block	

to ensure the patient's comfort and acceptance. Regardless of the sedation technique chosen, the goal of sedation is to provide maximum patient comfort while maintaining meaningful patient contact throughout the procedure.

In **Table 7.1** we suggest some premedication protocols for common nerve block procedures. More information on the doses of sedatives and analgesics are suggested in the chapters for each individual block procedure.

TIP

▶ The choice of medication, the dose, and the mode of administration should take into consideration the block technique, individual patient's characteristics, response to drugs, and overall medical status of the patient

Precision

The two main factors for effective neuronal blockade are successful localization of the nerve(s) and the ability to maintain the needle in the same position while the local anesthetic is injected. Although most trainees learn relatively quickly how to accurately place the needle in the intended position, learning to maintain this position throughout the injection takes a more concentrated effort.

We teach all our trainees to use a two-hand, immobile technique. With this technique, the palpating hand firmly press the desired anatomic location and while the fingers are anchored on the patient's body to prevent moving the fingers and changing the depth of palpation. The hand holding the needle is then positioned over the palpating hand with the free fingers supported by the palpating hand or the patient's body **(Fig. 7-2)**.

The exact position of the hands during block performance is demonstrated for each individual block technique in the respective chapters.

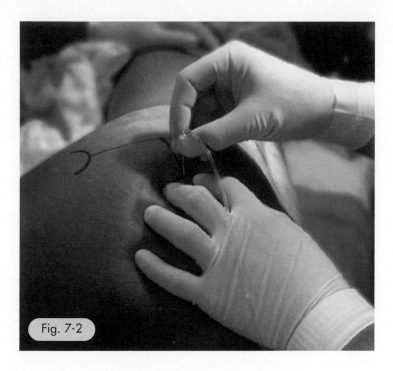

Fig. 7-2

Equipment

The proper selection of equipment, such as needles of the appropriate length and a properly functioning nerve stimulator is very important for successful block performance. Insulated needles are preferred over needles without electrical insulation because of their superior stimulating characteristics. It should be noted that there are differences in needle design among various manufacturers, resulting in clinically significant differences in stimulating characteristics, ease of advancement, and internal resistance. Although paresthesia techniques are still taught at some centers, we have completely abandoned this practice and teach only the techniques with nerve stimulators. Paresthesia techniques can be used with some upper-extremity blocks.

However, modern lower-extremity and continuous nerve blocks cannot be successfully practiced without nerve stimulation. Nerve stimulators also provide useful information on needle position, allow for objective, logical needle redirection, and serve as an excellent educational tool for a better understanding of functional anatomy. In our practice, we use nerve stimulators with a remote (foot) control, which allows quick, frequent control of the current by a single anesthesiologist. A hand or foot remote-controlled nerve stimulator is useful in teaching programs because it allows the instructor to control the current while keeping the hands on the patient sterile during resident training.

Local Anesthetic Selection

Selection of the type, dose, and volume of local anesthetic plays an important role in successful neuronal blockade. The choice of local anesthetics is discussed in detail with specific block techniques. Adequate volume and concentration are important to ensure a fast onset and a complete blockade. However, unnecessarily high doses and concentra-tions should be avoided, particularly in older and ill patients in whom inadvertent intravascular injection of local anesthetic carries a much higher risk than in young, fit patients. High pressures and fast, forceful injections should be avoided to decrease the risk of massive inadvertent channeling of local anesthetic into the systemic circulation.

Intraoperative Management

Sedation appropriately adjusted for patient comfort is almost always beneficial and improves the quality of the anesthesia achieved with peripheral nerve blocks. Most surgeons prefer patients to be lightly asleep during surgery so that they can better concentrate on the technical aspects of the operation. Similarly, the majority of patients also prefer not to be "aware" of activities in the operating room. For outpatients, after completion of the block, sedation is maintained throughout the surgical procedure and adjusted to the patient's comfort. In outpatients, this is most often accomplished using an intravenous infusion of propofol in a dose of 10 to 30 μg/kg/min (20 to 30 mL/h) while patients are breathing spontaneously. A face mask is routinely applied and oxygen delivered (5 to 6 L/min). On completion of the procedure, the infusion is discontinued. After surgery, most patients are fully alert and able to meaningfully discuss the findings with the surgeon in the operating room while a wound dressing is being applied. On arrival at the recovery room, most ambulatory surgery patients are fast-tracked to the postanesthesia care unit and prepared for discharge.

We avoid the use of narcotics at any point during the intraoperative treatment of patients receiving regional anesthesia. For inpatients, a combination of small boluses of midazolam and propofol is a good choice. A small proportion of regional anesthetics inevitably fail to provide adequate operating conditions because of inadequate anesthesia or difficulties in achieving adequate sedation. Because anesthesia of the skin is often the last to occur, local infiltration by the surgeon, when possible, and deeper levels of sedation at the beginning of the procedure are often all that is required for the procedure to proceed while the block is "setting up." However, when anesthesia is deemed incomplete for the planned surgery, we often induce a light general anesthetic and control the airway instead of resorting to oversedation and intravenous narcotics.

Because most operating rooms are kept cold, all patients undergoing surgery under regional anesthesia should be kept warmed by using forced air or warm blankets **(Fig. 7-3)**. Failure to prevent shivering can result in uncontrolled patient movement, tremors, and consequent failure of an otherwise successful block placement.

Significant noise levels are often present in operating rooms because of discussions among the staff, handling of instruments, or the use of various pneumatic instruments. In a study on noise levels during various orthopedic surgery procedures, we recorded levels higher than 100 dB when pneumatic drills and saws were being used. Such noise is invariably nox-

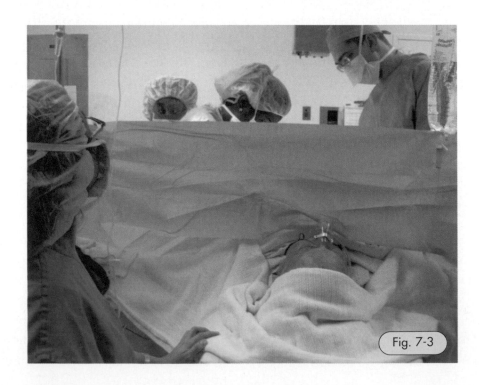

Fig. 7-3

ious to the patient and requires that much higher doses of sedative be used. Therefore, shielding the patient's ears from the unwanted noise should be done routinely to help reduce patient anxiety. This can be accomplished using blankets **(Fig. 7-3)**, ear plugs or headphones with or without music.

During the administration and conductance of regional anesthesia, incremental doses (boluses) of sedatives, narcotics, intravenous sedation, and antibiotics are routinely administered, and there is often a tendency to overadminister intravenous (IV) fluids. Overhydration should be avoided because of the possibility of difficulties intraoperatively when patients need to void. For this reason, it is advisable to use an electronic infusion pump or a micro-drip intravenous infusion set.

Postoperative Management

On completion of the surgical procedure, it is important to discuss with the surgeons, patient, and nursing staff the expected duration of the motor and sensory blockade to prevent unnecessary concerns by anyone involved in treating the patient. In addition, a proper multimodal pain management protocol must be developed and discussed thoroughly with the patient to avoid severe pain when the block(s) wears off. For inpatients, this is perhaps best accomplished by prescribing intravenous patient-controlled analgesia (IV PCA) or oral analgesics. This applies even to patients who may receive continuous nerve block infusion catheters. For outpatients, such a plan most often consists of a combination of an oral nonsteroidal anti-inflammatory regimen and an oral acetaminophen-codeine prescription.

Clear instructions regarding care of the insensate extremity should also be given to patients to prevent secondary injuries, which may occur when the anesthetized extremity is not handled with care.

APPENDIX

TABLE 7.2
Choice of Peripheral Nerve Block Technique for Common Surgical Procedures

SURGICAL PROCEDURE	PERIPHERAL NERVE BLOCK TECHNIQUE	COMMENTS
Neck surgery		
• Neck lymph node biopsy • Carotid endarterectomy • Postoperative pain management after neck surgery (e.g., radical neck dissection)	• Superficial cervical plexus block • Deep or superficial cervical plexus block	• Because cervical plexus block is a "blind" technique, the success rate can be significantly increased by performing both superficial and deep cervical plexus blocks routinely for carotid endarterectomy. • It should be remembered that cervical plexus block needs to be supplemented intraoperatively during carotid endarterectomy because the carotid artery receives neuronal input from glossopharyngeal nerve. This is best accomplished with a carotid "sheath" block by the surgeon when the carotid artery is exposed. • Cutaneous coverage from the opposite side is blocked by a subcutaneous injection of local anesthetic along the line connecting the thyroid cartilage to just above the sternal notch.

(continued on next page)

APPENDIX / 85

TABLE 7.2 (continued)

Choice of Peripheral Nerve Block Technique for Common Surgical Procedures

SURGICAL PROCEDURE	PERIPHERAL NERVE BLOCK TECHNIQUE	COMMENTS
Upper extremity surgery		
• Shoulder arthroscopy • Rotator cuff repair • Shoulder arthroplasty • Shoulder stabilization • Fracture of the humerus neck repair	• Interscalene brachial plexus block	• Interscalene brachial plexus block provides complete anesthesia of the shoulder joint. • Cutaneous coverage of the area over the shoulder varies and may require subcutaneous injection of local anesthetic if cutaneous coverage proves inadequate. • Surgeons should be encouraged to routinely infiltrate the site of the arthroscopic port insertion with local anesthetic.
• Surgery on the lower arm • Surgery on the elbow • Forearm surgery • Hand surgery	• Infraclavicular block • Supraclavicular block • Infraclavicular/axillary block • Infraclavicular/axillary block	• Both techniques are excellent choices for lower arm, elbow, forearm, and hand surgery. • Neither is an optimal choice for shoulder surgery. • The main advantages of supra and infraclavicular block techniques over an axillary block are a higher success rate and routine blockade of the musculocutaneous nerve (better tourniquet coverage). • The main disadvantage of a supraclavicular block is the risk of pneumothorax.
• Hand surgery	• Infraclavicular block • Axillary block • Intravenous regional anesthesia (Bier block)	• When prolonged tourniquet application is not required, an axillary block is a simple, effective technique to use for hand surgery. • Double- and multiple-injection techniques have been proposed to increase the success rate of an axillary blockade. • When arterial puncture (axillary artery) occurs on needle advancement, injection of one-half of the total volume behind and in front of the artery increases the success rate.

TABLE 7.2 (continued)

Choice of Peripheral Nerve Block Technique for Common Surgical Procedures

SURGICAL PROCEDURE	PERIPHERAL NERVE BLOCK TECHNIQUE	COMMENTS
Upper extremity surgery (continued)		
• Hand surgery • Surgery on the digits	• Wrist block • Digital block • Intravenous regional anesthesia (Bier block)	• Wrist and digital blocks are simple, highly effective anesthetic techniques for surgery on the digits and hands not requiring a tourniquet. • A tourniquet on the forearm, when required, is well tolerated and can be used to avoid the need for a more proximal neuronal blockade for short procedures. • Intravenous regional anesthesia (Bier block) should be limited to surgery of short duration (30–45 min) because of tourniquet pain that becomes difficult to manage.
Surgery on the chest and abdominal wall		
• Thoracotomy • Mid-CABG • Surgery on the chest wall • Mastectomy • Reconstructive breast surgery	• Intercostal nerve block • Paravertebral blocks	• Paravertebral blocks can be used for any of the listed surgical applications. • Paravertebral blocks are preferred to intercostal blocks because of the lower risk of systemic toxicity, higher success rate, and longer duration of blockade. • For breast surgery, paravertebral levels T1 through T6 are necessary; when surgery extends to the clavicle, local anesthetic infiltration or superficial cervical blockade is also necessary. • For axillary node surgery, paravertebral level T1 is also required; surgical manipulation should be gentle to avoid irritation of the brachial plexus in the axilla.
• Inguinal hernia repair • Colostomy closure • Uncomplicated appendectomy • Pain management after hip surgery	• Thoracolumbar paravertebral block	• Paravertebral levels T9 through L1 must be blocked. • The groin, part of the hip and knee, the anterolateral and medial thigh, also and the medial skin below the knee are anesthetized. • Distribution of anesthesia is unilateral. • 15% epidural spread may occur.

TABLE 7.2 (continued)

Choice of Peripheral Nerve Block Technique for Common Surgical Procedures

SURGICAL PROCEDURE	PERIPHERAL NERVE BLOCK TECHNIQUE	COMMENTS
Lower extremity surgery		
• Knee arthroscopy • Patella tendon and anterior cruciate ligament repair • Saphenous vein stripping • Open reduction internal fixation of patella fracture • Pain management after hip and knee surgery	• Lumbar plexus block • Femoral nerve block	• With the lumbar plexus block, the groin, portion of the hip and knee, the anterolateral and medial thigh, and the medial skin below knee are also anesthetized. • Femoral nerve block combined with a genitofemoral nerve block is an excellent choice for saphenous vein stripping. • For complete anesthesia of the knee and lower leg, femoral or lumbar plexus blocks must be combined with a sciatic block. • When choosing a femoral versus a lumbar plexus block, lumbar plexus block should be chosen when anesthesia of the lumbar plexus (lateral femoral cutaneous nerve, obturator nerve) is sought. • A femoral nerve block does not reliably result in lumbar plexus blockade regardless of volume used.
• Above and below knee amputations • Any surgery on the tibia and/or fibula • Achilles tendon repair • Foot surgery • Pain management after surgery on the lower extremity	• Sciatic nerve block	• Combined with a lumbar plexus or femoral block results in complete anesthesia of the lower extremity. • Can be combined with a saphenous block or "low-volume" femoral block to achieve complete anesthesia of the leg below the knee. • A femoral nerve block is not an adequate supplement for surgery above the knee because the obturator nerve and lateral femoral cutaneous nerve of the thigh are not anesthetized and may be important for complete anesthesia; a lumbar plexus block is a better choice.
• Ankle surgery • Foot surgery • Achilles tendon repair • Short saphenous vein stripping	• Popliteal nerve block or ankle block	• When surgery involves the medial aspect of the lower leg, a saphenous nerve block is needed. • Success rate is volume-dependent. • A popliteal block is chosen over an ankle block for more proximal, more extensive surgery and surgery requiring the use of a tourniquet.

SUGGESTED READINGS

- Dickerman D, Vloka JD, Koorn R, Hadžić A. Excessive noise levels during orthopedic surgery. *Reg Anesth* 1997;22:97.

- Hadžić A, Vloka JD, Koenigsamen J. Training requirements for peripheral nerve blocks. *Curr Opin Anesthesiol* 2002;15:669–673.

- Hadžić A, Vloka JD, Kuroda MM, et al. The practice of peripheral nerve blocks in the United States: a national survey. *Reg Anesth Pain Med* 1998;23:241–246.

- New York School of Regional Anesthesia. www.nysora.com, October 18, 2001.

- Karaca P, Hadžić A, Vloka, JD. Specific nerve blocks: an update. *Curr Opin Anaesthesiol* 2000;13:549–555.

- Kopacz DJ, Bridenbaugh LD. Are anesthesia residency programs failing regional anesthesia? The past, present, and future. *Reg Anesth* 1993;18:84–87.

- Kopacz DJ, Neal J, Pollock J. The regional anesthesia "learning curve": what is the minimum number of epidural and spinal blocks to reach consistency? *Reg Anesth* 1996;21:182–190.

- Vloka, JD, Hadžić A, Santos A. Lower extremity nerve blocks for ambulatory surgery. *Curr Anesthesiol Rep* 2000;2(4):327–332.

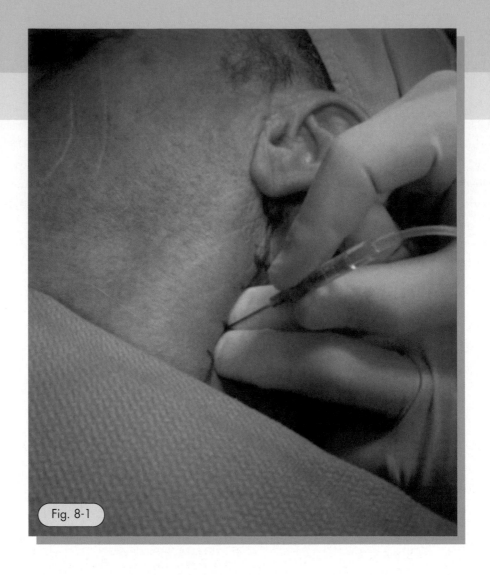

Fig. 8-1

BLOCK AT A GLANCE

- Deep and superficial cervical plexus blocks

- Indications: carotid endarterectomy, neck surgery

- Landmarks: mastoid process, sternocleidomastoid muscle
  C6 transverse process

- Equipment, *superficial:* 1½-in, 25-gauge needle

- Equipment, *deep:* 1½-in, 22-gauge, short-bevel needle

- Local anesthetic: 15 to 20 mL

- Complexity level: intermediate (deep), basic (superficial)

DEEP CERVICAL PLEXUS BLOCK

General Considerations

A deep cervical plexus block is essentially a paravertebral block of the C2 through C4 spinal nerves as they emerge from the foramina of their respective vertebrae. Blockade of the deep cervical plexus also results in blockade of the superficial cervical plexus. A deep cervical block is often present when a larger volume of local anesthetic is used in an interscalene brachial plexus block. In our practice, the most common clinical uses for this block are carotid endarterectomy and the removal of cervical lymph nodes.

Regional Anesthesia Anatomy

The cervical plexus is formed by the anterior divisions of the four upper cervical nerves. The plexus is situated on the anterior surface of the four upper cervical vertebrae, resting on the levator anguli scapulae and scalenus medius muscle and covered by the sternocleidomastoid muscle. The dorsal and ventral roots combine to form spinal nerves as they exit through the intervertebral foramen. The anterior rami of C2 through C4 form the cervical plexus (the C1 root is a primarily motor nerve and is not blocked by this technique). The cervical plexus lies in the plane just behind the sternocleidomastoid muscle, giving off both superficial (superficial cervical plexus) and deep branches (deep cervical plexus) **(Fig. 8-2)**. The branches of the superficial cervical plexus supply innervation to the skin and superficial structures of the head, neck, and shoulder. The deep branches of the cervical plexus innervate the deeper structures of the neck, including the muscles of the anterior neck and the diaphragm (phrenic nerve). The third and fourth cervical nerves typically send a branch to the spinal accessory nerve or directly into the deep surface of the trapezius to supply sensory fibers to this muscle. The fourth cervical nerve may send a branch downward to join the fifth cervical nerve and participates in formation of the brachial plexus.

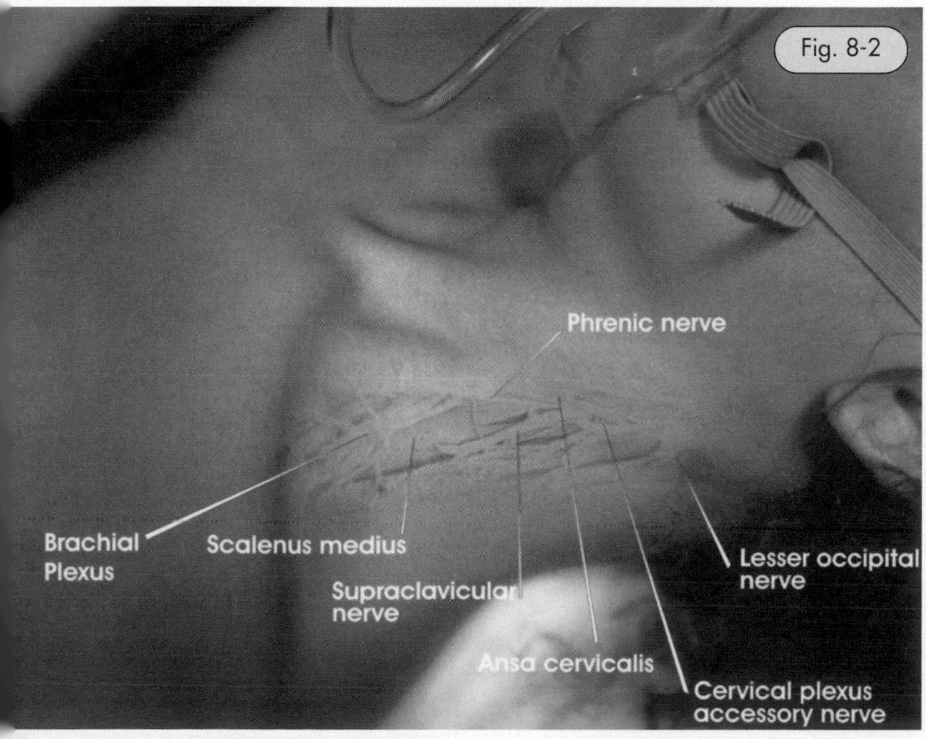

Fig. 8-2

Brachial Plexus

Scalenus medius

Supraclavicular nerve

Ansa cervicalis

Phrenic nerve

Lesser occipital nerve

Cervical plexus accessory nerve

TABLE 8.1
Deep Cervical Plexus Branches

Internal branches	• Communicating branches • Muscular branches • Hypoglossal communicating branches • Phrenic
External branches	• Communicating branches • Muscular branches

The deep branches of the cervical plexus can be classified as internal and external **(Table 8.1).**

Distribution of Anesthesia

Cutaneous innervation of both the deep and the superficial cervical plexus blocks includes the skin of the anterolateral neck and the ante- and retroauricular areas **(Fig. 8-3).**

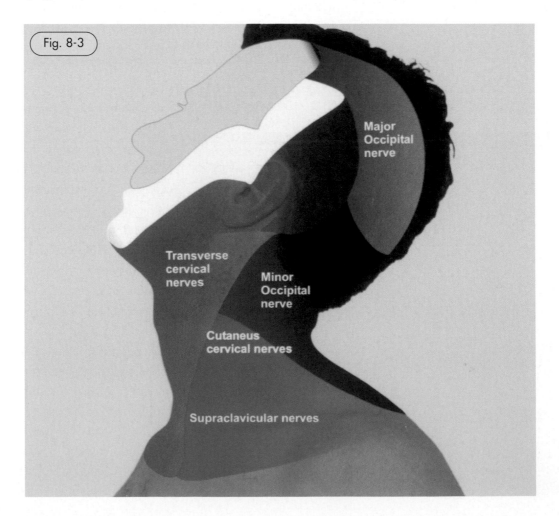

Fig. 8-3

Major Occipital nerve

Transverse cervical nerves

Minor Occipital nerve

Cutaneus cervical nerves

Supraclavicular nerves

Patient Positioning

The patient is in a supine or semi-sitting position with the head facing away from the side to be blocked **(Fig. 8-4)**.

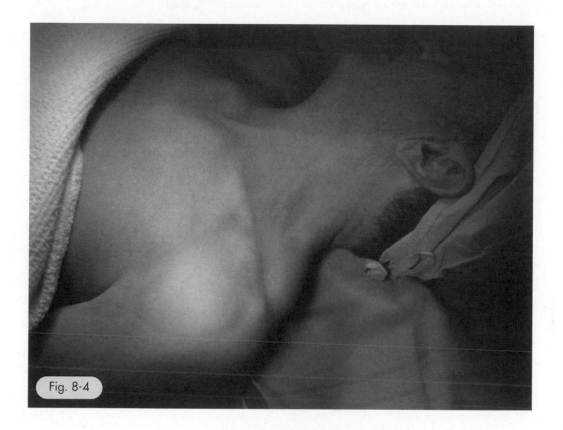

Fig. 8-4

Equipment

A standard regional anesthesia tray is prepared with the following equipment **(Fig. 8-5)**:

- Sterile towels and gauze packs

- 20-mL syringe(s) with local anesthetic

- Sterile gloves and marking pen

- 1½-in, 25-gauge needle for skin infiltration

- 1½-in, 22-gauge, short-bevel needle

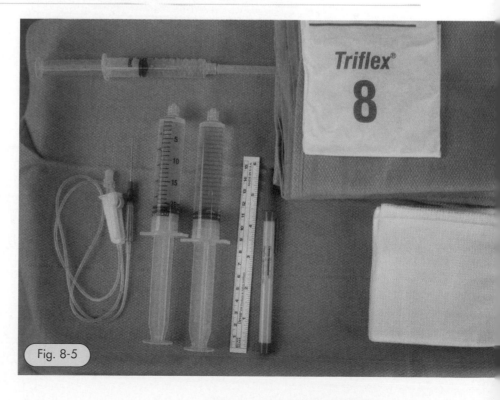

Fig. 8-5

Surface Landmarks

The following surface anatomy landmarks are helpful for estimating the location of the transverse processes: mastoid process, transverse process of the sixth cervical vertebra (C6), and the posterior border of the sternocleidomastoid muscle **(Fig. 8-6)**.

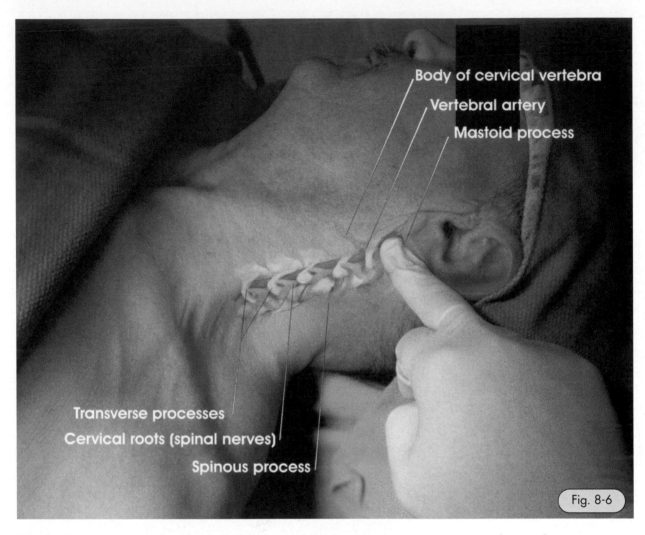

Relationship of anatomic landmarks to the cervical nerves, transverse processes, and carotid artery.

> **TIP**
>
> ▶ The proportions of the shoulder girdle, size of the neck, prominence of the muscles, and other areas vary among patients. When in doubt, always perform a "reality check" and estimate the three bony landmarks: sternal notch, clavicle, and mastoid process.

Anatomic Landmarks

The following three landmarks for a deep cervical plexus block are identified and marked (**Fig. 8-7**):

1. Mastoid process

2. Chassaignac tubercle transverse (process of the C6)

3. Posterior border of the sternocleidomastoid muscle

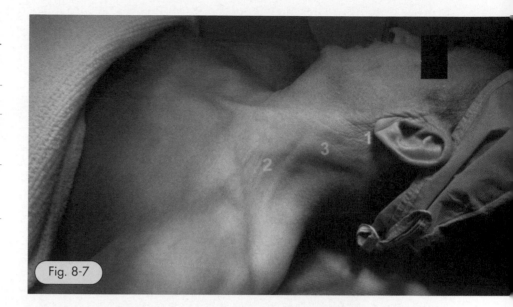

Fig. 8-7

TIPS

The anatomic landmarks for this block can be accentuated by asking the patient to:

▶ Turn the head slightly away from the side to be blocked

▶ Lift the head up (tensing the sternocleidomastoid muscles)

▶ Reach for the knee with the hand on the ipsilateral side

To estimate the line of needle insertion overlying the transverse processes, the mastoid process and the the transverse of C6 process are identified and marked. The C6 transverse process is easily palpated behind the clavicular head of the sternocleidomastoid muscle at the level just below the cricoid cartilage (**Fig. 8-8**).

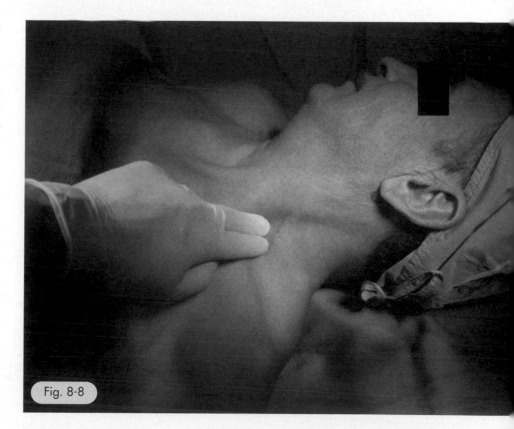

Fig. 8-8

Next, a line is drawn connecting the mastoid process to the Chassaignac tubercle of the C6 transverse process **(Fig. 8-9)**. The palpating hand is best positioned just behind the posterior border of the sternocleidomastoid muscle. Once this line is drawn, the insertion sites over C2 through C4 are labeled as follows: C2 through C4 are located on the mastoid process–C6 line about 2, 4, and 6 cm caudal from the mastoid process, respectively **(Fig. 8-10)**.

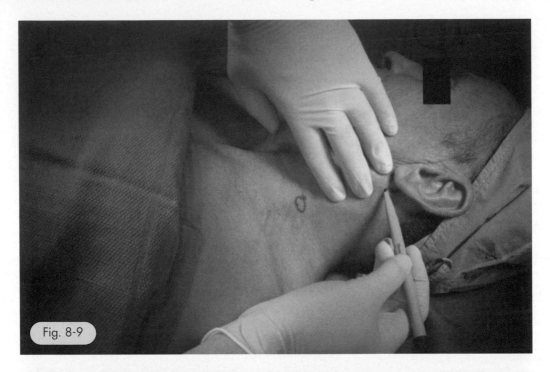

Fig. 8-9

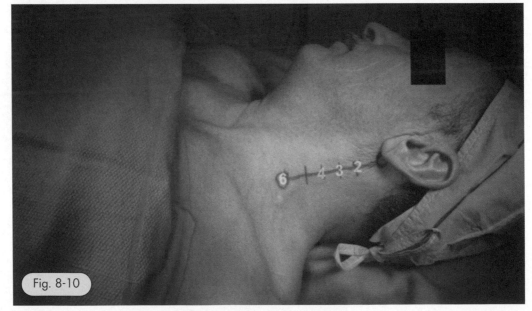

Fig. 8-10

TIP

▶ It should be noted that the distances specified for spacing along the transverse processes at various levels are at best approximations. However, once contact is made with the transverse processes at the first two levels, the spacing between the two neighboring ones follows a similar pattern.

Local Anesthetic Skin Infiltration

After cleaning the skin with an antiseptic solution, local anesthetic is infiltrated subcutaneously along the line estimating the position of the transverse processes **(Fig. 8-11)**. The local anesthetic is best infiltrated over the entire length of the line rather than at the projected insertion sites. This allows reinsertion of the needle slightly caudally or cranially when the transverse process is not contacted, without the need to infiltrate the skin at a new insertion site.

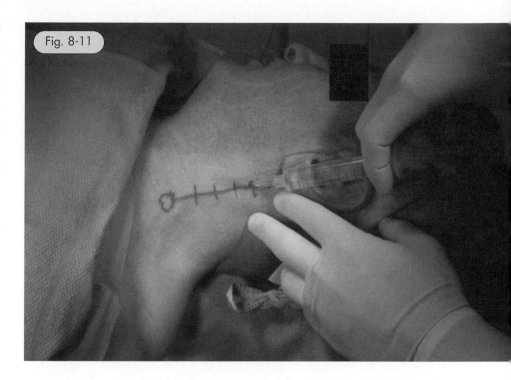

Fig. 8-11

Needle Insertion

A needle connected via flexible tubing to a syringe containing local anesthetic is inserted between the palpating fingers and is advanced at an angle perpendicular to the skin plane **(Fig. 8-12)**. The needle should never be oriented cephalad. A slightly caudal orientation of the needle is important to prevent inadvertent insertion of the needle toward the cervical spinal cord. The needle is advanced slowly until the transverse process is contacted. At this point, the needle is withdrawn 1 to 2 mm and firmly stabilized, and 4 mL of local anesthetic is injected after obtaining negative results from an aspiration test for blood. The needle is then removed, and the entire procedure is repeated at consecutive levels.

TIPS

▶ The transverse process is typically contacted at a depth of 1 to 2 cm in most patients. This distance can be further shortened by exerting pressure on the skin during needle advancement.

▶ The needle should never be advanced beyond 2.5 cm to avoid the risk of cervical cord injury or carotid or vertebral artery puncture.

▶ Paresthesia is often elicited close to the transverse process, but it should not be relied on or actively sought because of its nonspecific radiating pattern.

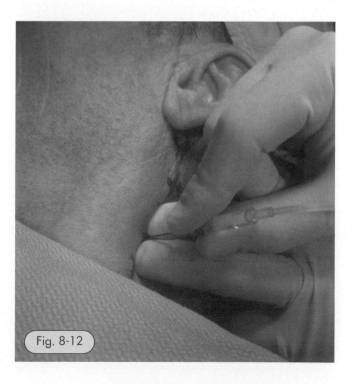

Fig. 8-12

Failure to Contact the Transverse Process on the First Needle Pass

When insertion of the needle does not result in contact with the transverse process within 2 cm, the following maneuvers are used:

1. While avoiding skin movement, keep the palpating hand in the same position and the skin between the fingers stretched.

2. Withdraw the needle to the skin, redirect it 15° inferiorly, and repeat the procedure **(Fig. 8-13)**.

3. Withdraw the needle to the skin, reinsert it 1 cm caudal, and repeat the above procedure.

TIPS

▶ When these maneuvers fail to result in contact with the transverse process, the needle should be withdrawn and the landmarks reassessed.

▶ Redirecting the needle cephalad in an attempt to contact the transverse process should be avoided because it carries a risk of cervical cord injury when the needle is advanced too deep.

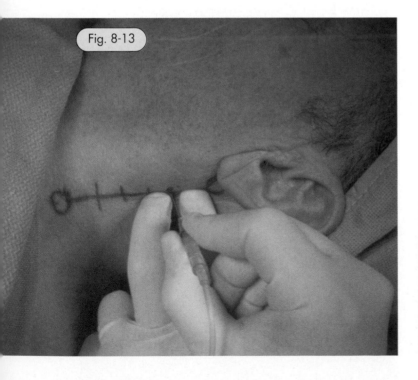

Fig. 8-13

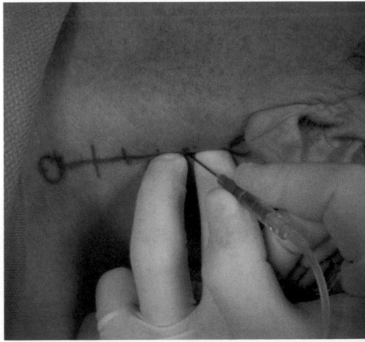

Choice of Local Anesthetic

A deep cervical plexus block requires 3 to 5 mL of local anesthetic per level to ensure a reliable blockade. With possible exception of patients with significant respiratory disease (blockade of the phrenic nerve), most patients benefit from the use of a long-acting local anesthetic **(Table 8-2)**.

TABLE 8.2
Choice of Local Anesthetic For Deep Cervical Plexus Block

ANESTHETIC	ONSET (min)	DURATION OF ANESTHESIA (h)	DURATION OF ANALGESIA (h)
1.5% Mepivacaine (HCO_3 + epinephrine)	10–15	2.0–2.5	3–6
2% Lidocaine (plus HCO_3 + epinephrine)	10–15	2–3	3–6
0.5% Ropivacaine	10–20	3–4	4–10
0.25% Bupivacaine (+ epinephrine)	10–20	3–4	4–10

Block Dynamics and Perioperative Management

Although the placement of a deep cervical block may be associated with moderate patient discomfort, excessive sedation should be avoided. During neck surgery, airway management may be difficult because the anesthesiologist must share access to the head and neck with the surgeon. Surgeries like carotid endarterectomy may require the patient to be fully conscious, oriented, and cooperative during the entire procedure. In addition, excessive sedation and the consequent lack of patient cooperation can result in restlessness and create difficulty for the surgeon. The onset time for this block is 10 to 15 minutes. The first sign is decreased sensation in the area of distribution of the respective components of the cervical plexus. It should be noted that because of the complex arrangement of the neuronal coverage of the various layers in the neck area, as well as cross-coverage from the contralateral side, the anesthesia achieved with a cervical plexus block is rarely complete. While this should not discourage the use of this block, it does require an understanding surgeon who is willing to supplement the block with a local anesthetic if and when necessary.

TIP

► Carotid surgery also requires blockade of the glossopharyngeal nerve branches. This is easily accomplished intraoperatively by injecting local anesthetic inside the carotid artery sheath.

SUPERFICIAL CERVICAL PLEXUS BLOCK

Regional Anesthesia Anatomy

TABLE 8.3 Superficial Cervical Plexus Branches	
Ascending branches	• Occipitalis major • Auricularis magnus • Superficialis colli • Phrenic • Suprasternal • Supraclavicular
Descending branches	• Supraacromial

The superficial cervical plexus innervates the skin of the anterolateral neck through the anterior primary rami of C2 through C4. The nerves emerge as four distinct nerves from the posterior border of the sternocleidomastoid muscle **(Table 8-3, Fig. 8-14)**. The lesser occipital nerve is usually a direct branch from the main stem of the second cervical nerve. The larger remaining part of this stem then joins part of the third cervical nerve to form a trunk that arises as the greater auricular and transverse cervical nerves. Another part of the third cervical nerve runs downward to join a major part of the fourth cervical nerve to form the supraclavicular trunk, which then divides into three groups of supraclavicular nerves.

Distribution of Anesthesia

The superficial cervical plexus innervates the skin of the anterolateral neck **(see Fig. 8-3 p. 92)**.

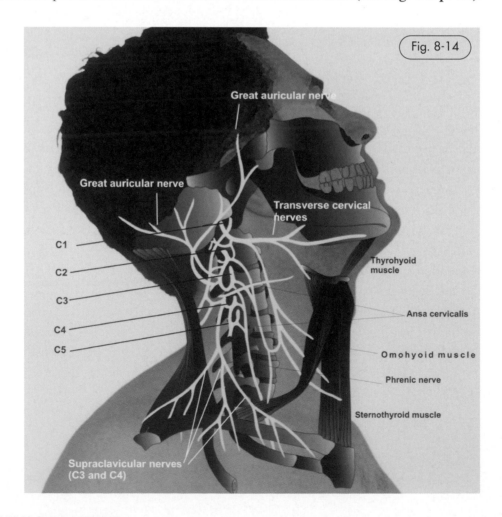

Fig. 8-14

Great auricular nerve

Great auricular nerve

Transverse cervical nerves

Thyrohyoid muscle

C1

C2

C3

C4

C5

Ansa cervicalis

Omohyoid muscle

Phrenic nerve

Sternothyroid muscle

Supraclavicular nerves (C3 and C4)

Patient Positioning

The patient is in the same position as for the deep cervical plexus block, with the head facing away from the side to be blocked **(Fig. 8-15)**.

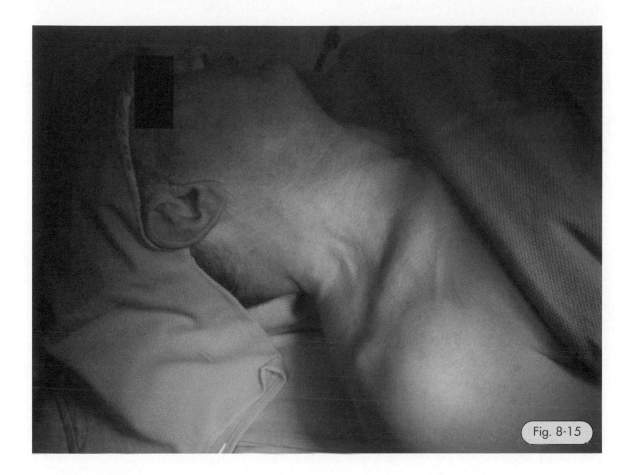

Fig. 8-15

Equipment

A standard regional anesthesia tray **(see Fig. 8-5, p. 93)** is prepared with the following equipment:

- Sterile towels and gauze packs

- 20-mL syringe(s) containing local anesthetic

- Sterile gloves, a marking pen

- 1½-in, 25-gauge needle for block infiltration

- 1½-in, 22-gauge, short-bevel needle

Surface Landmarks

The following surface anatomy landmarks are helpful in estimating the location of the posterior border of the sternocleidomastoid muscle and in estimating the site of needle injection **(Fig. 8-16)**:

1. Mastoid process

2. Tubercle of the C6 transverse process

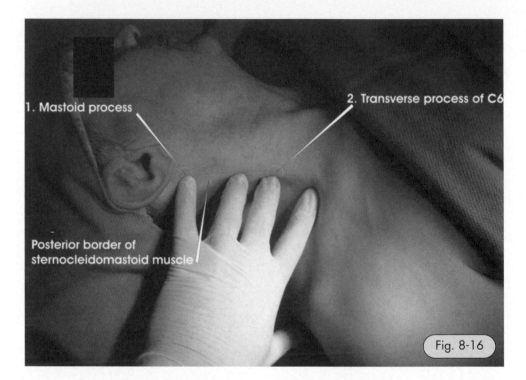

1. Mastoid process

2. Transverse process of C6

Posterior border of sternocleidomastoid muscle

Fig. 8-16

The fingers of the palpating hand should be stretched to outline the posterior border of the clavicular head of the sternocleidomastoid muscle and to help visualize the line connecting the mastoid process with the C6 transverse process.

Anatomic Landmarks

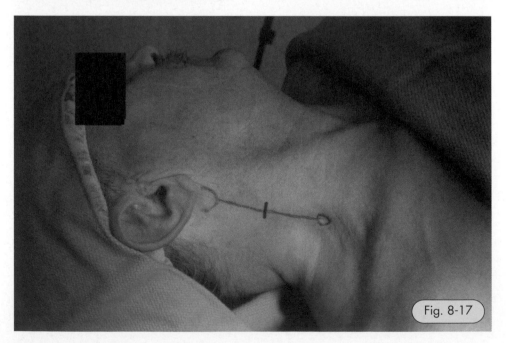

Fig. 8-17

A line extending from the mastoid to C6 is drawn **(Fig. 8-17)**. The site of needle insertion is marked at the midpoint of the line connecting the mastoid process with the Chassaignac tubercle of the C6 transverse process. This is where the branches of the superficial cervical plexus emerge behind the posterior border of the sternocleidomastoid muscle.

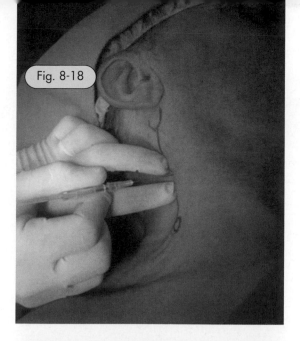

Fig. 8-18

Needle Insertion

After cleansing the skin with an antiseptic solution, a skin wheal is raised at the site of needle insertion using a 25-gauge needle. Next, using a "fan" technique with superior-inferior needle redirections, the local anesthetic is injected along the posterior border of the sternocleidomastoid muscle 2 to 3 cm below and above the needle insertion site **(Fig. 8-18)**. This technique should be adequate to achieve blockade of all four major branches of the superficial cervical plexus.

GOAL

The goal of the injection is to infiltrate the local anesthetic subcutaneously and behind the sternocleidomastoid muscle. Deep needle insertion (e.g., greater than 1 to 2 cm) should be avoided to minimize the risk of subarachnoid injection.

TIPS

▶ The transverse process should never be sought with the superficial cervical plexus technique.

▶ Paresthesia is occasionally elicited during needle insertion. However, it is nonspecific and should not be routinely sought or relied upon.

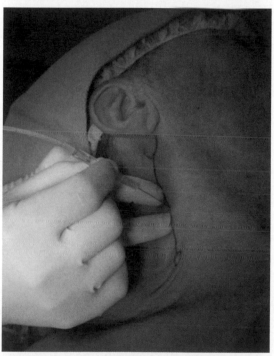

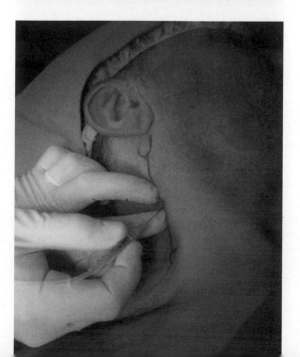

Choice of Local Anesthetic

A superficial cervical plexus block requires 10 to 15 mL of local anesthetic (3 to 5 mL per each redirection and injection) **(Table 8-4)**.

Most patients benefit from the use of a long-acting local anesthetic. Because a motor block is not sought with this technique, some anesthesiologists suggest using a low concentration of local anesthetic (e.g., 0.2% ropivacaine or 0.25% bupivacaine). Although a low concentration may suffice when the needle is ideally placed in the vicinity of the cervical plexus nerves, a higher concentration results in faster onset, a higher success rate and a longer duration of blockade.

TABLE 8.4
Choice of Local Anesthetic For Superficial Cervical Plexus Block

ANESTHETIC	ONSET (min)	DURATION OF ANESTHESIA (h)	DURATION OF ANALGESIA (h)
1.5% Mepivacaine (HCO_3 + epinephrine)	10–15	2.0–2.5	3–6
2% Lidocaine (HCO_3 + epinephrine)	10–15	2–3	3–6
0.5% Ropivacaine	10–20	3–4	4–10
0.25% Bupivacaine (+ epinephrine)	10–20	3–4	4–10

Block Dynamics and Perioperative Management

A superficial cervical plexus block is associated with minor patient discomfort. Small doses of midazolam 1 to 2 mg for sedation and alfentanil 250 to 500 µg for analgesia just before needle insertion, should result in a comfortable, cooperative patient during block injection. Similar to that of the deep cervical plexus blockade, a degree of cross-coverage from the cervical plexus branches from the opposite side of the neck should be expected. The onset time for this block is 10 to 15 minutes, and the first sign is decreased sensation in the area of the distribution of the respective components of the cervical plexus. Excessive sedation should be avoided before and during head and neck procedures because if airway management becomes necessary, it may prove difficult because access to the head and neck is shared with the surgeon.

TIP

▶ A subcutaneous midline injection of local anesthetic extending from the thyroid cartilage distally to the suprasternal notch will block the branches crossing from the opposite side. This injection can be considered a "field" block. It is very useful for preventing pain from surgical skin retractors on the medial aspect of the neck.

Complications and How to Avoid Them

TABLE 8.5
Complications of Cervical Plexus Blocks and Techniques on How to Avoid Them

Infection	• Low risk. • A strict aseptic technique should be used.
Hematoma	• Avoid multiple needle insertions, particularly in patients undergoing anticoagulant therapy. • Keep a 5-min steady pressure on the site if the carotid artery is inadvertently punctured.
Phrenic nerve blockade	• Phrenic nerve blockade (diaphragmatic paresis) invariably occurs with a deep cervical plexus block. • A deep cervical block should be carefully considered in patients with significant respiratory disease. • A bilateral deep cervical block may be contraindicated in patients with significant respiratory disease • Blockade of the phrenic nerve does not occur following a superficial cervical plexus block.
Local anesthetic toxicity	• Central nervous system toxicity is the most common serious consequence of a cervical plexus block. • This complication occurs because of the rich vascularity of the neck, including vertebral and carotid artery vessels; it is usually caused by inadvertent intravascular injection rather than absorption of local anesthetic. • Gentle and frequent aspiration should be performed during the injection.
Nerve injury	• Local anesthetic should never be injected against resistance or when the patient complains of severe pain on injection.
Spinal anesthesia	• This complication may occur with injection of a large volume of local anesthetic inside the dural sleeve surrounding the nerves of the cervical plexus. • Avoidance of high volume and pressure during injection are the best measures to avoid this complication. • It should be noted that negative results from an aspiration test for cerebrospinal fluid does not rule out the possibility of intrathecal spread of local anesthetic.

SUGGESTED READINGS

Deep Cervical Plexus Block

- Aunac S, Carlier M, Singelyn F, De Kock M. The analgesic efficacy of bilateral combined superficial and deep cervical plexus block administered before thyroid surgery under general anesthesia. *Anesth Analg* 2002; 95:746–750.
- Benzon HT, Raja SN, Borsook D, Molloy RE, Strichartz G. *Essentials of Pain Medicine and Regional Anesthesia.* Philadelphia, Pa: Churchill Livingstone; 1999.
- Brown DL. *Atlas of Regional Anesthesia.* Philadelphia, Pa: WB Saunders; 1992.
- Carling A, Simmonds M. Complications from regional anaesthesia for carotid endarterectomy. *Br J Anaesth* 2000;84:797–800.
- Davies MJ, Silbert BS, Scott DA, Cook RJ, Mooney PH, Blyth C. Superficial and deep cervical plexus block for carotid artery surgery: A prospective study of 1000 blocks. *Reg Anesth* 1997;22:442–446.
- Emery G, Handley G, Davies MJ, Mooney PH. Incidence of phrenic nerve block and hypercapnia in patients undergoing carotid endarterectomy under cervical plexus block. *Anaesth Intensive Care* 1998;26: 377–831.
- Johnson TR. Transient ischaemic attack during deep cervical plexus block. *Br J Anaesth* 1999;83:965–967.
- Kulkarni RS, Braverman LE, Patwardhan NA. Bilateral cervical plexus block for thyroidectomy and parathyroidectomy in healthy and high risk patients. *J Endocrinol Invest* 1996;19:714–718.
- Lo Gerfo P, Ditkoff BA, Chabot J, Feind C. Thyroid surgery using monitored anesthesia care: An alternative to general anesthesia. *Thyroid* 1994;4:437–439.
- Masters RD, Castresana EJ, Castresana MR. Superficial and deep cervical plexus block: Technical considerations. *AANA J* 1995;63:235–243
- Murphy TM. Somatic blockade of head and neck. In: Cousins MJ, Bridenbaugh PO, eds. *Neuronal Blockade in Clinical Anesthesia and Management of Pain.* Philadelphia, Pa: Lippincott-Raven, 1988;489–514.
- Pandit JJ, Bree S, Dillon P, Elcock D, McLaren ID, Crider B. A comparison of superficial versus combined (superficial and deep) cervical plexus block for carotid endarterectomy: A prospective, randomized study. *Anesth Analg* 2000;91:781–786.
- Stoneham MD, Wakefield TW. Acute respiratory distress after deep cervical plexus block. *J Cardiothorac Vasc Anesth* 1998;12:197–198.
- Stoneham MD, Doyle AR, Knighton JD, Dorje P, Stanley JC. Prospective, randomized comparison of deep or superficial cervical plexus block for carotid endarterectomy surgery. *Anesthesiology* 1998;89: 907–912.
- Winnie AP, Ramamurthy S, Durrani Z, Radonjic R. Interscalene cervical plexus block: A single-injection technique. *Anesth Analg* 1975;54:370–375.

Superficial Cervical Plexus Block

- Aunac S, Carlier M, Singelyn F, De Kock M. The analgesic efficacy of bilateral combined superficial and deep cervical plexus block administered before thyroid surgery under general anesthesia. *Anesth Analg* 2002;95: 746–750.
- Diedone N, Gomola A, Bonnichon P, Ozier YM. Prevention of postoperative pain after thyroid surgery: A double-blinded randomized study of bilateral superficial cervical plexus blocks. *Anesth Analg* 2001;92: 1538.
- Jankovic D, Wells C. *Regional Nerve Blocks.* 2nd ed. Wissenchafts-Verlag Berlin, Germany: Blackwell Scientific Publications, 2001.
- Masters RD, Castresana EJ, Castresana MR. Superficial and deep cervical plexus block: Technical considerations. *AANA J* 1995;63:235–243.
- Mulroy MF. *Regional Anesthesia: An Illustrated Procedural Guide.* 3rd ed. Philadelphia, Pa: Lippincott; 2002.
- Murphy TM. Somatic blockade of head and neck. In: Cousins MJ, Bridenbaugh PO, eds. *Neuronal Blockade in Clinical Anesthesia and Management of Pain.* Philadelphia, Pa: Lippincott-Raven, 1988;489–514.
- Pandit JJ, Bree S, Dillon P, Elcock D, McLaren ID, Crider B. A comparison of superficial versus combined (superficial and deep) cervical plexus block for carotid endarterectomy: a prospective, randomized study. *Anesth Analg* 2000;91:781–786.

- Stoneham MD, Doyle AR, Knighton JD, Dorje P, Stanley JC. Prospective, randomized comparison of deep or superficial cervical plexus block for carotid endarterectomy surgery. *Anesthesiology* 1998;89:907–912.

- Winnie AP, Ramamurthy S, Durrani Z, Radonjic R. Interscalene cervical plexus block: A single-injection technique. *Anesth Analg* 1975;54:370–375.

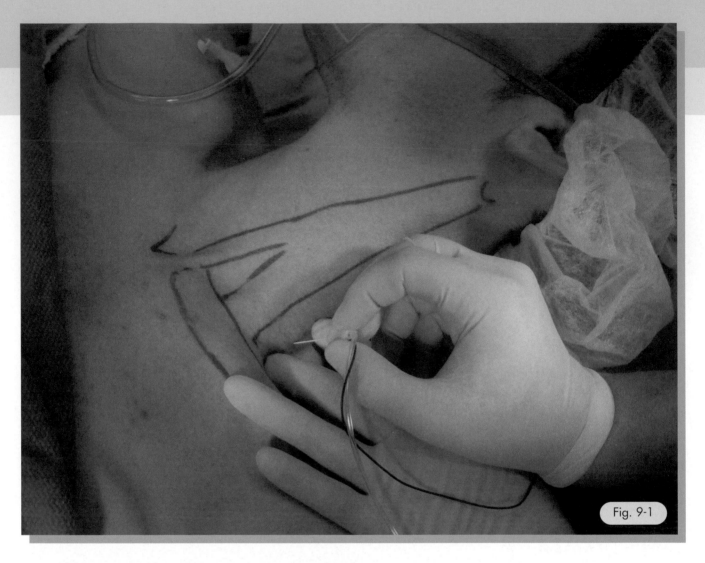

Fig. 9-1

BLOCK AT A GLANCE

- Indications: shoulder, arm, and elbow surgery

- Landmarks: clavicular head of the sternocleidomastoid muscle, clavicle, external jugular vein

- Nerve stimulation: twitch of the pectoralis, deltoid, arm, forearm, or hand muscles at 0.2 to 0.4 mA current

- Local anesthetic: 35 to 40 mL

- Complexity level: intermediate

INTERSCALENE
BRACHIAL PLEXUS BLOCK

SINGLE-SHOT TECHNIQUE

General Considerations

An interscalene block relies on dispersion of a large volume of local anesthetic within the interscalene groove to accomplish blockade of the brachial plexus. In our practice, we use a low approach technique which consists of inserting the needle more distal than in the commonly described procedure performed at the level of the cricoid cartilage. At the lower neck, the interscalene groove is more shallow and easier to identify, and the distribution of anesthesia is also adequate for elbow and forearm surgery. In addition, the needle insertion is much more lateral, which makes vascular puncture rare and performance of the block easier for trainees. We use this low approach to interscalene block routinely for shoulder, arm, and forearm surgery. In our practice the most common indications for this procedure are shoulder surgery and the insertion of arteriovenous grafts for hemodialysis.

Regional Anesthesia Anatomy

The brachial plexus supplies innervation to the shoulder and the upper limb and consists of a branching network of nerves derived from the anterior rami of the lower four cervical and the first thoracic spinal nerves. Starting from their origin and descending distally, the components of the plexus are named roots, trunks, divisions, and cords. The five roots of the cervical and the first thoracic spinal nerves (anterior rami) give rise to three trunks (superior, middle, and inferior) that emerge between the medial and anterior scalene muscles to lie on the floor of the posterior triangle of the neck **(Fig. 9-2)**. The roots of the plexus lie deep to the prevertebral fascia, whereas the trunks are covered by its lateral extension, the axillary sheath. Each trunk divides into an anterior and a posterior division behind the clavicle, at the apex of the axilla **(Fig. 9-3)**. Within the axilla, the divisions combine to produce

the three cords, which are named lateral, medial, and posterior according to their relationship to the axillary artery. From there on, individual nerves are formed as these neuronal elements descend distally **(Table 9-1)**.

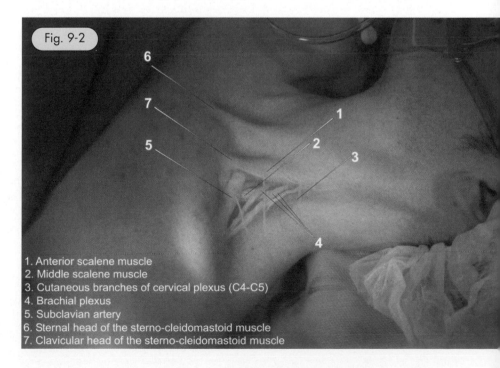

Fig. 9-2

1. Anterior scalene muscle
2. Middle scalene muscle
3. Cutaneous branches of cervical plexus (C4-C5)
4. Brachial plexus
5. Subclavian artery
6. Sternal head of the sterno-cleidomastoid muscle
7. Clavicular head of the sterno-cleidomastoid muscle

TABLE 9.1
Distribution of the Brachial Plexus

NERVE(S)	SPINAL SEGMENT(S)	DISTRIBUTION
Nerves to subclavius	C4 through C6	Subclavius muscle
Dorsal scapular nerve	C5	Rhomboid muscles and levator scapulae muscle
Long thoracic nerve	C5 through C7	Serratus anterior muscle
Suprascapular nerve	C5, C6	Supraspinatus and infraspinatus muscles
Pectoralis nerve (medial and lateral)	C5 through T1	Pectoralis muscles
Subscapular nerves	C5, C6	Subscapularis and teres major muscles
Thoracodorsal nerve	C6 through C8	Latissimus dorsi muscle
Axillary nerve	C5 and C6	Deltoid and teres minor muscles; skin of shoulder
Radial nerve	C5 through T1	Extensor muscles of the arm and forearm (triceps brachii, extensor carpi radialis, extensor carpi ulnaris) and brachioradialis muscle; digital extensors and abductor pollicis muscle; skin over posterolateral surface of the arm
Musculocutaneous nerve	C5 through C7	Flexor muscles of the arm (biceps brachii, brachialis, nerve coracobrachialis); skin over lateral surface of the forearm
Median nerve	C6 through T1	Flexor muscles of the forearm (flexor carpi radialis, palmaris longus); pronator quadratus and pronator teres muscles; digital flexors (through the palmar interosseous nerve); skin over anterolateral surface of the hand
Ulnar nerve	C8, T1	Flexor carpi ulnaris muscle, adductor pollicis muscle, and small digital muscles; skin over medial surface of the hand

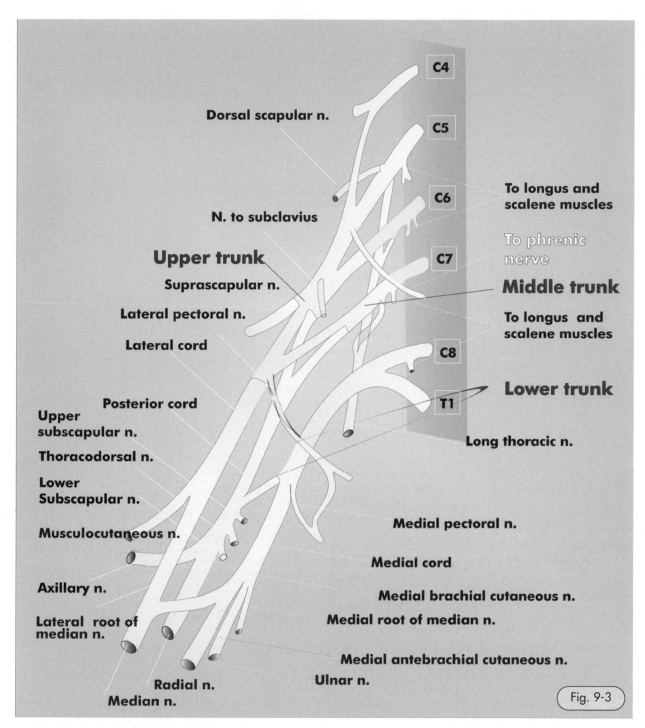

Organization of the brachial plexus.

Distribution of Anesthesia

The interscalene approach to brachial plexus blockade results in consistent anesthesia of the shoulder, arm, and elbow **(Fig. 9-4)**. This block is not recommended for hand surgery; more distal approaches to the brachial plexus should be used instead (e.g., infraclavicular, axillary). Note that the labeled areas without a color shade are not anesthetized consistently with an interscalene brachial plexus block.

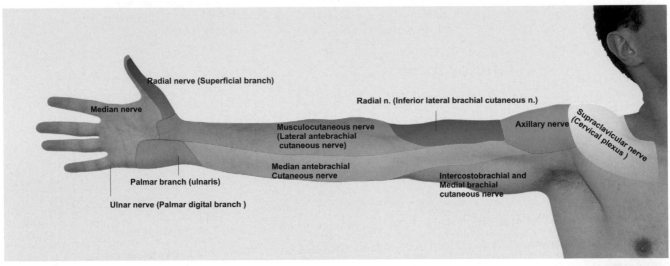

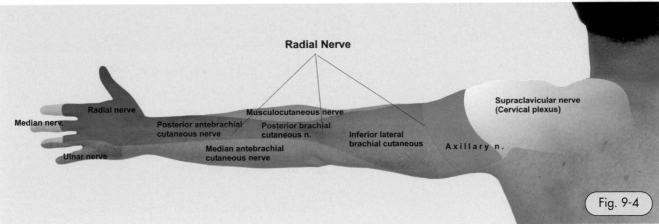

Fig. 9-4

Patient Positioning

The patient is in a supine or semi-sitting position with the head facing away from the side to be blocked **(Fig. 9-5)**. The arm should rest on the bed or on an arm board to allow detection of responses to nerve stimulation. The removal of a cast prior to performance of the block is beneficial for detecting twitches but not essential, as the responses to nerve stimulation are usually mixed (stimulation of the cords and trunks rather than specific nerves).

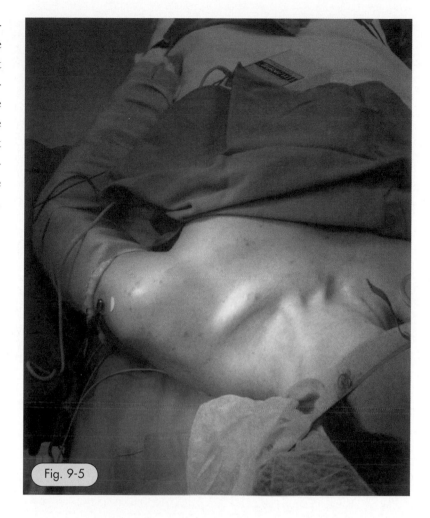

Fig. 9-5

Equipment

A standard regional anesthesia tray is prepared with the following equipment **(Fig. 9-6)**:

- Sterile towels and gauze packs

- 20-mL syringes containing local anesthetic

- Sterile gloves, marking pen, and surface electrode

- 1½-in, 25-gauge needle for skin infiltration

- 3- to 5-cm, short-bevel 22-gauge, insulated stimulating needle

- Peripheral nerve stimulator

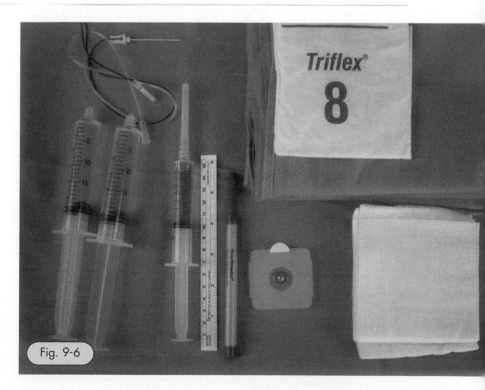

Fig. 9-6

Surface Landmarks

The following surface anatomy landmarks are helpful for identifying the interscalene groove in patients undergoing an interscalene brachial plexus block (**Fig. 9-7**):

1. Sternal notch

2. Clavicle

3. Sternal head of the ster-
    nocleidomastoid muscle

4. Clavicular head of the ster-
    nocleidomastoid muscle

5. Mastoid process

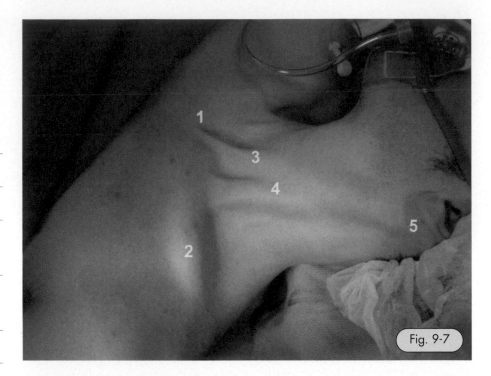

Fig. 9-7

TIP

▶ The proportions of the shoulder girdle, size of the neck and prominence of the muscles, vary greatly among patients. For this reason, when in doubt, always perform a "reality check" by estimating the three bony landmarks: sternal notch, clavicle, and mastoid process.

Anatomic Landmarks

When preparing to perform an interscalene brachial plexus block, the following three land-marks should always be marked with a pen (**Fig. 9-8**):

1. Clavicle

2. Posterior border of the
    clavicular head of the ster-
    nocleidomastoid muscle

3. External jugular vein

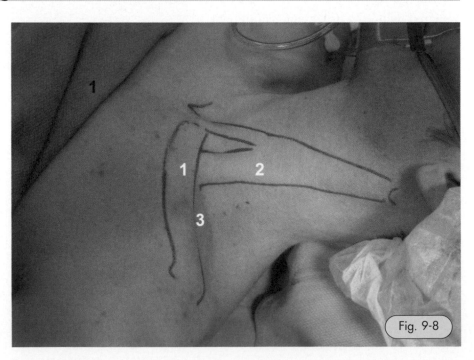

Fig. 9-8

Maneuvers to Accentuate the Landmarks for Interscalene Block

1. Ask the patient to slightly face away from the side to be blocked. This maneuver tenses the sternocleidomastoid muscles and makes this landmark much more prominent **(Fig. 9-9)**.

2. Ask the patient to reach for the ipsilateral knee on the side to be blocked or passively pull patient's wrist toward the knee. This maneuver flattens the skin of the neck and helps to identify both the scalene muscles and the external jugular vein **(Fig. 9-9)**.

3. Ask the patient to lift the head off the table with the patient's head facing away. This maneuver tenses the sternocleidomastoid muscles and helps to identify the posterior border of the clavicular head of the sternocleidomastoid muscle **(Fig. 9-7)**.

4. While palpating the interscalene groove, ask the patient to sniff forcefully. Sniffing tenses the accessory respiratory muscles (scalene muscles), and the fingers of the palpating hand often fall into the scalene groove.

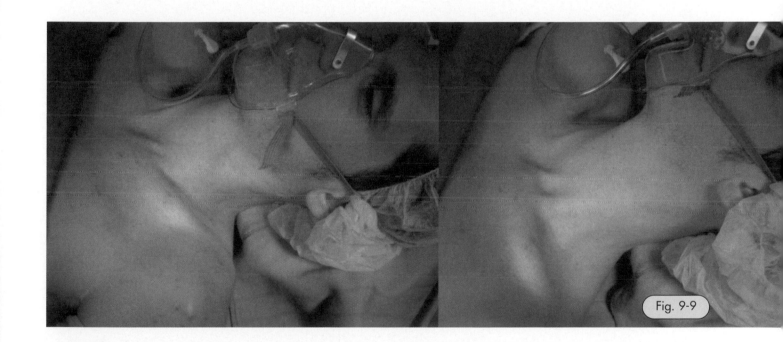

Fig. 9-9

TIPS

▶ All anatomic landmarks outlined under "Surface Landmarks" are important in estimating the site for needle insertion. However, in most patients, the clavicle, clavicular head of the sternocleidomastoid muscle, and external jugular vein are all that is really important.

▶ An argument can be made that the external jugular vein is not a consistent landmark and that it has a highly variable course. Although this is certainly true, the interscalene groove is almost always immediately in *front* of or *behind* the external jugular vein.

▶ In patients with difficult anatomy, the clavicle and external jugular vein often prove to be the most reliable landmarks.

Local Anesthetic Skin Infiltration

After cleaning the skin with an antiseptic solution, local anesthetic is infiltrated subcutaneously at the determined needle insertion site **(Fig. 9-10)**. This is typically the most uncomfortable part of the entire block procedure.

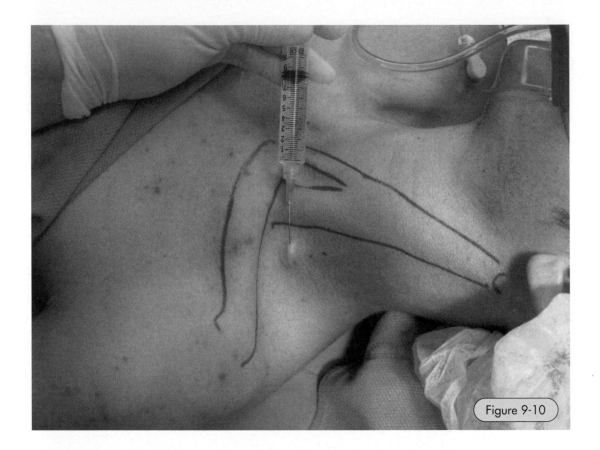

Figure 9-10

TIPS

▶ Care should be taken to infiltrate local anesthetic into the subcutaneous tissue plane *only* because the brachial plexus is very shallow at this location. A deeper needle insertion could easily result in injection into the brachial plexus sheath and consequent difficulty in obtaining the twitch response.

▶Local anesthetic is best infiltrated *tangentially* rather than at a single insertion point **(Fig. 9-10)**. This ensures a superficial injection and allows for needle repositioning during the block performance if required.

Hand Position

The fingers of the palpating hand should be gently but firmly pressed between the anterior and middle scalene muscles to shorten the skin–brachial plexus distance **(Fig. 9-11)**. The skin over the neck is highly movable, and care should be taken to stabilize the fingers as well as to distend the skin between the two fingers to ensure accuracy in needle advancement and redirection. The palpating hand should not be moved during the entire block procedure to allow for precise redirection of the angle of needle insertion when necessary.

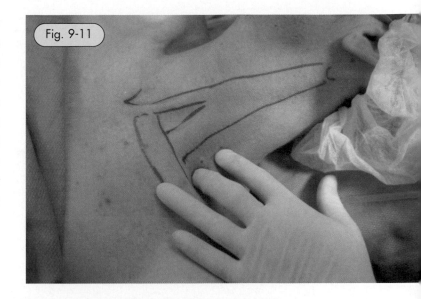

Fig. 9-11

TIPS

▶ To ensure proper position of the palpating hand, first feel the posterior border of the clavicular head of the sternocleidomastoid muscle. The patient should be asked to lift the head up to ensure accurate palpating of this landmark. Then, slowly move the palpating fingers posteriorly until they locate the interscalene groove muscles.

▶ The mistake most commonly made when identifying the interscalene groove is inserting the needle too anteriorly **(Fig. 9-12)**. If the insertion site seems to be too anterior, the chances are that it is. Go back to the posterior border of the clavicular head of the sternocleidomastoid muscle and reassess the anatomy.

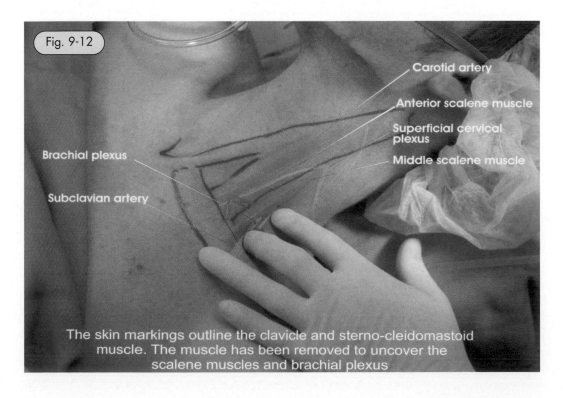

Fig. 9-12

Carotid artery

Anterior scalene muscle

Superficial cervical plexus

Middle scalene muscle

Brachial plexus

Subclavian artery

The skin markings outline the clavicle and sterno-cleidomastoid muscle. The muscle has been removed to uncover the scalene muscles and brachial plexus

Needle Advancement

A needle connected to the nerve stimulator is inserted between the palpating fingers 3–4 cm above the clavicle and advanced at an angle almost perpendicular to the skin plane **(Fig. 9-13)**. The needle must never be oriented cephalad. A slight caudal orientation is the single best measure for preventing inadvertent insertion of the needle toward the cervical spinal cord. The nerve stimulator should be initially set to deliver 0.8 mA (2 Hz, 100–300 µs). The needle is advanced slowly until stimulation of the brachial plexus is obtained. This typically occurs at a depth of 1 to 2 cm in almost all patients. Once appropriate twitches of the brachial plexus are elicited, 35 to 40 mL of local anesthetic is injected slowly with intermittent aspiration to rule out intravascular injection.

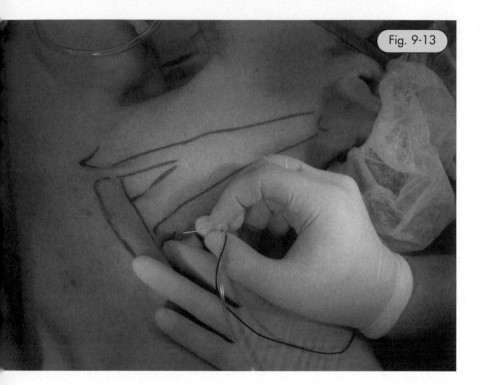

Fig. 9-13

TIPS

▶ The needle should never be advanced beyond 2.5 cm to avoid the risk of complications (cervical cord injury, pneumothorax, vascular puncture).

▶ *Never inject* when resistance (high pressure) on injection of local anesthetic is met. In such cases, do not move the palpating hand from its position; instead, remove and flush the needle before repeating the procedure.

GOAL

The goal is stimulation of the brachial plexus with a current intensity of 0.2 to 0.4 mA (100–300 µsec). The following twitches all result in the same success rate:

- *Pectoralis muscle*
- *Deltoid muscle*
- *Triceps muscles*
- *Biceps muscle*
- *Any twitch of the hand or forearm*

TIPS

▶ A controversy exists as to whether nerve stimulation or a paresthesia technique is better, safer, and more precise in an interscalene brachial plexus block. The truth is that because of the superficial position of the brachial plexus in the interscalene groove, either technique can be used. In our practice, however, we use only the nerve stimulation technique. This permits appropriate sedation and results in a much more pleasant experience for the patient and educational experience for the residents.

▶ Stimulation of the brachial plexus with a higher current (e.g., greater than 1.0 mA) results in an exaggerated response and unnecessary discomfort for the patient. In addition, an unpredictably strong response often causes dislodgement of the needle and a withdrawal reaction by the patient.

► A controversy exists about the optimal motor response to nerve stimulation in the brachial plexus. In our large series of procedures, there is no difference in the success rate for various twitches as long as stimulation is obtained using a similar current intensity (0.2 to 0.4 mA).

►Local anesthetic should not be injected when stimulation is obtained at a current intensity of less than 0.2 mA. Coupled with the *forceful injection* of large volumes of local anesthetic, this carries a risk of injec-

tion under pressure within the epidural sleeve and the consequent spread of local anesthetic toward the subarachnoid space (total spinal anesthesia).

►Care should always be taken to avoid attributing diaphragmatic and trapezius twitches to stimulation of the brachial plexus. Misinterpretation of these twitches is one of the most common causes of block failure.

► When in doubt, palpate the muscle that appears to be twitching to ensure the proper response.

Failure to Obtain Brachial Plexus Stimulation on the First Needle Pass

When insertion of the needle does not result in upper extremity muscle stimulation, the following maneuvers can be used **(Fig. 9-14)**:

A. Keep the palpating hand in the same position and the skin between the fingers stretched **(Fig. 9-14A)**.

B. Withdraw the needle to skin level, redirect it 15° posteriorly, and repeat the needle advancement **(Fig. 9-14B)**.

C. Withdraw the needle to skin level, redirect it 15° anteriorly, and repeat the needle insertion **(Fig. 9-14C)**.

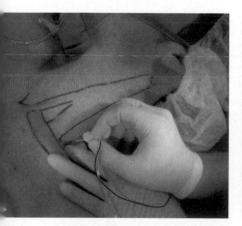
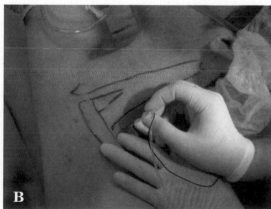
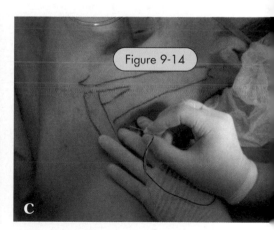

Figure 9-14

► When these maneuvers fail to result in a motor response, carefully and methodically reposition the palpating hand 1 cm posteriorly or anteriorly using an intuitive approach and repeat steps A through C.

► Failure to stimulate after following the above steps should prompt needle withdrawal and reassessment of the landmarks **(see also Table 9.2 for more tips)**.

► Keep in mind that failure to obtain brachial plexus stimulation is most commonly a result of inserting the needle too anteriorly.

► Do not forget to ascertain that the nerve stimulator is properly functional and connected.

► Increasing the current intensity to more than 1.0 mA is more likely to result in patient discomfort than in helping to localize the brachial plexus.

TABLE 9.2
Common Problems During Nerve Localization and the Corrective Action

RESPONSE OBTAINED	INTERPRETATION	PROBLEM	ACTION
Local twitch of the neck muscles	Direct stimulation of the anterior scalene or sternocleidomastoid muscle	Needle pass is in the wrong plane; usually anteriorly and medially to the plexus	Withdraw the needle to skin level and reinsert it 15° posteriorly
Needle contacts bone at 1- to 2-cm depth; no twitches are seen	Needle stopped by the transverse process (or 1st rib)	Needle is inserted too posteriorly; the needle is contacting the anterior tubercles of the transverse process	Withdraw needle to skin level and reinsert it 15° anteriorly
Twitches of the diaphragm	Results from stimulation of the phrenic nerve	Needle is inserted too anteriorly	Withdraw needle and reinsert it 15° posteriorly
Arterial blood noticed in the tubing	Puncture of the carotid artery (most common)	Needle insertion and angulation are too anterior	Withdraw needle and keep a steady pressure for 2–3 minutes; reinsert it 1–2 cm posteriorly
Pectoralis muscle twitch	Brachial plexus stimulation (C4 through C5)	None	Accept and inject local anesthetic
Twitch of the scapula	Twitch of the serratus anterior muscle; stimulation of the thoracodorsal nerve	Needle position is posterior and deep to the brachial plexus	Withdraw needle to skin level and reinsert it anteriorly
Trapezius muscle twitches	Accessory nerve stimulation	Needle is posterior to the brachial plexus	Withdraw needle and reinsert it anteriorly
Twitch of pectorals, deltoid, triceps, biceps, forearm, and hand muscles	Stimulation of the brachial plexus	None	Accept and inject local anesthetic

Choice of Local Anesthetic

Interscalene block technique requires a relatively large volume of local anesthetic to achieve anesthesia of the entire plexus. The choice of the type and concentration of local anesthetic should be based on whether the block is planned for surgical anesthesia or for pain management. Because of the highly vascular area and the potential for inadvertent intravascular injection, the local anesthetic solution should be injected slowly with frequent aspiration.

Table 9.3 outlines some commonly used local anesthetic solutions and their dynamics with this block.

TABLE 9.3
Choice of Local Anesthetic For Interscalene Block

ANESTHETIC	ONSET (min)	DURATION OF ANESTHESIA (h)	DURATION OF ANALGESIA (h)
2-Chloroprocaine <3% (HCO$_3$ + epinephrine)	5–10	1.5	2.0
1.5% Mepivacaine (+ HCO$_3$)	10–20	2–3	2–4
1.5% Mepivacaine (HCO$_3$ + epinephrine)	5–15	2.5–4	3–6
2% Lidocaine (+ HCO$_3$)	10–20	2.5–3	2–5
2% Lidocaine (HCO$_3$ + epinephrine)	5–15	3–6	5–8
0.5% Ropivacaine	15–20	6–8	8–12
0.75% Ropivacaine	5–15	8–10	12–18
0.5% Bupivacaine (+ epinephrine)	20–30	8–10	16–18

TIPS

▶ Always assess the risk/benefit ratio of using large volumes and concentrations of long-acting local anesthetic for interscalene brachial plexus block.

▶ Smaller volumes and concentrations can be used successfully for analgesia (e.g., 15 to 20 mL).

Block Dynamics and Perioperative Management

When stimulation with a low-intensity current and slow needle advancement are used, an interscalene brachial plexus block is associated with minimal patient discomfort. Thus, excessive sedation is not only unnecessary, but also disadvantageous because patient cooperation during landmark assessment and block performance is beneficial. Besides, the administration of benzodiazepines tends to decrease the tonus of the interscalene and sternocleidomastoid muscles, making palpation and identification of these landmarks difficult. We typically use small doses of midazolam (e.g., 1 to 2 mg) so that the patient is comfortable and cooperative during nerve localization.

The onset time of this block is short. The first sign of the blockade is a loss of coordination of the shoulder and arm muscles. This sign is seen sooner than the onset of a sensory blockade or a temperature change and, when observed within 1 to 2 minutes after injection, is highly predictive of a successful brachial plexus blockade. In fact, this is the single test that we perform before allowing the surgeon to proceed with preparations for surgery. In patients undergoing shoulder arthroscopic procedures, it is important to note that the arthroscopic portals are often inserted outside the cutaneous distribution of the interscalene block. Local infiltration at the site of the incision by the surgeon is all that is needed because the entire shoulder joint and deep tissues are anesthetized with the interscalene block alone.

TIPS

▶ Many patients develop a hoarse voice, mild ipsilateral ptosis (Horner syndrome), and nasal congestion following an interscalene block. A proper explanation and reassurance are all that such patients need.

▶ An interscalene block inevitably results in ipsilateral diaphragmatic paralysis (a phrenic nerve block). The significance of this is often debated, and avoidance of this block is suggested in patients with chronic respiratory disease such as chronic obstructive lung disease and bronchial asthma.

▶ We avoid the use of this block only in patients whose breathing involves the use of accessory respiratory muscles.

▶ Appropriate intravenous sedation, communication with the patient, lifting drapes off the patient's face, and shielding the ears from noise are all necessary ingredients for success with interscalene blocks in patients undergoing shoulder surgery.

CONTINUOUS INTERSCALENE BLOCK

A continuous interscalene block is an advanced regional anesthesia technique, and adequate experience with the single-injection technique is necessary. Paradoxically, although a single-injection interscalene block is one of the easiest intermediate techniques to perform and master, placement of the catheter is perhaps one of the more technically challenging procedures. It is difficult mostly because of the shallow position of the brachial plexus and problems in stabilizing the needle during catheter advancement. In addition, there is a difference in the stimulating characteristics of smaller-caliber, single-injection and larger-caliber, often Tuohy-style-tip needles. The technique is otherwise similar to the single-injection procedure except that the needle is inserted at a lower angle to allow for threading of the catheter. This procedure provides excellent analgesia in patients following shoulder, arm, and elbow surgery.

Patient Positioning

The patient is in the same position as for the single-injection technique. However, it is imperative that the anesthesiologist assumes an ergonomic position to allow maneuvering during catheter insertion. It is also important that all equipment, including the catheter, be immediately available and prepared in advance because small movements of the needle that might occur while trying to prepare the catheter may result in dislodging the needle from its position in the brachial plexus sheath.

Equipment

A standard regional anesthesia tray is prepared with the following equipment (**Fig. 9-15**):

- Sterile towels and gauze packs

- 20-mL syringes containing local anesthetic

- Sterile gloves, marking pen, and surface electrode

- 1½-in, 25-gauge needle for skin infiltration

- 3- to 5-cm, insulated stimulating needle (Tuohy-style or Quincke-tip)

- Catheter

- Peripheral nerve stimulator

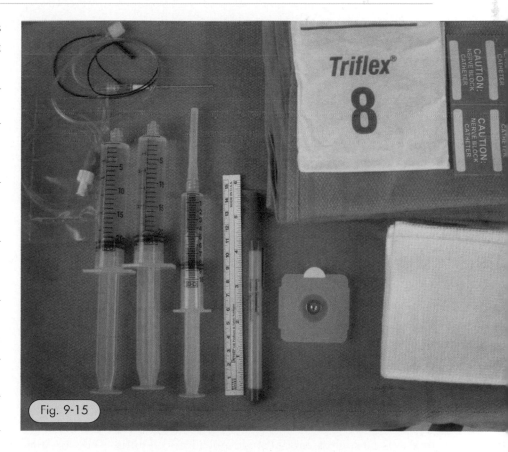
Fig. 9-15

Landmarks

The landmarks for a continuous interscalene brachial plexus block are similar to those for the single-shot technique **(Fig. 9-16)**:

1. Clavicle

2. Clavicular head of the sternocleidomastoid muscle

3. External jugular vein

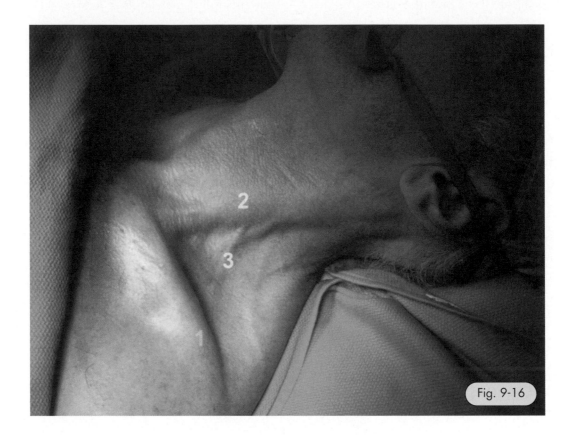

Fig. 9-16

Local Anesthetic Infiltration and Needle Insertion

The subcutaneous tissue at the projected site of needle insertion is anesthetized with local anesthetic. The block needle is then attached to a nerve stimulator (0.08 mA, 2 Hz, 100–300 μs) and to a syringe with local anesthetic. With this technique, it is imperative that the palpating hand firmly stabilizes the skin to facilitate needle insertion and insertion of the catheter **(Fig. 9-17)**. A 3 to 5 cm block needle is inserted at a slightly caudal angle and advanced until the brachial plexus twitch is elicited at 0.2 to 0.5 mA. Precautions should be taken to avoid inserting the needle through the external jugular vein because this invariably results in prolonged oozing from the site of puncture. This can be avoided by retracting the external jugular vein and inserting the needle slightly in *front* of or *posteriorly* to the external jugular vein. Additionally, making a small skin nick before inserting the needle can be helpful in preventing uncontrolled needle insertion as the skin is penetrated. The initial volume of local anesthetic (20 to 40 mL) is always injected through the needle before advancing the catheter. While paying meticulous attention to the position of the needle, the catheter is inserted about 5 cm beyond the tip of the needle **(Fig. 9-18)**.

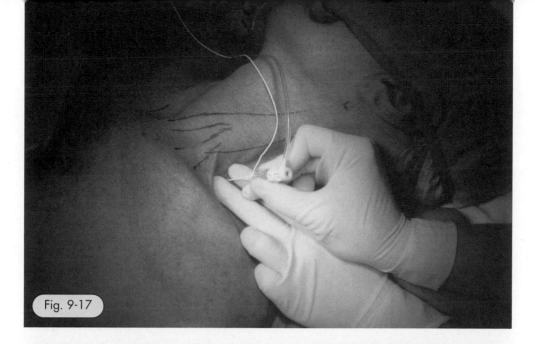

Fig. 9-17

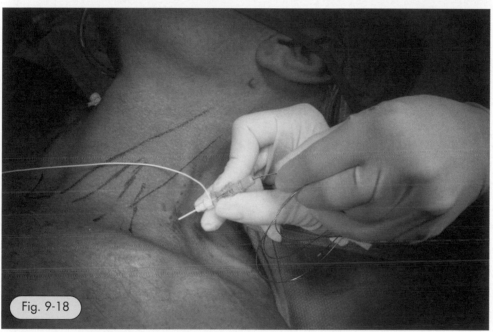

Fig. 9-18

TIPS

► The most difficult aspect of this technique is stabilization of the needle for catheter insertion after the brachial plexus is localized.

► When the needle encounters the brachial plexus at a very shallow location, it is best to have an assistant advance the catheter to ensure that the needle does not move from its original position.

► A slightly caudal orientation of the needle may be required to facilitate catheter insertion.

► It is difficult to advance some needles through the skin, particularly those with blunt tips. For this reason, it is some-

times best to create a small skin nick with a scalpel or the side of a sharp-tipped, 18-gauge needle before attempting to insert these needles through the skin.

► Continuous nerve blocks require the use of larger-gauge needles, and thus, the risk of large vessels puncturing has greater implications.

► In patients with less than ideal landmarks, it may be prudent to first use a single-shot needle to localize the brachial plexus and determine the needle insertion point and proper angulation before inserting a large-gauge continuous block needle.

The catheter is secured using a benzoin skin preparation, followed by application of a clear dressing **(Fig. 9-19)**. The infusion port should be clearly marked "continuous interscalene block," and the catheter should be carefully checked for intravascular placement before administering a bolus or infusion of local anesthetics.

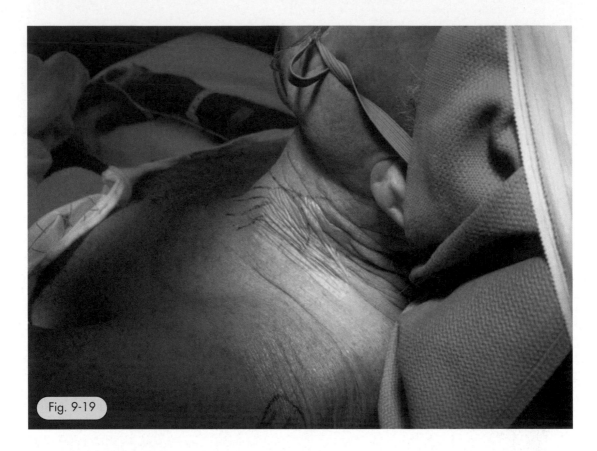

Fig. 9-19

Continuous Infusion

Continuous infusion is initiated after an initial bolus of dilute local anesthetic is administered through a catheter. For this purpose, we routinely use 0.2% ropivacaine 15 to 20 mL. Diluted bupivacaine or levobupivacaine is also suitable but may result in greater motor blockade. The infusion is maintained at 5 mL/h when a dose of patient-controlled analgesia (PCA) (4 mL every 30 minutes) is planned.

TIPS

▶ Breakthrough pain in patients undergoing continuous infusion is always managed by administering a bolus of local anesthetic. Increasing the rate of infusion alone is rarely adequate.

▶ For patients on the ward, a higher concentration of a shorter-acting, epinephrine-containing local anesthetic (e.g., 1% mepivacaine or lidocaine with 1:300,000 epinephrine) is useful and safe to test the position of the catheter.

▶ When the bolus injection through the catheter fails to result in a blockade after 30 minutes, the catheter should be considered dislodged and should be removed.

▶ Every patient undergoing a continuous interscalene block should be prescribed an immediately available alternative pain management protocol because incomplete analgesia and catheter dislodgment can occur. For inpatients, this is probably best done using backup intravenous PCA.

TABLE 9.4
Complications and How to Avoid Them

Infection	• A strict aseptic technique is used.
Hematoma	• Avoid insertion of the needle through external jugular vein. • Avoid multiple needle insertions, particularly in patients undergoing anticoagulant treatment. • Keep a 5-min steady pressure if the carotid artery is inadvertently punctured. • Use a single-injection needle to localize the brachial plexus in patients with difficult anatomy. • In the absence of spontaneous bleeding, the use of anticoagulant therapy should not be regarded as a contraindication for this block.
Vascular puncture	• Vascular puncture is not common with this technique. • Steady pressure of 5-min duration should be maintained if the carotid artery is punctured (rare).
Local anesthetic toxicity	• Systemic toxicity most commonly occurs during or shortly after the injection of local anesthetic; it is most commonly caused by inadvertent intravascular injection or channeling of forcefully injected local anesthetic into small veins or lymphatic channels that were cut during needle manipulation. • Large volumes of long-acting anesthetic should be reconsidered in older and frail patients. • Careful, frequent aspiration should be performed during the injection. • Avoid fast, forceful injection of local anesthetic.
Nerve injury	• Never inject local anesthetic when pressure is encountered on injection. • Local anesthetic should never be injected when the patient complains of severe pain or exhibits a withdrawal reaction on injection.
Total spinal anesthesia	• When stimulation is obtained with a current intensity of <0.2 mA, the needle should be pulled back to achieve the same response with a current >0.2 mA before injecting local anesthetic to avoid injection into the dural sleeves and consequent epidural or spinal spread.
Horner syndrome	• The occurrence of ipsilateral ptosis, hyperemia of the conjunctiva, and nasal congestion is common and depends on the site of injection (it is less common with the low interscalene approach) and the total volume of local anesthetic injected. • The patient should be instructed on the occurrence of this syndrome and reassured about its benign nature.
Diaphragmatic paralysis	• Invariably present; avoid interscalene blockade or the use of a large volume of local anesthetic in patients who have severe chronic respiratory disease and use accessory respiratory muscles during breathing at rest.

SUGGESTED READINGS

Interscalene Block: Single-injection

- Agostoni M, Marchesi M, Fanelli G, Reineke R. Analgesic brachial plexus block for reduction of shoulder dislocation. *Reg Anesth* 1996;21:37.

- Borgeat A, Ekatodramis G, Kalberer F, Benz C. Acute and nonacute complications associated with interscalene block and shoulder surgery: a prospective study. *Anesthesiology* 2001;95:875–880.

- Brown DL, Bridenbaugh LD. The upper extremity: somatic block. In: Cousins MJ, Bridenbaugh PO, eds. *Neuronal Blockade in Clinical Anesthesia and Management of Pain.* Philadelphia, Pa: Lippincott-Raven, 1988;345–371.

- Chelly JE. *Peripheral Nerve Blocks: A Color Atlas.* Philadelphia, Pa: Lippincott, 1999.

- Coleman MM, Peng P. Pectoralis major in interscalene brachial plexus blockade. *Reg Anesth Pain Med* 1999;24: 190–191.

- Hadžić A, Vloka JD, Kuroda MM, Koorn R, Birnbach DJ. The practice of peripheral nerve blocks in the United States: a national survey. *Reg Anesth Pain Med* 1998;23: 241–246.

- Long TR, Wass CT, Burkle CM. Perioperative interscalene blockade: an overview of its history and current clinical use. *J Clin Anesth* 2002;14:546–556.

- Maurer K, Ekatodramis G, Rentsch K, Borgeat A. Interscalene and infraclavicular block for bilateral distal radius fracture. *Anesth Analg* 2002;94:450–452.

- Raj PP. *Textbook of Regional Anesthesia.* London, England: Churchill Livingstone; 2002.

- Silverstein WB, Saiyed MU, Brown AR. Interscalene block with a nerve stimulator: a deltoid motor response is a satisfactory endpoint for successful block. *Reg Anesth Pain Med* 2000;25:356–359.

- White JL. Catastrophic complications of interscalene nerve block. *Anesthesiology* 2001;95:1301.

- Winnie AP. Interscalene brachial plexus block. *Anesth Analg* 1970;49:455–466.

- Winnie AP. *Plexus Anesthesia, Perivascular Techniques of Brachial Plexus Block.* 2nd ed. Philadelphia, Pa: WB Saunders; 1990.

- Wong GY, Brown DL, Miller GM, Cahill DR. Defining the cross-sectional anatomy important to interscalene brachial plexus block with magnetic resonance imaging. *Reg Anesth Pain Med* 1998;23:77–80.

Continuous Interscalene Block

- Borgeat A, Ekatodramis G, Kalberer F, Benz C. Acute and nonacute complications associated with interscalene block and shoulder surgery: a prospective study. *Anesthesiology* 2001;95:875–880.

- Chelly JE, Casati A, Fanelli G. *Continuous Peripheral Nerve Block Techniques: An Illustrated Guide.* London, England: Mosby International; 2001.

- Coleman MM, Chan VW. Continuous interscalene brachial plexus block. *Can J Anaesth* 1999;46:209–214.

- Klein SM, Grant SA, Greengrass RA, Nielsen KC, Speer KP, White W, Warner DS, Steele SM. Interscalene brachial plxus block with a continuous catheter insertion system and a disposable infusion pump. *Anesth Analg* 2000;91:1473–1478.

- Lehtipalo S, Koskinen LO, Johansson G, Kolmodin J, Biber B. Continuous interscalene brachial plexus block for postoperative analgesia following shoulder surgery. *Acta Anaesthesiol Scand* 1999;43:258–264.

- Maurer K, Ekatodramis G, Hodler J, Rentsch K, Perschak H, Borgeat A. Bilateral continuous interscalene block of brachial plexus for analgesia after bilateral shoulder arthroplasty. *Anesthesiology* 2002; 6:762–764.

- Pere P, Pitkanen M, Rosenbergh PH, et al. Effect of continuous interscalene brachial plexus block on diaphragm motion and on ventilatory function. *Acta Anaesthesiol Scand* 1992;36:53–57.

- Rawal N, Allvin R, Axelsson K, Hallen J, Ekback G, Ohlsson T, Amilon A. Patient-controlled regional analgesia (PCRA) at home: controlled comparison between bupivacaine and ropivacaine brachial plexus analgesia. *Anesthesiology* 2002;96:1290–1296.

- Singelyn FJ, Seguy S, Gouverneur JM. Interscalene brachial plexus analgesia after open shoulder surgery: continuous versus patient-controlled infusion. *Anesth Analg* 1999; 89:1216–1220.

- White JL. Catastrophic complications of interscalene nerve block. *Anesthesiology* 2001;95:1301
- Winnie AP. Interscalene brachial plexus block. *Anesth Analg* 1970;49:455–466.
- Winnie AP. *Plexus Anesthesia, Perivascular Techniques of Brachial Plexus Block.* 2nd ed. Philadelphia, Pa: WB Saunders, 1990.
- Wong GY, Brown DL, Miller GM, Cahill DR. Defining the cross-sectional anatomy important to interscalene brachial plexus block with magnetic resonance imaging. *Reg Anesth Pain Med* 1998;23:77–80

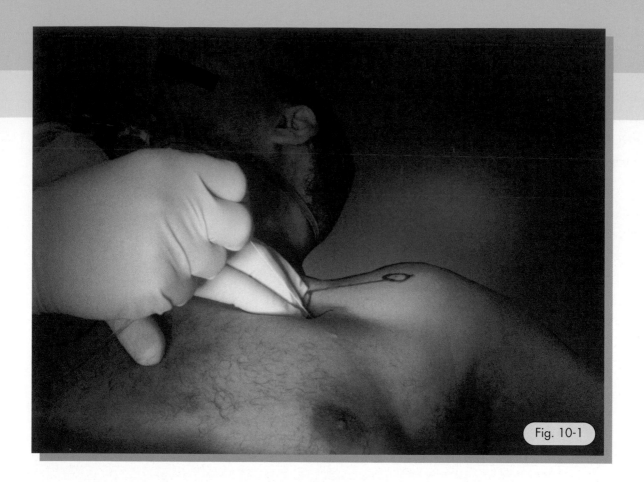

Fig. 10-1

BLOCK AT A GLANCE

- Indications: elbow, forearm, hand surgery

- Landmarks: medial clavicular head, coracoid process

- Needle: 10 cm

- Nerve stimulation: hand twitch at 0.2 to 0.3 mA

- Local anesthetic: 30 to 45 mL

- Complexity level: intermediate

10 INFRACLAVICULAR
BRACHIAL PLEXUS BLOCK

GENERAL CONSIDERATIONS

The infraclavicular block is a blockade of the brachial plexus below the level of the clavicle and in the proximity of the coracoid process; it is an intermediate nerve block technique. Experience with basic brachial plexus techniques and nerve stimulation is necessary for its efficient implementation. This block is uniquely well-suited for hand, wrist, elbow, and distal arm surgery. It also provides excellent analgesia for an arm tourniquet.

Regional Anesthesia Anatomy

Anatomic Highlights

The boundaries of the infraclavicular fossa are the pectoralis minor and major muscles anteriorly, ribs medially, clavicle and the coracoid process superiorly, and humerus laterally **(Fig. 10-2)**. At this location, the brachial plexus is most commonly composed of cords. The sheath surrounding the plexus is delicate. It also contains the subclavian or axillary artery and vein. Axillary and musculocutaneus nerves leave the sheath at or before the coracoid process in 50% of patients **(Table 10.1 and Fig. 10-3)**. Consequently, deltoid and biceps twitches should not be accepted as reliable signs of brachial plexus identification.

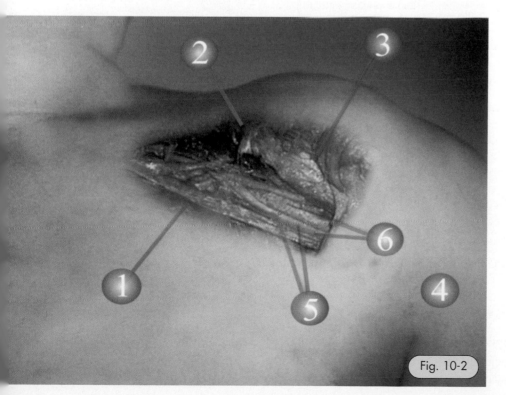

Fig. 10-2

Anatomic structures of importance.

1. Pectoralis muscle (shown cut to expose brachial plexus)

2. Clavicle (removed)

3. Coracoid process

4. Humerus

5. Brachial plexus

6. Subclavian or axillary artery and vein

TABLE 10.1

Distribution of the Branches of the Brachial Plexus

Chest	• Anterior thoracic
Shoulder	• Subscapular • Axillary
Arm, forearm, shoulder, hand	• Musculocutaneous • Internal cutaneous • Lesser internal cutaneous • Median • Ulnar • Radial (musculospiral)

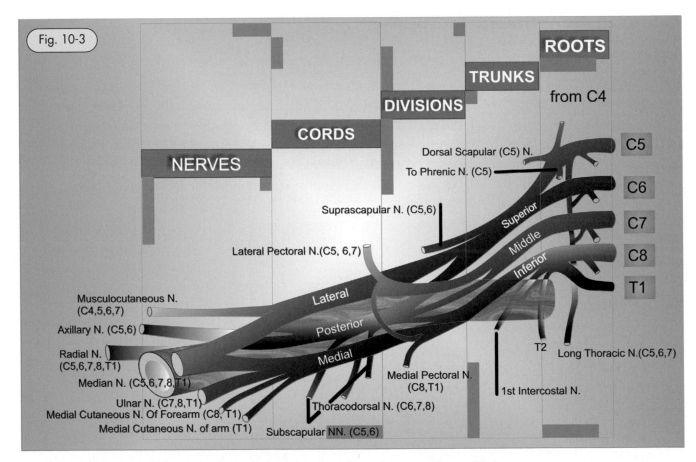

The organization of the brachial plexus below the clavicle is shown in **Figure 10-3**.

Distribution of Anesthesia

A typical distribution of anesthesia following an infra-clavicular brachial plexus block includes the hand, wrist, forearm, elbow, and distal arm **(Fig. 10-4)**. The skin of the axilla and proximal medial arm (unshaded areas) is not anesthetized (intercostobrachial and medium cutaneous brachial nerves).

Fig. 10-4

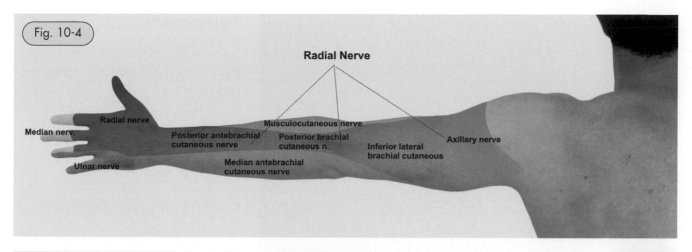

Radial Nerve

Radial nerve

Median nerv.

Ulnar nerve

Posterior antebrachial
cutaneous nerve

Median antebrachial
cutaneous nerve

Musculocutaneous nerve

Posterior brachial
cutaneous n.

Inferior lateral
brachial cutaneous

Axillary nerve

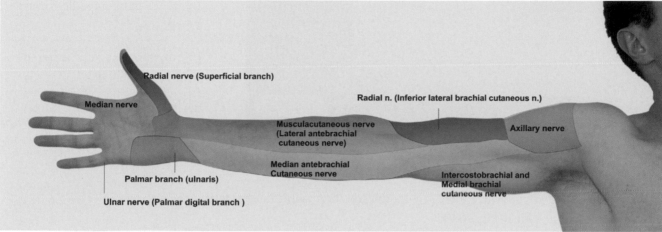

Radial nerve (Superficial branch)

Median nerve

Palmar branch (ulnaris)

Ulnar nerve (Palmar digital branch)

Musculacutaneous nerve
(Lateral antebrachial
cutaneous nerve)

Median antebrachial
Cutaneous nerve

Radial n. (Inferior lateral brachial cutaneous n.)

Axillary nerve

Intercostobrachial and
Medial brachial
cutaneous nerve

SINGLE-INJECTION INFRACLAVICULAR BLOCK

Patient Positioning

The patient is in the supine position with the head facing away from the side to be blocked **(Fig. 10-5)**. The anesthesiologist also stands opposite the side to be blocked to assume an ergonomic position during the block performance. It is best to keep the patient's arm abducted and flexed at the elbow to keep the relationship of the landmarks to the brachial plexus constant. After a certain level of comfort with the technique is reached, the arm can be in any position during the block performance. The arm should be supported at the wrist to allow a clear, unobstructed view of twitches of the hand.

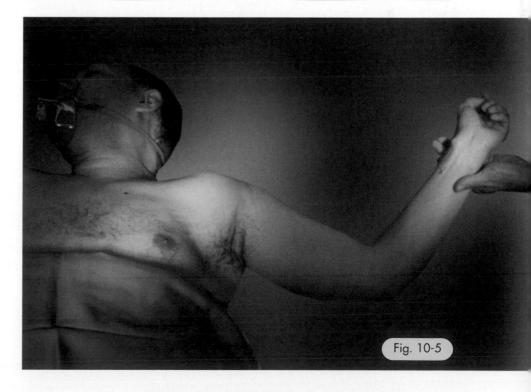

Fig. 10-5

Equipment

A standard regional anesthesia tray is prepared with the following equipment **(Fig. 10-6)**:

- Sterile towels and gauze packs

- 20-mL syringes containing local anesthetic

- Sterile gloves, marking pen, surface electrode

- 1½-in, 25-gauge needle for skin infiltration

- 10-cm, short-bevel, insulated stimulating needle

- Peripheral nerve stimulator

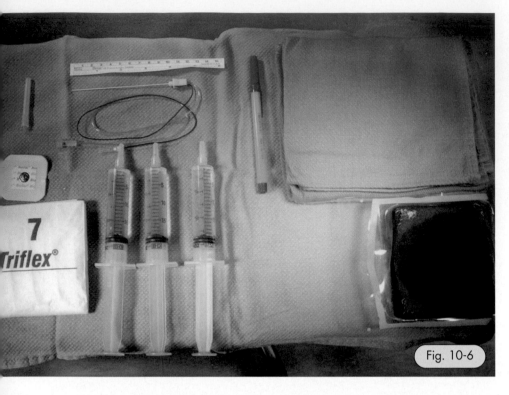

Fig. 10-6

Surface Landmarks

The following surface anatomy landmarks are useful in estimating the site for an infra-clavicular block **(Fig. 10-7)**:

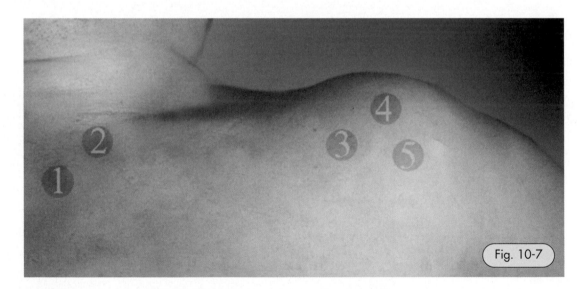

Fig. 10-7

1. Sternoclavicular joint

2. Medial end of the clavicle

3. Coracoid process

4. Acromioclavicular joint

5. Head of the humerus

Anatomic Landmarks

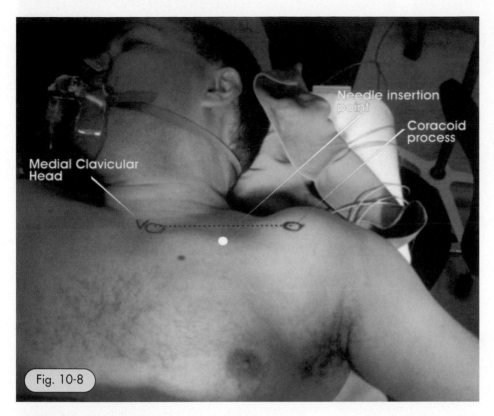

Fig. 10-8

Landmarks for an infraclavicular block include (**Fig. 10-8**):

1. Medial clavicular head

2. Coracoid process

3. Midpoint of line connecting landmarks 1 and 2

The needle insertion site is marked approximately 3 cm caudal to the midpoint of landmark 3.

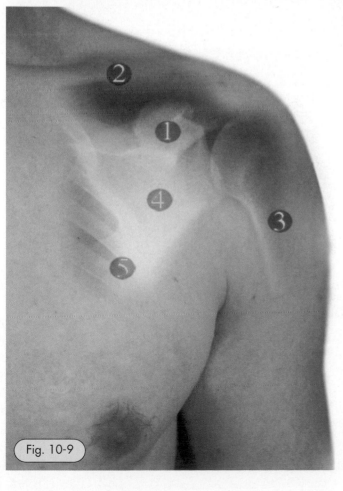

Fig. 10-9

An x-ray film demonstrating the relevant anatomy (**Fig. 10-9**):

1. Coracoid process

2. Clavicle

3. Humerus

4. Scapula

5. Rib cage.

TIPS

▶ Coracoid process is identified by palpating the bony prominence just medial to the shoulder, while the arm is elevated and lowered.

▶ As the arm is lowered, the coracoid process meets the fingers of the palpating hand (**Fig. 10-10**).

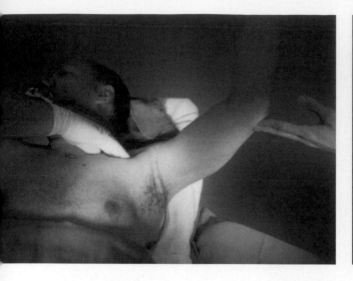
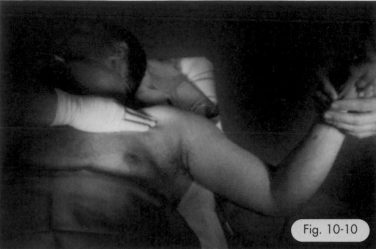

Fig. 10-10

Local Anesthetic Skin Infiltration

The needle insertion site is infiltrated with local anesthetic using a 25-gauge needle **(Fig. 10-11)**.

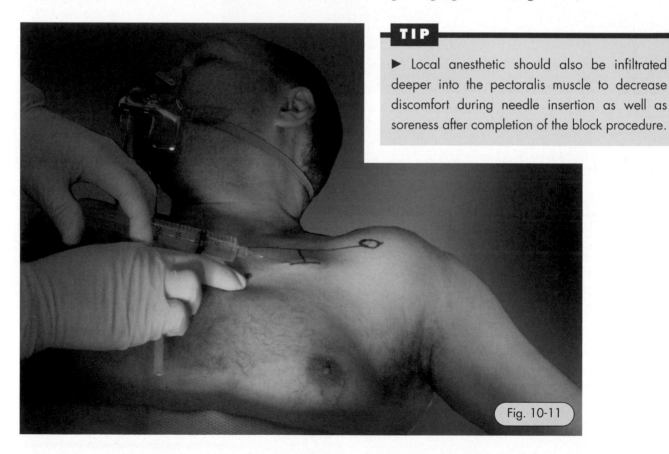

TIP

▶ Local anesthetic should also be infiltrated deeper into the pectoralis muscle to decrease discomfort during needle insertion as well as soreness after completion of the block procedure.

Fig. 10-11

Needle Insertion

A 10-cm, 22-gauge, insulated needle, attached to a nerve stimulator, is inserted at a 45° angle to the skin and advanced parallel to the line connecting the medial clavicular head with the coracoid process **(Fig. 10-12)**. The nerve stimulator is initially set to deliver 1.5 mA. A local twitch of the pectoralis muscle is typically elicited as the needle is advanced beyond the subcutaneus tissue. Once these twitches disappear, the needle advancement should be slow and methodical while the patient is observed for a twitch of the brachial plexus.

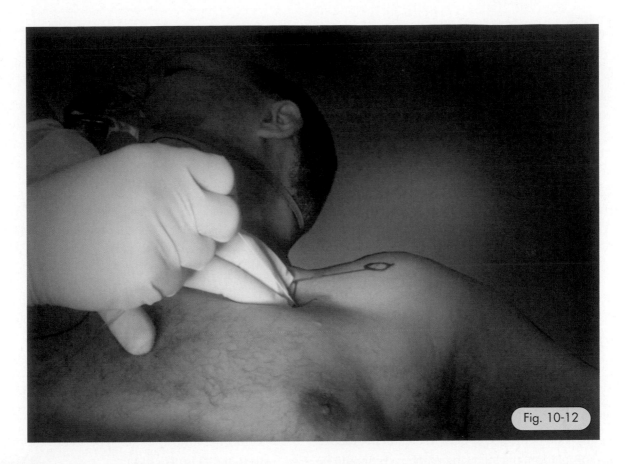

Fig. 10-12

▶ When the pectoralis muscle twitch is absent despite an appropriately deep needle insertion, the landmarks should be checked as the needle has most likely been inserted too cranially (underneath the clavicle).

▶ The bevel of the needle should be facing downward to facilitate nerve stimulation and reduce the risk of vascular puncture (subclavian or axillary artery and vein).

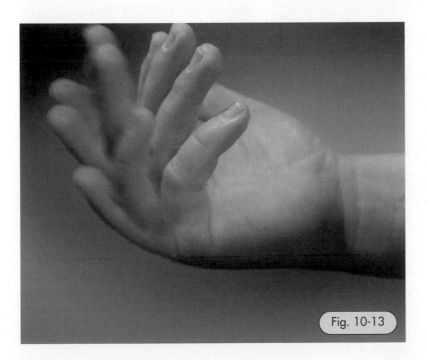

Fig. 10-13

GOAL

The goal is to achieve a hand twitch (preferably the medial nerve) using a current of 0.2 to 0.3 mA (Fig. 10-13).

► Twitches from the biceps or deltoid muscles should not be accepted because the musculocutaneous or axillary nerve may exit the brachial sheath before the coracoid process.

► Hand stabilization and precision are crucial in this block, as the sheath of the brachial plexus is thin at this location and small movements of the needle may result in injection of local anesthetic outside the sheath. This in turn will result in a weak block with a slow onset.

► A twitch of the pectoralis muscle usually indicates too shallow a placement of the needle. As contractions of the pectoralis muscle cease, the needle should be slowly advanced until twitches of the brachial

plexus are elicited, which usually occurs at a depth of 5 to 8 cm.

► After the twitches of the pectoralis muscle cease, the stimulating current should be lowered to below 1.0 mA to decrease patient discomfort. The needle is then slowly advanced or withdrawn until hand twitches are obtained at 0.2 to 0.3 mA.

► The success rate with this block decreases when local anesthetic is injected after obtaining stimulation with a current intensity above 0.3 mA.

► In the absence of a medial nerve response, stimulation of the radial or ulnar nerve can also be accepted as long as the twitch of the hand is unambiguosly documented.

Failure to Obtain Nerve Stimulation on the First Needle Pass

When insertion of the needle does not result in brachial plexus stimulation, the following maneuvers should be undertaken **(Figs. 10-14A–C)**:

A. Keep the palpating hand in the same position, with the palpating finger firmly seated in the

pectoralis and the skin between the fingers stretched **(Fig. 10-14A)**.

B. Withdraw the needle to skin level, redirect it 10° cephalad, and repeat the procedure **(Fig. 10-14B)**.

C. Withdraw the needle from the skin, redirect it 10° caudal, and repeat the procedure **(Fig. 10-14C)**.

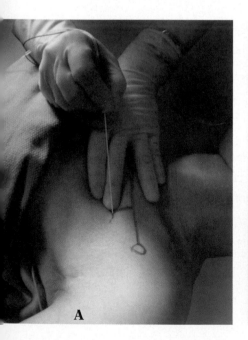

A

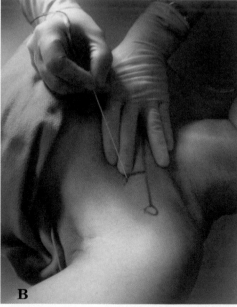

B

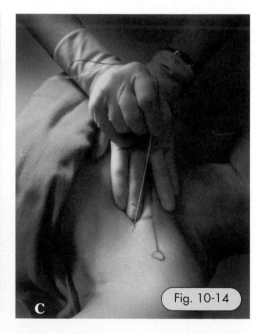

C

Fig. 10-14

▶ If these maneuvers fail to result in a motor response, withdraw the needle and assess the landmarks.

▶ Check that the nerve stimulator is properly connected and delivering the set stimulus.

▶ Insert the needle 2 cm laterally and repeating the above steps.

Interpreting Responses to Nerve Stimulation

Some common responses to nerve stimulation and the course of action needed to obtain the proper response are listed in **Table 10.2**.

TABLE 10.2
Common Problems During Nerve Localizations and Corrective Actions

STIMULATION	MOTOR RESPONSE	EXPLANATION	CORRECTIVE ACTION
Pectoralis muscle, direct muscle stimulation	Arm adduction	Too shallow a placement of needle	Continue advancing the needle
Subscapularis muscle	Local twitch resembling latissimus twitch	Too deep a placement of needle	Withdraw the needle to skin level and reinsert in another direction (superior or inferior)
Axillary nerve	Deltoid muscle	Needle placed too inferiorly	Withdraw the needle to skin level and reinsert with a superior orientation
Musculocutaneous nerve	Biceps twitch	Needle placed too superiorly	Withdraw the needle to skin level and reinsert with a light caudal orientation

Block Dynamics and Perioperative Management

Adequate sedation and analgesia are crucial during nerve localization to ensure patient comfort and to facilitate the interpretation of responses to nerve stimulation. For instance, midazolam 2 to 6 mg intravenously (IV) can be used to achieve sedation. A short-acting narcotic (e.g., alfentanil 250 to 750 µg) is added just before insertion of the needle. A typical onset time for this block is 5 to 15 minutes, depending on the local anesthetic chosen. Waiting beyond 20 minutes will not result in further enhancement of the blockade. The first sign of an impending successful blockade is loss of muscle coordi-

nation within minutes after the injection. This loss can be easily tested by asking the patient to touch his/her nose, paying close attention that they do not miss the nose and injure an eye. The loss of motor coordination typically occurs before sensory blockade can be documented. In case of inadequate skin anesthesia, despite the apparently timely onset of the blockade, local infiltration by the surgeon at the site of the incision is often all that is needed to allow the surgery to proceed. Before and after surgery, both the patient and the surgeon should be informed about the expected duration of the blockade.

Choice of Local Anesthetic

A relatively large volume of local anesthetic is required to achieve anesthesia of the entire brachial plexus. The choice of type and concentration of local anesthetic should be based on whether the block is intended for surgical anesthesia or pain management. Because of the high vascular content of the area and the potential for inadvertent intravascular injection, the local anesthetic solution should be injected slowly with frequent aspiration. Some commonly used local anesthetic solutions and their dynamics with this block are listed in **Table 10.3.**

TABLE 10.3

Choice of Local Anesthetic For Infraclavicular Block

ANESTHETIC	ONSET (min)	DURATION OF ANESTHESIA (h)	DURATION OF ANALGESIA (h)
3% 2-chloroprocaine (HCO^3 + epinephrine)	5–10	1.5	2
1.5% Mepivacaine (HCO^3 + epinephrine)	5–15	2.5–4	3–6
2% Lidocaine (HCO^3 + epinephrine)	5–15	3–6	5–8
0.5% Ropivacaine	15–20	6–8	8–12

TIP

▶ Always assess the risk/benefit ratio of using large volumes and concentrations of long-acting local anesthetic for a infraclavicular brachial plexus block.

CONTINUOUS INFRACLAVICULAR BLOCK

A continuous infraclavicular block is an advanced regional anesthesia technique, and considerable experience with the single-injection technique is necessary for its safe, successful implementation. The use of a catheter significantly increases the utility of an infraclavicular block. The brachial plexus is encountered at a relatively deep location, which decreases the chance of inadvertent catheter dislodgement. Additionally, the catheter insertion site is easily approached for maintenance and inspection. Typically, the initial dose of local anesthetic is injected through the needle, followed by infusion of a more dilute local anesthetic through the catheter at a desired rate. This technique can be utilized for prolonged surgery on the hand, wrist, elbow, or distal arm and for surgery at the same anatomic location requiring prolonged postoperative pain management or a sympathetic block.

Patient Positioning

The patient is in the same position as for the single-injection technique **(see Fig. 10-5)**. However, it is imperative that the anesthesiologist be in an ergonomic position to allow for maneuvering during catheter insertion. It is also important that all the equipment, including the catheter, be immediately available and prepared in advance because small movements of the needle while trying to prepare the catheter may result in dislodging the needle from its position in the brachial plexus sheath.

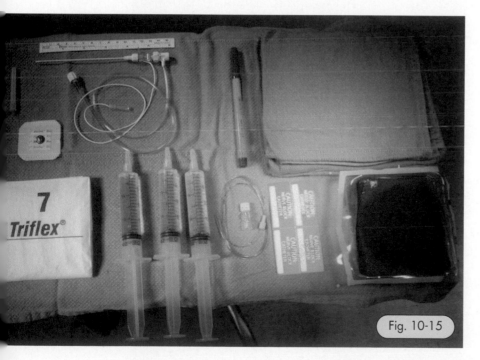

Fig. 10-15

Equipment

A standard regional anesthesia tray is prepared with the following equipment **(see Fig. 10-15)**:

- Sterile towels and gauze packs

- 20-mL syringes containing local anesthetic

- Sterile gloves, marking pen, and surface electrode

- 1½-in, 25-gauge needle for skin infiltration

- 10-cm, insulated stimulating needle (Tuohy-style or Quincke tip)

- Catheter

- Peripheral nerve stimulator

Landmarks

The landmarks are the same as for the single-injection technique **(Fig. 10-16)**:

1. Medial clavicular head

2. Coracoid process

3. Midpoint of line connecting landmarks 1 and 2.

Elevating and raising the arm while palpating for the bony prominence of the coracoid process determines the exact location of the coracoid process **(Fig. 10-17)**. The point of needle insertion is labeled 3 cm caudal to the midpoint between the medial clavicular head and the coracoid process.

TIPS

▶ Inserting the needle too medially should be carefully avoided, as well as inserting the needle at too steep an angle, which carries a risk of pneumothorax.

▶ With proper technique, the risk of pneumothorax is almost negligible.

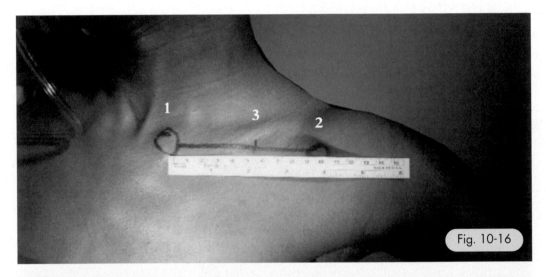

Fig. 10-16

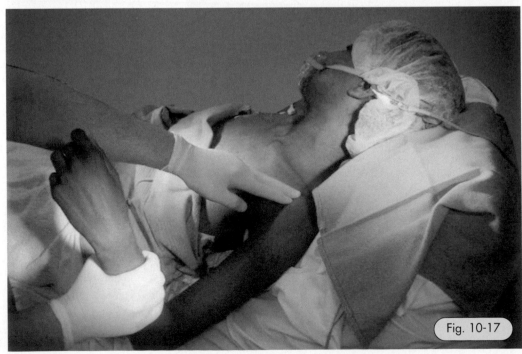

Fig. 10-17

Needle Insertion

The subcutanoues tissue at the projected site of needle insertion is anesthetized with local anethetic. The block needle is then attached to the nerve stimulator (1.5 mA, 2 Hz, 100–300 μs) and to a syringe containing local anesthetic. The fingers of the left hand should be firmly positioned on the pectoralis muscle, and the needle inserted at a 45° angle to the horizontal plane and approximately parallel to the medial clavicular head–coracoid process line **(Fig. 10-18)**. As the needle is advanced beyond the subcutaneous tissue, direct stimulation of the pectoralis muscle is obtained as it enters the body of the muscle. Stimulation of the brachial plexus is encountered soon after the pectoralis muscle twitches cease. The desired response is that of the medial nerve, indicated by rhythmic flexion of the wrist and fingers **(see Fig. 10-13)**. Once the medial nerve response is obtained at a current of 0.2 – 0.4 mA the initial dose of local anesthetic is injected (30 to 45 mL). The catheter is then inserted, making sure that the needle remains firmly seated in the position in which stimulation of the brachial plexus was obtained. The catheter tip should be advanced about 5 cm beyond the needle tip. To prevent it from being dislodged, the needle is carefully withdrawn as the catheter is simultaneously advanced. The most important aspect of this technique is stabilization of the needle for catheter insertion after the brachial plexus is localized.

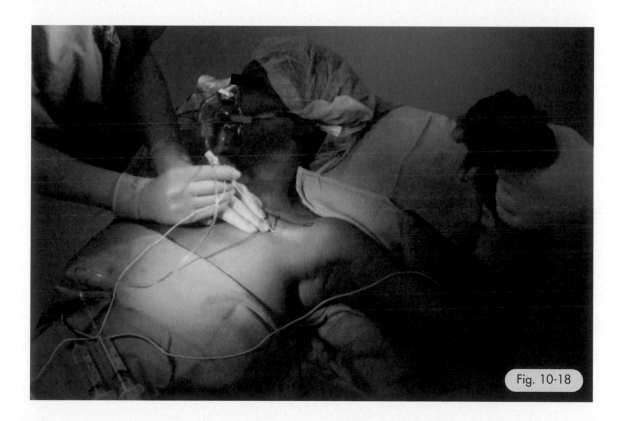

Fig. 10-18

TIPS

▶ This block should be avoided in patients with coagulopathy because the combination of a large-diameter needle and the inability to apply pressure in case of accidental puncture of the infraclavicular vessels (subclavian or axillary artery and vein) carries a risk of hematoma.

▶ The stimulation characteristics of current in Tuohy-style needles appear to be somewhat different from those of single-injection needles. This is likely due to the larger needle diameter and the coating on the needle tip. A slight needle rotation or angle change can make a significant difference in the ability to stimulate.

▶ A slight caudal orientation of the needle may be required to facilitate insertion of the catheter.

▶ It is difficult to advance some needles through the skin, particularly those with blunt tips. For this reason, it is sometimes best to create a small skin nick with a scalpel or the side of a sharp-tipped, 18-gauge needle before attempting to insert such a needle through the skin.

The catheter is checked for inadvertent intravascular placement and secured to the chest **(Fig. 10-19)**. Several techniques for securing it to the skin have been proposed. We find that a benzoin preparation followed by application of a clear dressing is the simplest and sufficiently efficacious. The infusion port should be clearly marked "continuous infraclavicular block."

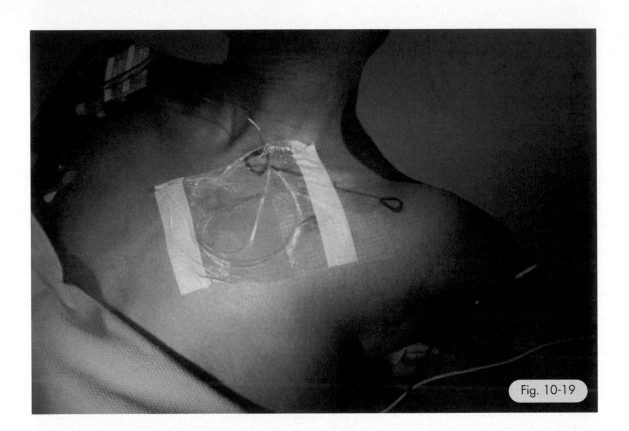

Fig. 10-19

Management of a Continuous Infusion Catheter

The catheter is activated by injecting a bolus of local anesthetic (10 to 15 mL) followed by an infusion at 8 mL/h **(Fig. 10-20)**. A patient-controlled analgesia (PCA) dose of 3 to 5 mL every 30 minutes can be added for breakthrough pain, in which case, the basal infusion should be decreased to 5 mL/min. For continuous infusion, we typically use 0.2% ropivacaine.

Patients should be seen and instructed on the use of PCA at least twice a day. During each visit, the insertion site should be checked for erythema and swelling and the extent of motor and sensory blockade documented. The infusion and PCA dose should then be adjusted accordingly. When the patient complains of breakthrough pain, the extent of the blockade should be checked first. A bolus of dilute local anesthetic (e.g., 10 to 15 mL of 0.2 – 0.5% ropivacaine) can be injected to reactivate the catheter. Increasing the infusion rate alone never results in improvement in analgesia. When the bolus fails to result in blockade after 30 minutes, the catheter should be considered to have migrated and should be removed. Every patient receiving a continuous nerve block infusion should be prescribed an immediately available alternative pain management protocol because incomplete analgesia and catheter dislodgment can occur. For inpatients, this is best done using backup IV PCA.

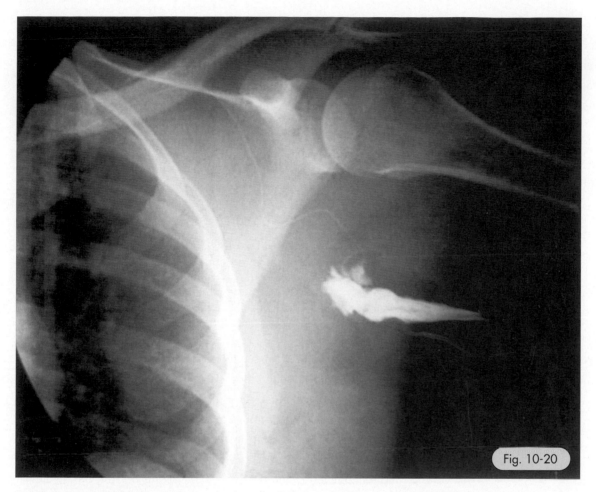

Fig. 10-20

Disposition of radiopaque dye in the brachial plexus sheath after the injection of 2 mL through an infraclavicular catheter.

TIPS

► Breakthrough pain in patients undergoing continuous infusion is always managed by administering a bolus of local anesthetic. Increasing the rate of infusion alone is never adequate.

► For patients on the ward, a higher concentration of a shorter-acting, epinephrine-containing local anesthetic (e.g., 1% mepivacaine or lidocaine with 1:300,000 epinephrine) is useful and safe to both manage the breakthrough pain and test the position of the catheter.

TABLE 10.4

Complications and How to Avoid Them

Hematoma	• Avoid multiple needle insertions through the pectoralis muscle. • Apply firm pressure over the site of needle insertion after needle withdrawal. • Avoid continuous infraclavicular block in patients with abnormal coagulation.
Systemic toxicity	• Limit the volume and dose of long-acting local anesthetic. • Carefully review risks and benefits of using long-acting local anesthetics for each and every patient and/or operation. • Inject local anesthetic with frequent aspiration to rule out intravascular injection, while carefully assessing the patient for signs of local anesthetic toxicity. • Inject local anesthetic slowly and avoid high pressures during injection to reduce the risk of channeling of local anesthetic to smaller veins and/or lymphatic channels that may have been punctured during needle advancement.
Nerve injury	• Make sure the nerve stimulator is fully functional and connected properly. • Use the nerve stimulator to confirm the needle position. This technique requires deep needle insertion, and the use of paresthesia is not acceptable. • Advance the needle slowly when the twitches of the pectoralis muscle cease. • Do not inject against high pressures. Instead, withdraw the needle, check its patency by flushing it, and repeat the procedure. • Stop injecting immediately when the patient complains of pain on injection.
Pneumothorax	• This is an often-feared, but exceedingly rare complication. • The needle direction is actually away from the chest cavity (as opposed to interscalene or supraclavicular blocks). • Attention should be paid to the site and angle of needle insertion to ensure that the needle is in a plane away from the chest wall.

SUGGESTED READINGS

Infraclavicular Block: Single-injection Technique

• Brown DL, Bridenbaugh LD. The upper extremity. Somatic block. In: Cousins MJ, Bridenbaugh PO, eds. *Neuronal Blockade in Clinical Anesthesia and Management of Pain*. Philadelphia, Pa: Lippincott-Raven, 1988;345–371.

• Greher M, Retzl G, Niel P, Kamolz L, Marhofer P, Kapral S. Ultrasonographic assessment of topographic anatomy in volunteers suggests a modification of the infraclavicular vertical brachial plexus block. *Br J Anaesth* 2002;88:632–636.

• Hadžić A, Vloka JD, Kuroda MM, Koorn R, Birnbach DJ. The practice of peripheral nerve blocks in the United States: A national survey. *Reg Anesth Pain* 1998; 23:241–246.

• Ilfeld BM, Morey TE, Enneking FK. Continuous infraclavicular brachial plexus block for postoperative pain control at home: A randomized, double-blinded, placebo-controlled study. *Anesthesiology* 2002;96:1297-1304.

• Klaastad O, Lilleas FG, Rotnes JS, Breivik H, Fosse E. Magnetic resonance imaging demonstrates lack of precision in needle placement by the infraclavicular brachial plexus block described by Raj et al. *Anesth Analg* 1999;88:593–598.

- Koscielniak-Nielsen ZJ, Rotboll Nielsen P, Risby Mortensen C. A comparison of coracoid and axillary approaches to the brachial plexus. *Acta Anaesthesiol Scand* 2000;44:274–279.
- Maurer K, Ekatodramis G, Rentsch K, Borgeat A. Interscalene and infraclavicular block for bilateral distal radius fracture. *Anesth Analg* 2002;94:450–452.
- Rodriguez J, Barcena M, Rodriguez V, Aneiros F, Alvarez J. Infraclavicular brachial plexus block effects on respiratory function and extent of the block. *Reg Anesth Pain Med* 1998;23:564–568.
- Raj PP. Infraclavicular approaches to brachial plexus anesthesia. *Tech Reg Anesth Pain Management* 1997;1:169–177.
- Raj PP, Pai U, Rawal N. Techniques of regional anesthesia in adults. In: Raj PP, ed. *Clinical Practice of Regional Anesthesia.* New York, NY: Churchill Livingstone, 1991;276–300.
- Whiffler K. Coracoid block—a safe and easy technique. *Br J Anaesth* 1981;53:845–848.
- Wilson JL, Brown DL, Wong GY, Ehman RL, Cahill DR. Infraclavicular brachial plexus block: parasagittal anatomy important to the coracoid technique. *Anesth Analg* 1998; 87:870–873.

Infraclavicular Block: Continuous Technique

- Chelly JE, Casati A, Fanelli G. *Continuous Peripheral Nerve Block Technique: An Illustrated Guide.* London; Mosby International; 2001.
- Greher M, Retzl G, Niel P, Kamolz L, Marhofer P, Kapral S. Ultrasonographic assessment of topographic anatomy in volunteers suggests a modification of the infraclavicular vertical brachial plexus block. *Br J Anaesth* 2002;88:632–636.
- Ilfeld BM, Morey TE, Enneking FK. Continuous infraclavicular brachial plexus block for postoperative pain control at home: a randomized, double-blinded, placebo-controlled study. *Anesthesiology* 2002;96:1297–1304.
- Klaastad O, Lilleas FG, Rotnes JS, Breivik H, Fosse E. Magnetic resonance imaging demonstrates lack of precision in needle placement by the infraclavicular brachial plexus block described by Raj et al. *Anesth Analg* 1999;88:593–598.
- Koscielniak-Nielsen ZJ, Rotboll NP, Risby MC. A comparison of coracoid and axillary approaches to the brachial plexus. *Acta Anaesthesiol Scand* 2000;44:274–279.
- Rodriguez J, Barcena M, Rodriguez V, Aneiros F, Alvarez J. Infraclavicular brachial plexus block effects on respiratory function and extent of the block. *Reg Anesth Pain Med* 1998;23:564–568.
- Raj PP. Infraclavicular approaches to brachial plexus anesthesia. *Tech Reg Anesth Pain Mangagement* 1997; 1:169–177.
- Raj PP, Pai U, Rawal N. Techniques of regional anesthesia in adults. In: Raj PP, ed. *Clinical Practice of Regional Anesthesia.* New York, NY: Churchill Livingstone, 1991;276–300.
- Whiffler K. Coracoid block—a safe and easy technique. *Br J Anaesth* 1981; 53:845–848.
- Wilson JL, Brown DL, Wong GY, Ehman RL, Cahill DR. Infraclavicular brachial plexus block: parasagittal anatomy important to the coracoid technique. *Anesth Analg* 1998;87:870–873.

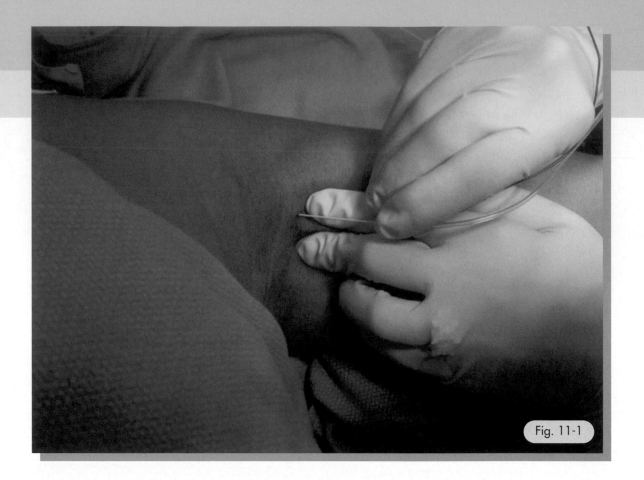

Fig. 11-1

BLOCK AT A GLANCE

- Indications: forearm and hand surgery

- Landmarks: artery pulse

- Needle: 3 to 5 cm

- Any of the following three end points: nerve stimulation, hand twitch at 0.2 to 0.4 mA current; paresthesia, hand; perivascular blood aspiration (axillary artery)

- Local anesthetic: 35 to 40 mL

- Complexity level: basic

GENERAL CONSIDERATIONS

The axillary brachial plexus block was first described by Halstead in New York City at St. Luke's–Roosevelt Hospital Center in 1884. The axillary brachial plexus block is a basic nerve block technique and one of the most commonly practiced blocks. An axillary block is an excellent choice for elbow, forearm, and hand surgery.

Anatomy

The brachial plexus innervates of the upper limb. It consists of nerves derived from the anterior rami of the lower four cervical and the first thoracic spinal nerves (**Fig. 11-2**). The five roots (anterior rami) give rise to three trunks (superior, middle, and inferior) that emerge anteriorly between the scalenus medius and scalenus to lie on the floor of the posterior triangle of the neck. The roots of the brachial plexus lie deep in the prevertebral fascia. The trunks are covered by its lateral extension, the axillary sheath. Each trunk divides into an anterior and a posterior division behind the clavicle at the apex of the axilla. Within the axilla, they combine to produce the three cords, which are named the lateral, medial, and posterior, respectively, according to their relationship to the axillary artery. Each cord ends near the lower border of the pectoralis minor by dividing into two terminal branches. Other branches of the plexus arise from the neck and axilla directly from the roots, trunks, and cords. The anterior divisions form the lateral and medial cords, with branches that supply the flexor muscle of the arm, forearm, and hand and the skin overlying the flexor compartments. The three posterior divisions unite to form the posterior cord. The cord branches supply the extensor musculature of the shoulder, arm, and forearm and the skin of the posterior surface of the limb.

Fig. 11-2

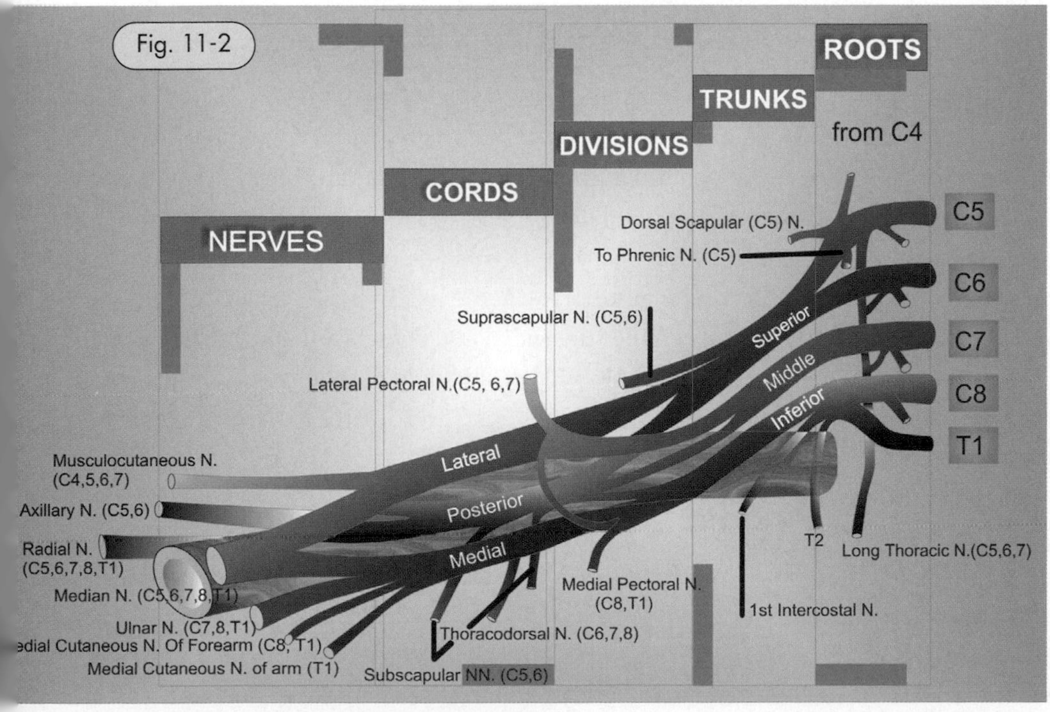

ROOTS

TRUNKS

DIVISIONS

from C4

CORDS

NERVES

Dorsal Scapular (C5) N.

To Phrenic N. (C5)

Suprascapular N. (C5,6)

Lateral Pectoral N.(C5, 6,7)

Superior

Middle

Inferior

C5

C6

C7

C8

T1

Musculocutaneous N. (C4,5,6,7)

Axillary N. (C5,6)

Radial N. (C5,6,7,8,T1)

Median N. (C5,6,7,8,T1)

Ulnar N. (C7,8,T1)

Medial Cutaneous N. Of Forearm (C8, T1)

Medial Cutaneous N. of arm (T1)

Lateral

Posterior

Medial

Subscapular NN. (C5,6)

Thoracodorsal N. (C6,7,8)

Medial Pectoral N. (C8,T1)

1st Intercostal N.

T2

Long Thoracic N.(C5,6,7)

The arrangement of the individual nerves and their relationship to the axillary artery are important in axillary blockade **(Fig. 11-3)**. The medial nerve is positioned superiorly and medially. The ulnar nerve is inferior and medial. The musculocutaneous nerve is superior and lateral, and the radial nerve is inferior and lateral. At this level, the musculocutaneous nerve is outside the brachial plexus sheath.

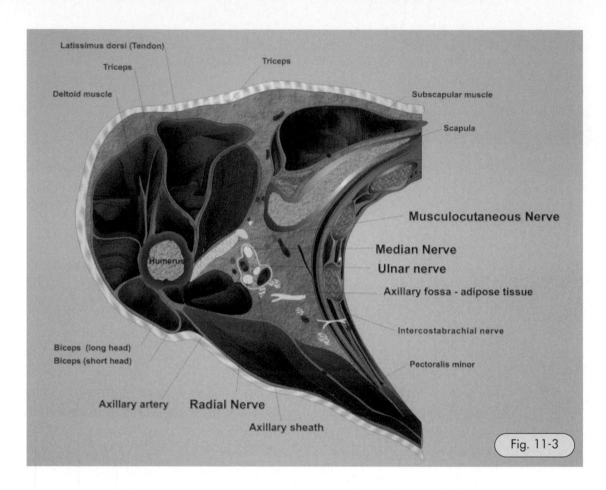

Fig. 11-3

Musculocutaneous Nerve

The musculocutaneous nerve is a terminal branch of the lateral cord. It pierces the coracobrachialis muscle and lies between biceps and brachialis, supplying both these muscles. The nerve continues distally as the lateral cutaneous nerve of the forearm, which pierces the deep fascia between the biceps and brachioradialis to lie superficially over the cubital fossa.

Medial Nerve

The medial and ulnar nerves traverse the entire length of the arm, but neither produces any branches above the elbow joint. The medial nerve derives its fibers from the lateral and medial cords. In the upper part of the arm, it lies lateral to the brachial artery. However, at the midarm level, it crosses anteriorly to the vessels and finally lies medial to the brachial artery, in a position in which it continuous its path through the cubital fossa. The medial nerve enters the forearm from the cubital fossa between the two heads of the pronator teres. It crosses anteriorly to the ulnar artery and descends between the superficial and deep flexors. At the wrist, it is remarkably superficial, lying medial to the tendon of flexor carpi radialis just deep to the palmaris longus tendon.

Ulnar Nerve

The ulnar nerve is a terminal branch of the medial cord. Together with the medial cutaneous nerve of the forearm, it initially lies medial to the brachial artery but leaves the artery at midarm through the intermuscular septum. It enters the posterior compartment to lie between the septum and the medial head of triceps. The ulnar nerve passes behind the medial epicondyle and enters the forearm between the two heads of flexor carpi ulnaris. Lying on the flexor digitorum profundus and covered by the flexor carpi ulnaris, it traverses the medial side of the anterior compartment, accompanied in the lower part of the forearm by the ulnar artery. The ulnar nerve emerges near the wrist lateral to the flexor carpi ulnaris tendon and crosses superficially to the flexor retinaculum with the ulnar artery on its lateral side. It terminates in the hand by dividing into superficial and deep branches. The ulnar nerve supplies the elbow joint and provides branches to the flexor carpi ulnaris and the medial part of the flexor digitorum profundus. It also provides a palmar cutaneous nerve that supplies the skin on the medial aspect of the palm and dorsal cutaneous branches that innervate part of the medial part of the dorsum of the hand.

Radial Nerve

The radial nerve, a terminal branch of the posterior cord, leaves the axilla by passing below the teres major and between the humerus and the long head of the triceps. It passes between the medial and lateral heads of the triceps in the posterior compartment and then leaves the posterior compartment by piercing the lateral intermuscular septum to reach the lateral part of the cubital fossa in front of the elbow joint. In the arm, the radial nerve supplies branches to the medial and lateral heads of the triceps and to the brachioradialis and extensor radialis longus. Cutaneous branches innervate the lateral aspect of the arm and the posterior aspect of the forearm. The branch to the long head of the triceps usually arises in the axilla.

Distribution of Anesthesia

An axillary brachial plexus block (including a musculocutaneous nerve block) provides anesthesia to the to the arm, elbow, forearm, and hand **(Fig. 11-4)**. It should be noted that the unshaded areas are not covered by the axillary brachial plexus block.

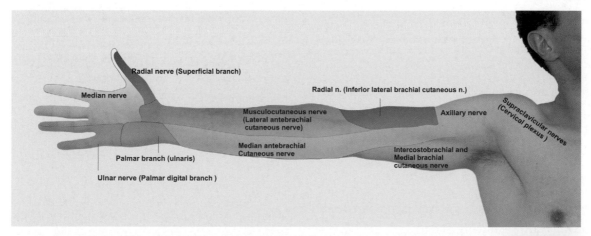

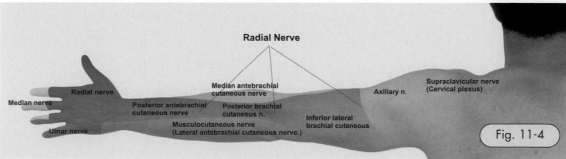

Fig. 11-4

Patient Positioning

The patient is in the supine position with the head facing away from the side to be blocked. The arm on the side of the block placement should be abducted and form a roughly 90° angle in the elbow joint **(Fig. 11-5)**.

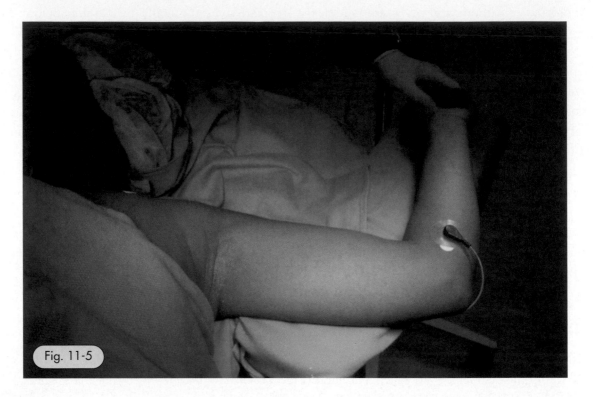

Fig. 11-5

TIPS

► Excessive abduction in the shoulder joint should be avoided because it makes palpation of the axillary artery pulse difficult.

► Excessive abduction can also result in stretching and "fixing" of the brachial plexus. Such stretching of the

plexus components increases its vulnerability during needle advancement. Stretching may increase the risk of nerve injury because the plexus components are fixed and are more likely to be penetrated by the needle rather than "roll" away from the advancing needle.

Equipment

A standard regional anesthesia tray is prepared with the following equipment **(Fig. 11-6)**:

- Sterile towels and gauze packs

- 20-mL syringes containing local anesthetic

- Sterile gloves, marking pen, and surface electrode

- 1-in, 25-gauge needle for skin infiltration

- 3- to 5-cm, short-bevel, insulated stimulating needle

- Three-way stopcock

- Peripheral nerve stimulator

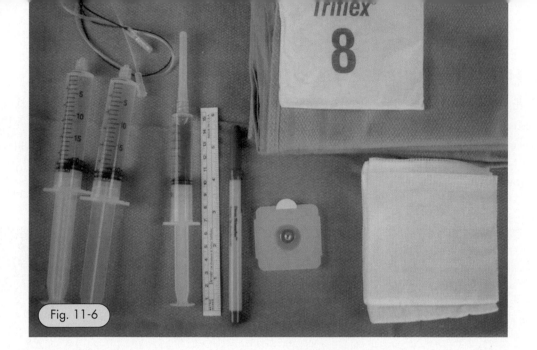

Fig. 11-6

Surface Landmarks

Surface landmarks for the axillary brachial plexus block include **(Fig. 11-7)**:

1. Pulse of the axillary artery

2. Coracobrachialis muscle

3. Pectoralis major muscle

TIPS

▶ In some patients, palpation of the axillary artery may prove difficult, a common scenario in young, athletic men.

▶ In this case, the approximate location of the brachial plexus can be estimated by percutaneous nerve stimulation. The nerve stimulator is set to deliver 4 to 5 mA, and a blunt probe or an "alligator" clip is firmly applied over the skin in front of the palpating fingers until twitches of the brachial plexus are elicited.

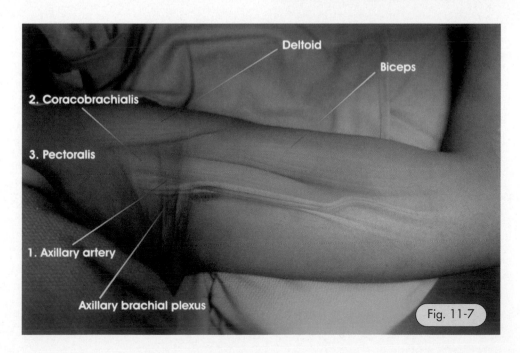

Fig. 11-7

Anatomic Landmarks

After thorough skin preparation, the pulse of the axillary artery is palpated high in the axilla **(Fig. 11-8)**. Once the pulse is felt, it should be straddled between the index and the middle finger and firmly pressed against the humerus to prevent "rolling" of the axillary artery during block performance. At this point, movement of the palpating hand and the patient's arm should be minimized because the axillary artery is highly movable in the adipose tissue of the axillary fossa.

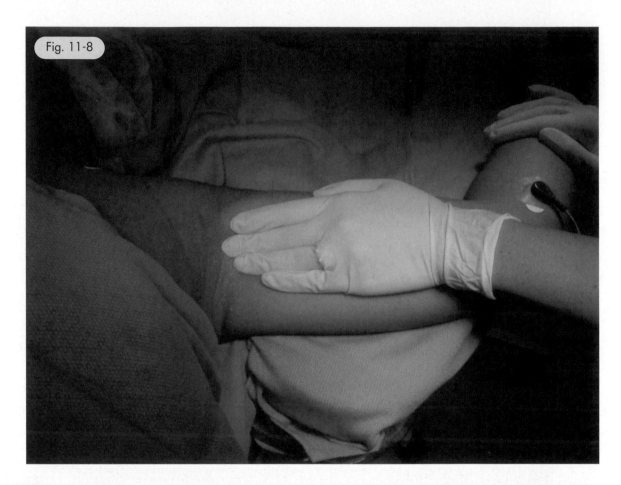

Fig. 11-8

TIPS

► When the location of the artery and the plexus is not immediately apparent, the patient should be asked to adduct the arm against resistance during palpation of the artery, which tenses the pectoralis and coracobrachialis muscles.

► This maneuver is helpful to identify the groove between the coracobrachialis and pectoralis muscles where the arterial pulse is easily detected.

► The position of the brachial plexus can be also estimated using percutaneous nerve stimulation with a current output of 0.4 to 0.5 mA. A blunt probe or an alligator clip is applied over the skin in front of the palpating fingers until twitches of the brachial plexus are elicited. At this point, the probe is replaced by a needle directed toward the estimated direction of the brachial plexus sheath.

Local Anesthetic Infiltration and Needle Insertion

After cleaning the skin with an antiseptic solution, local anesthetic is infiltrated subcutaneously at the determined needle insertion site. The anesthesiologist should assume a sitting position by the patient's side. This avoids strain and hand movement during block performance and facilitates axillary block placement.

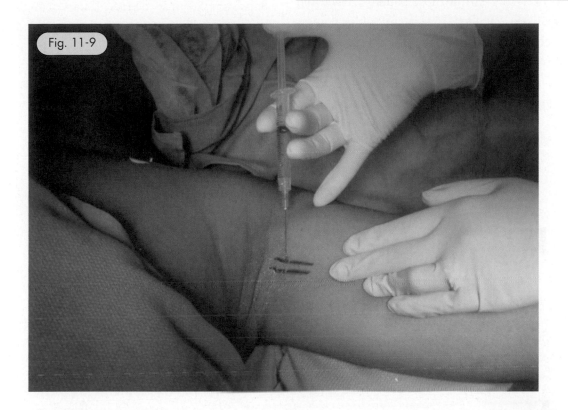

Fig. 11-9

Hand Position

The index and middle fingers of the palpating hand should be firmly pressed against the arm, straddling the pulse of the axillary artery at the midaxillary fossa level **(Fig. 11-10)**. This maneuver shortens the distance between the needle insertion site and the brachial plexus block by compressing the subcutaneous tissue. Also, it helps to stabilize the position of the artery and needle during performance of the block. The palpating hand should not be moved during the entire procedure to allow for precise redirection of the angle of needle insertion when necessary.

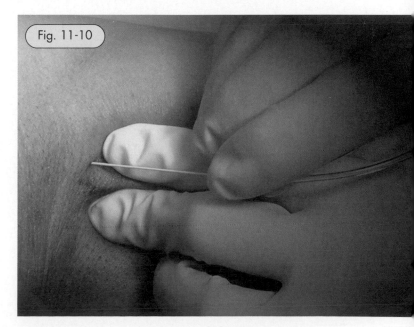

Fig. 11-10

Needle Advancement

A needle connected to the nerve stimulator is inserted just in front of the palpating fingers and advanced at an angle 45° cephalad **(Fig. 11-11)**. The nerve stimulator should be initially set to deliver l-mA current. The needle is advanced slowly until stimulation of the brachial plexus, or paresthesia is obtained. Typically, this occurs at a depth of 1 to 2 cm in most patients. Once the sought response is obtained, 35 to 40 mL of local anesthetic is injected slowly with intermittent aspiration to rule out intravascular injection.

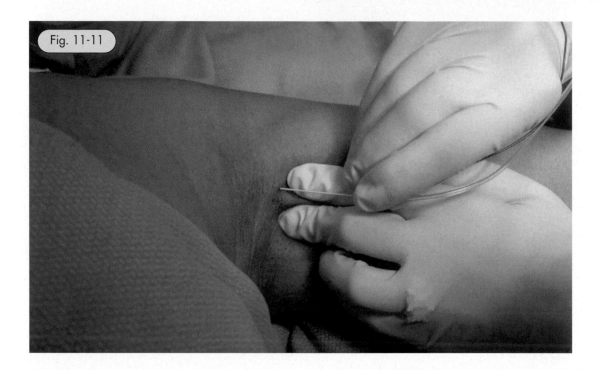

Fig. 11-11

GOALS

• We use a nerve stimulator technique and look for a single nerve response (hand twitch at 0.2- to 0.4-mA current output). On obtaining such a response, we then inject the entire volume of local anesthetic. Although multiple stimulation techniques (stimulating and injecting each major nerve of the brachial plexus separately) may increase the success rate, it also increases the complexity and the time required to complete the block. However, when the axillary artery is punctured before the plexus is stimulated (rare), we do not continue searching for stimulation, but resort to the transarterial technique and inject two-thirds of the total volume of the local anesthetic posteriorly and one-third anteriorly to the axillary artery (Table 11.1).

TABLE 11.1

An Algorithm That Can be Followed When Localizing the Brachial Plexus in the Axilla

Paresthesia in the hand distribution	Inject entire volume of local anesthetic. Do not inject if paresthesia increases at the beginning of injection.
Nerve stimulation (hand twitch) at 0.2–0.4 mA	Inject entire volume of local anesthetic.
Arterial blood obtained	Inject two-thirds volume behind and one-third in front of the artery.
Venous blood obtained	Disregard and continue searching for nerve stimulation.

Failure to Obtain Axillary Brachial Plexus Stimulation on the First Needle Pass

When insertion of the needle does not result in nerve stimulation, the following maneuvers should be made **(Fig. 11-12)**:

1. Keep the palpating hand in the same position and the skin between the fingers stretched.

2. Withdraw the needle to skin level, redirect it at angle of 15° to 30° laterally, and repeat the procedure.

3. Withdraw the needle to skin level, redirect it at angle of 15° to 30° medially, and repeat the procedure.

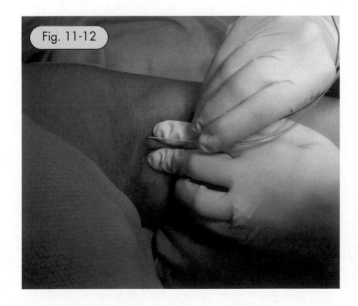

Fig. 11-12

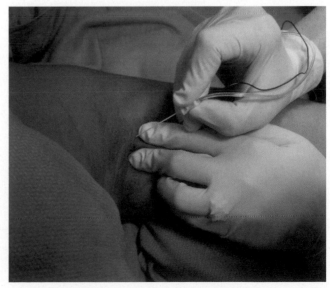

Musculocutaneous Nerve Block

The musculocutaneous nerve is not consistently blocked with the axillary brachial plexus block, because this nerve leaves the brachial plexus sheath proximally. Because of the large area covered by this nerve and its importance in achieving complete anesthesia of the forearm and biceps (see description earlier in this chapter), a block of the musculocutaneous nerve is often necessary for complete anesthesia. This is achieved with a separate injection by inserting the needle above the artery toward the coracobrachial muscle **(Figure 11-13)**. Nerve stimulation is used to produce twitches of the musculocutaneous nerve (biceps twitch). When twitches are observed, 5 mL of local anesthetic is injected.

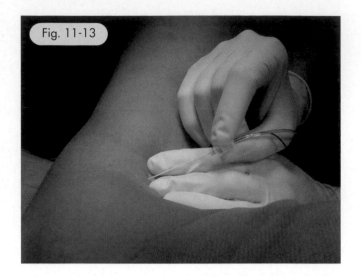

Fig. 11-13

Troubleshooting

Some common responses to nerve stimulation and the course of action to obtain the proper response are shown in **Table 11.2**.

TABLE 11.2

Some Common Responses to Nerve Stimulation and the Course of Action to Obtain the Proper Response

RESPONSE OBTAINED	INTERPRETATION	PROBLEM	ACTION
Local twitch of the arm muscles	Direct stimulation of the biceps or triceps muscles	Needle is inserted in a direction that is too superior or too inferior	Withdraw needle and redirect it accordingly
The needle contacts bone at a 2- to 3-cm depth; no twitches are seen	Needle stopped by the humerus	Brachial plexus was missed and the needle is inserted too deep	Withdraw needle to skin level and reinsert it at an angle 15°–30° superior or inferior
Twitches of the hand	Stimulation of the medial, radial, or ulnar nerve	Correct needle position	Accept, and inject local anesthetic
Arterial blood noticed in the tubing	Puncture of the axillary artery	Needle entered the lumen of the axillary artery	Inject two-thirds of the local anesthetic posterior to the artery, and one-third anterior to the artery
Paresthesia—no motor response	Contact of the needle with the brachial plexus branches	Equipment malfunction (stimulator, needle, electrode)	Carefully assess the distribution of the paresthesia and, if typical, inject local anesthetic

Choice of Local Anesthetic

The axillary brachial plexus requires a relatively large volume of local anesthetic (35 to 40 mL) to achieve complete anesthesia. The choice of the type and concentration of local anesthetic should be based on whether the block is planned for surgical anesthesia or pain management **(Table 11.3)**. Because of the highly vascular area and potential for inadvertent intravascular injection, the local anesthetic solution should be injected slowly with frequent aspiration.

TABLE 11.3

Some Commonly Used Local Anesthetic Solutions and Their Onset Times and Duration in Axillary Block

ANESTHETIC	ONSET (min)	DURATION OF ANESTHESIA (h)	ANALGESIA (h)
1.5% Mepivacaine (HCO_3 + epinephrine)	5–15	2.5–4	3–6
2% Lidocaine (HCO_3 + epinephrine)	5–15	3–6	5–8
0.5% Ropivacaine	15–20	6–8	8–12

Block Dynamics and Perioperative Management

An axillary brachial plexus block is associated with relatively minor patient discomfort. Intravenous midazolam 1 to 2 mg with alfentanil 250 to 500 µg at the time of needle insertion should produce a comfortable, cooperative patient during nerve localization. The onset time for this block is rather long (15 to 25 minutes). The first sign of the blockade is loss of coordination of the arm and forearm muscles. This sign is usually seen sooner than the onset of a sensory or temperature change. When it is observed within 1 to 2 minutes after injection, it is highly predictive of a successful brachial plexus blockade.

Complications and How to Avoid Them

TABLE 11.4
Complication of Axillary Block and Techniques to Avoid Them

Infection	• A strict aseptic technique is used.
Hematoma	• Avoid multiple needle insertions, particularly in patients undergoing anticoagulant therapy. • Keep a 5-min steady pressure if the axillary artery is punctured. • When using a continuous technique, use a single-injection needle to localize the brachial plexus in patients with difficult anatomy. • The use of antiplatelet therapy is not a contraindication for this block in the absence of spontaneous bleeding.
Vascular puncture	• A steady pressure of 5-min duration should be maintained if the axillary artery is punctured.
Local anesthetic toxicity	• Systemic toxicity most commonly occurs during or shortly after the injection of local anesthetic. It is most commonly caused by inadvertent intravascular injection or channeling of forcefully injected local anesthetic into small veins or lymphatic channels cut during needle manipulation. • The use of large volumes of long-acting anesthetic should be reconsidered in older and frail patients. • Careful, frequent aspiration should be performed during the injection. • Avoid fast, forceful injection of local anesthetic.
Nerve injury	• Never inject local anesthetic when pressure is encountered on injection. • Local anesthetic should never be injected when a patient complains of severe pain or exhibits a withdrawal reaction on injection. • When stimulation is obtained with a current intensity of <0.2 mA, needle should be pulled back to obtain the same response with the current >0.2 mA.

SUGGESTED READINGS

• Benhamou D. Axillary plexus block using multiple nerve stimulation: a European view. *Reg Anesth Pain Med* 2001;26:495.

• Bouaziz H, Narchi P, Mercier FJ, Labaille T, Zerrouk N, Girod J, Benhamou D. Comparison between conventional axillary block and a new approach at the mid-humeral level. *Anesth Analg* 1997;84:1058–1062.

• Carles M, Pulcini A, Macchi P, Duflos P, Raucoules-Aime M, Grimaud D. An evaluation of the brachial plexus block at the humeral canal using a neurostimulator (1417 patients): the efficacy, safety, and predictive criteria of failure. *Anesth Analg* 2001;92:194.

• De Jong RH. Axillary block of the brachial plexus. *Anesthesiology* 1961;22:215–225.

• Finucane BT, Yilling F. Safety of supplementing axillary brachial plexus blocks. *Anesthesiology* 1989;70:401–403.

• Hadžić A, Vloka JD, Kuroda MM, Koorn R, Birnbach DJ. The practice of peripheral nerve blocks in the

United States: a national survey. *Reg Anesth Pain Med* 1998;23:241.

- Hepp M, King R. Transarterial technique is significantly slower than the peripheral nerve stimulator technique in achieving successful block. *Reg Anesth Pain Med* 2000;25:660.

- Horlocker TT, Kufner RP, Bishop AT, Maxson PM, Schroeder DR. The risk of persistent paresthesia is not increased with repeated axillary block. *Anesth Analg* 1999;88:382.

- New York School of Regional Anesthesia. www.nysora.com, October 8, 2001.

- Klaastad O, Smedby O, Thompson GE, Tillung T, Hol PK, Rotnes JS, Brodal P, Breivik H, Hetland KR, Fosse ET. Distribution of local anesthetic in axillary brachial plexus block: a clinical and magnetic resonance imaging study. *Anesthesiology* 2002;96:1315–1324.

- Lanz E, Theiss D, Jankovic D. The extent of blockade following various techniques of brachial plexus block. *Anesth Analg* 1983;62:55–58.

- Mezzatesta JP, Scott DA, Schweitzer SA, Selander DE. Continuous axillary brachial plexus block for postoperative pain relief: intermittent bolus versus continuous infusion. *Reg Anesth* 1997;22:357–362.

- Partridge BL, Katz J, Benirschke K. Functional anatomy of the brachial plexus sheath: Implications for anesthesia. *Anesthesiology* 1987;66:743–747.

- Schroeder LE, Horlocker TT, Schroeder DR. The efficacy of axillary block for surgical procedures about the elbow. *Anesth Analg* 1996;83:747.

- Selander D. Axillary plexus block: paresthetic or perivascular. *Anesthesiology* 1987; 66:726.

- Selander D, et al. Catheter technique in axillary plexus block. *Acta Anaesthesiol Scand* 1977;21:324–329.

- Stan TC, Krantz MA, Solomon DL, Poulos JG, Chaouki K. The incidence of neurovascular complications following axillary brachial plexus block using a transarterial approach: a prospective study of 1,000 consecutive patients. *Reg Anesth* 1995;20:486.

- Thompson GE, Rorie DK. Functional anatomy of the brachial plexus sheaths. *Anesthesiology* 1983;59:117–122.

- Winnie A. *Plexus Anesthesia*. Vol 1: *Perivascular Techniques of Brachial Plexus Blocks*. Philadelphia, Pa: WB Saunders; 1984.

- Winnie AP, Radonjic R, Akkinemi SR, Durrani Z. Factors influencing the distribution of local anesthetics in the brachial plexus sheath. *Anesth Analg* 1979;58:225–234.

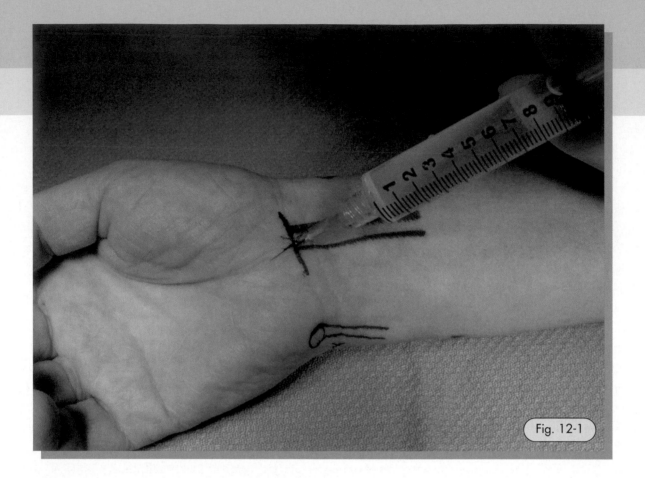

Fig. 12-1

BLOCK AT A GLANCE

- Indications: surgery on the hand and fingers

- Nerves: radial, ulnar, medial

- Needle: $1\frac{1}{2}$ inch

- Local anesthetic: 6 mL per nerve

- Never use an epinephrine-containing local anesthetic

- Complexity level: basic

GENERAL CONSIDERATIONS

A wrist block is a technique of blocking branches of the ulnar, medial, and radial nerves at the level of the wrist. It is a basic peripheral nerve block procedure that involves anesthesia of the terminal branches of the respective nerves. The technique is simple to perform, essentially devoid of systemic complications, and highly effective for a variety of procedures on the hand and fingers. As such, skill in performing a wrist block should be in the armamentarium of every anesthesiologist. Several different techniques of wrist blockade and their modifications have been suggested; in this chapter, we describe the one most commonly used at our institution. Wrist blocks are most commonly used for carpal tunnel and hand and finger surgery.

Regional Anesthesia Anatomy

Innervation of the hand is shared by the ulnar, medial, and radial nerves **(Fig. 12-2)**. The ulnar nerve supplies more intrinsic muscles than the medial nerve, which supplies digital branches to the skin of the medial $1^1/_2$ digits. A corresponding area of the palm is supplied by palmar branches that arise from the ulnar nerve in the forearm. The deep branch of the ulnar nerve accompanies the deep palmar arch and innervates the three hypothenar muscles, the two medial lumbricals, all the interossei, and the adductor pollicis. The ulnar nerve also innervates the palmar brevis.

The medial nerve traverses the carpal tunnel and terminates as digital and recurrent branches **(Fig. 12-2)**. The digital branches supply the skin of the lateral $3^1/_2$ digits and, usually, the two lateral lumbricals. A corresponding area of the palm is innervated by palmar branches that arise from the medial nerve in the forearm. The recurrent branch

of the medial nerve supplies the three thenar muscles. In the palm, the digital branches of the ulnar and medial nerves lie deep in the superficial palmar arch, but in the fingers they lie anterior to the digital arteries that arise from the superficial arch. Although there may be variability of innervation of the ring and middle fingers, the skin on the anterior surface of the thumb is always supplied by the medial nerve and that of the little finger by the ulnar nerve. The palmar digital branches of the medial and ulnar nerves also innervate the nail beds of their respective digits.

The radial nerve passes along the front of the radial side of the forearm. It arises first from the outer side the radial artery and beneath the supinator longus. About 3 inches above the wrist, it leaves the artery, pierces the deep fascia, and divides into two branches **(Fig. 12-2)**. The external branch, the smaller of the two, supplies the skin of the radial side and base of the thumb and joins the anterior branch of the musculocutaneous nerve. The internal branch communicates with the posterior branch of the musculocutaneous nerve. On the back of the hand, it forms an arch with the dorsal cutaneous branch of the ulnar nerve.

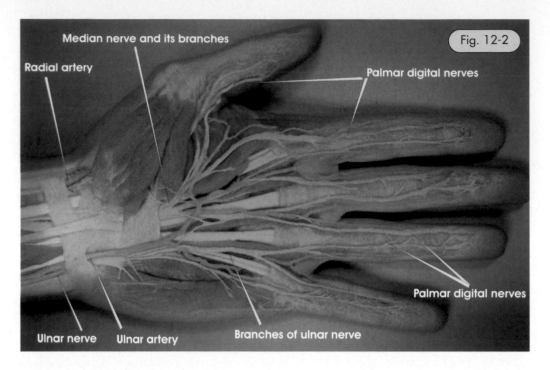

Fig. 12-2

Median nerve and its branches

Radial artery

Palmar digital nerves

Palmar digital nerves

Ulnar nerve   Ulnar artery   Branches of ulnar nerve

Distribution of Anesthesia

As previously mentioned, blockade of the ulnar, medial, and radial nerves results in anesthesia of the entire hand. The nerve contribution to innervation of the hand varies considerably; **(Fig. 12-3)** shows the most common arrangement.

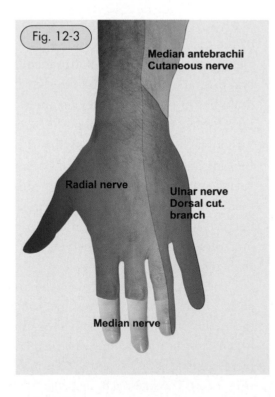

Fig. 12-3

Median antebrachii Cutaneous nerve

Radial nerve

Ulnar nerve Dorsal cut. branch

Median nerve

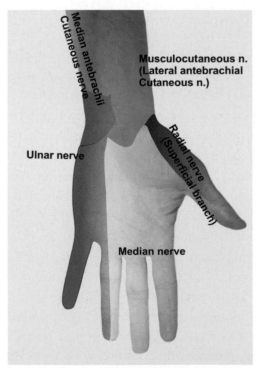

Median antebrachii Cutaneous nerve

Musculocutaneous n. (Lateral antebrachial Cutaneous n.)

Ulnar nerve

Radial nerve (Superficial branch)

Median nerve

Patient Positioning

The patient is in the supine position with the arm abducted. The wrist is best kept in slight dorsiflexion.

Equipment

A standard regional anesthesia tray is prepared with the following equipment:

- Sterile towels and gauze packs

- 10-mL syringe containing local anesthetic

- $1^1/_2$-in, 25-gauge needle

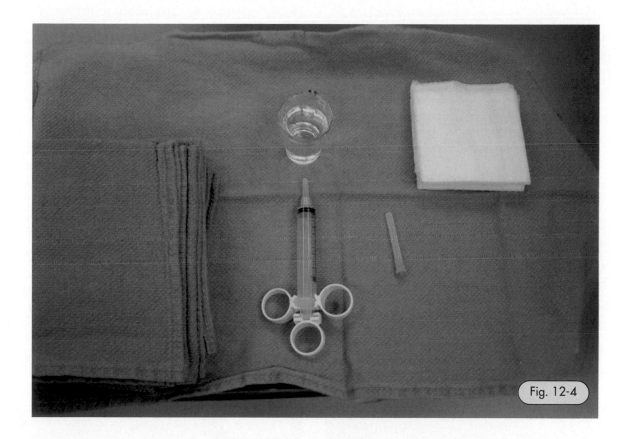

Fig. 12-4

Anatomic Landmarks

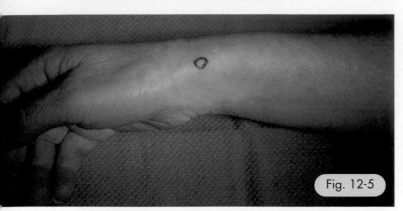

Fig. 12-5

The superficial branch of the radial nerve runs along the medial aspect of the brachioradialis muscle. It then passes between the tendon of the brachioradialis and radius to pierce the fascia on the dorsal aspect. Just above the styloid process of the radius (circle) **(Fig. 12-5)**, it produces digital branches for the dorsal skin of the thumb, index finger, and lateral half of the middle finger. Several of its branches pass superficially over the anatomic "snuff box."

The *medial nerve* is located between the tendons of the palmaris longus (white arrow) and the flexor carpi radialis (red arrow) **(Fig. 12-7)**. The palmaris longus tendon is usually the more prominent of the two; the medial nerve passes just lateral to it. The *ulnar nerve* passes between the ulnar artery and tendon of the flexor carpi ulnaris. The tendon of the flexor carpi ulnaris is superficial to the ulnar nerve **(Fig. 12-8)**.

TIP

▶ The position of the radial nerve in relationship to the radial artery is often confusing to trainees. The illustration in **(Fig. 12-6)** clarifies the course of the radial nerve branches at the wrist.

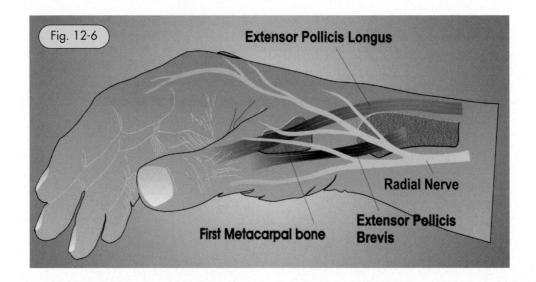

Fig. 12-6

Extensor Pollicis Longus

Radial Nerve

First Metacarpal bone

Extensor Pollicis Brevis

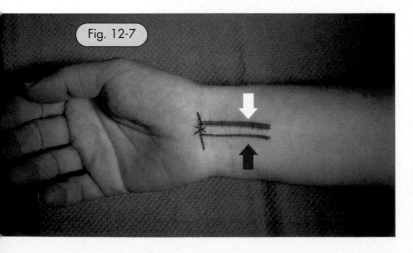

Fig. 12-7

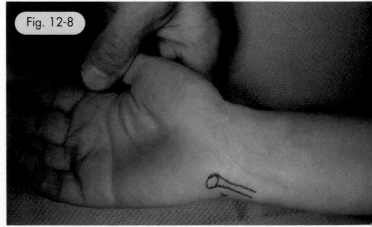

Fig. 12-8

Local Anesthetic Infiltration and Needle Insertion

The entire wrist area should be cleaned with a disinfectant solution.

Block of the Radial Nerve

The radial nerve is essentially a "field block" and requires more extensive infiltration because of its less predictable anatomic location and division into multiple smaller cutaneous branches. Five mililiters of local anesthetic should be injected subcutaneously just above the radial styloid, aiming medially **(Fig. 12-9)**. The infiltration is then extended laterally, using an additional 5 mL.

Block of the Ulnar Nerve

The ulnar nerve is anesthetized by inserting the needle under the tendon of the flexor carpi ulnaris muscle close to its distal attachment just above the styloid process of the ulna **(Fig. 12-10)**. The needle is advanced 5 to 10 mm to just past the tendon of the flexor carpi ulnaris. Three to 5 mL of local anesthetic solution is injected. A subcutaneous injection of 2 to 3 mL of local anesthesia just above the tendon of the flexor carpi ulnaris is also advisable in blocking the cutaneous branches of the ulnar nerve which often extend to the hypothenar area.

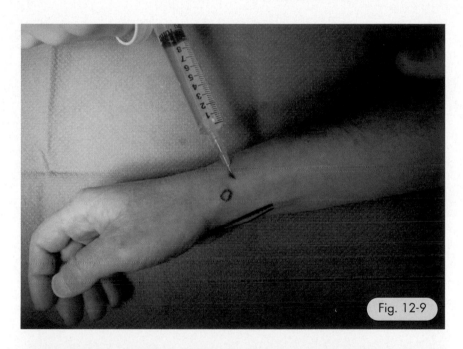

Fig. 12-9

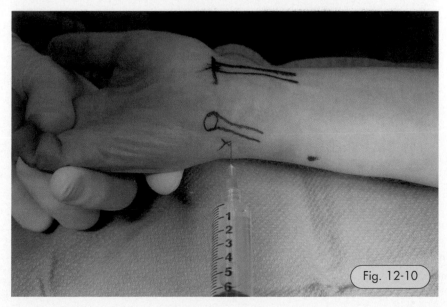

Fig. 12-10

Block of the Medial Nerve

The medial nerve is blocked by inserting the needle between the tendons of the palmaris longus and flexor carpi radialis **(Fig. 12-11)**. The needle is inserted until it pierces the deep fascia, and 3 to 5 mL of local anesthetic is injected. Although piercing of the deep fascia has been described to result in a fascial "click," it is more reliable to simply insert the needle until it contacts the bone. The needle is then withdrawn 2 to 3 mm, and the local anesthetic is injected.

TIP

▶A "fan" technique is recommended to increase the success rate of the medial block. After the initial injection, the needle is withdrawn back to skin level, redirected 30° laterally, and advanced again to contact the bone. After pulling back 1 to 2 mm from the bone, an additional 2 mL of local anesthetic is injected. A similar procedure is repeated with medial redirection of the needle.

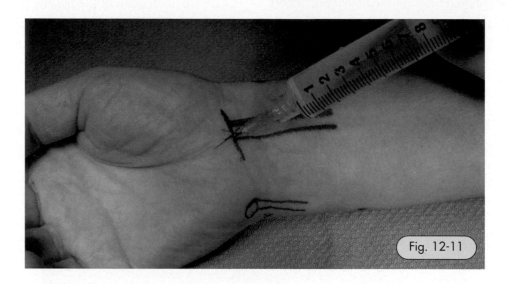

Fig. 12-11

Choice of Local Anesthetic

The choice of the type and concentration of local anesthetic for a wrist block is based on the desired duration **(Table 12.1)**.

TABLE 12.1
Onset Times and Durations for Some Commonly Used Local Anesthetic Mixtures

ANESTHETIC	ONSET (min)	DURATION OF ANESTHESIA (h)	DURATION OF ANALGESIA (h)
1.5% Mepivacaine (+ HCO₃)	15–20	2–3	3–5
2% Lidocaine (+ HCO₃)	10–20	2–5	3–8
0.5% Ropivacaine	15–30	4–8	5–12
0.75% Ropivacaine	10–15	5–10	6–24
0.5% Bupivacaine (or levobupivacaine)	15–30	5–15	6–30

Block Dynamics and Perioperative Management

This technique is associated with moderate patient discomfort because multiple insertions and subcutaneous injections are required. Appropriate sedation and analgesia (midazolam 2 to 4 mg and alfentanil 250 to 500 μg) are useful to ensure the patient's comfort. A typical onset time for a wrist block is 10 to 15 minutes, depending on the concentration and volume of local anesthetic used. Sensory anesthesia of the skin develops faster than the motor block. Placement of an Esmarch bandage or a tourniquet at the level of the wrist is well-tolerated and does not require additional blockade.

Complications and How to Avoid Them

Complications following a wrist block are typically limited to residual paresthesias due to inadvertent intraneuronal injection. Systemic toxicity is rare because of the distal location of the blockade.

TABLE 12.2
Complications of Wrist Block and Techniques to Avoid Them

Infection	• Should be very rare with the use of an aseptic technique.
Hematoma	• Avoid multiple needle insertions. • Use a 25-gauge needle and avoid puncturing superficial veins.
Vascular complications	• Do not use epinephrine for wrist and finger blocks.
Nerve injury	• Do not inject when the patient complains of pain or high pressure is detected on injection. • Do not reinject the medial and ulnar nerves.
Other	• Instruct the patient on care of the insensate hand.

SUGGESTED READINGS

- Brown DL, Bridenbaugh LD. The upper extremity: somatic block. In: Cousins MJ, Bridenbaugh PO, eds. *Neuronal Blockade in Clinical Anesthesia and Management of Pain.* Philadelphia, Pa: Lippincott-Raven, 1988;345–371.
- Delaunay L, Chelly JE. Blocks at the wrist provide effective anesthesia for carpal tunnel release. *Can J Anaesth* 2001;48:656–660.
- Derkash RS, Weaver JK, Berkeley ME, Dawson D. Office carpal tunnel release with wrist block and wrist tourniquet. *Orthopedics* 1996;19:589–590.
- Gebhard RE, Al-Samsam T, Greger J, Khan A, Chelly JE. Distal nerve blocks at the wrist for outpatient carpal tunnel surgery offer intraoperative cardiovascular stability and reduce discharge time. *Anesth Analg* 2002;95:351–355.
- Hahn MB, McQuillan PM, Sheplock GJ. *Regional Anesthesia: An Atlas of Anatomy and Techniques.* St. Louis, Mo: Mosby; 1996.
- Mulroy MF. *Regional Anesthesia: An Illustrated Procedural Guide.* 3rd ed. Philadelphia, Pa: Lippincott; 2002.
- Ramamurthy S, Hickey R. Anesthesia. In: Green DP, Hotchkiss RN, eds. *Operative Hand Surgery.* New York, NY: Churchill Livingstone, 1993;25–52

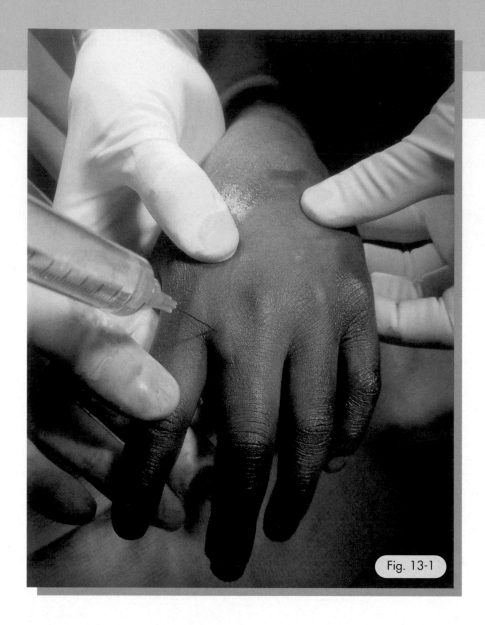

Fig. 13-1

BLOCK AT A GLANCE

- Indications: surgery on the fingers

- Nerves: digital nerves

- Local anesthetic: 2 to 3 mL per side

- Epinephrine-containing local anesthetic should not be used

- Complexity level: basic

GENERAL CONSIDERATIONS

A digital block is the technique of blocking the nerves of the digits to achieve anesthesia of the finger(s). This technique is simple to perform and essentially devoid of systemic complications. It is an effective, commonly used method of anesthesia for a wide variety of minor surgical procedures on the digits and should be in the armamentarium of every anesthesiologist. Several different techniques of digital blockade and their modifications are available. In this chapter, we describe the one that is most commonly used at our institution.

Regional Anesthesia Anatomy

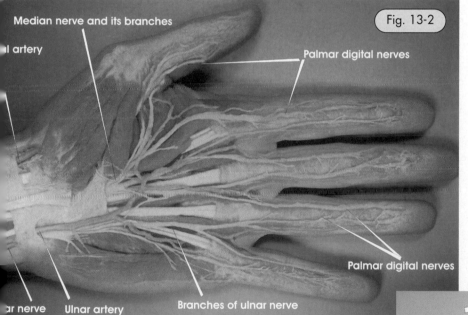

Fig. 13-2

Median nerve and its branches

l artery

Palmar digital nerves

Palmar digital nerves

ar nerve   Ulnar artery   Branches of ulnar nerve

The common digital nerves are derived from the medial and ulnar nerves and divide in the distal palm into the volar aspect, tip, and nail bed area **(Fig. 13-2)**. The main digital nerves, accompanied by digital vessels, run on the ventrolateral aspect of the finger immediately lateral to the flexor tendon sheath **(Fig. 13-3)**. Small dorsal digital nerves run on the dorsolateral aspect of the finger and innervate the back of the fingers as far as the proximal joint.

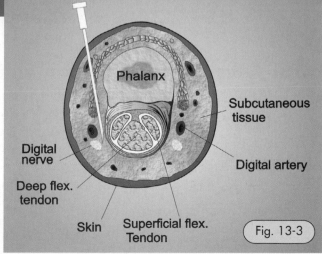

Phalanx

Subcutaneous tissue

Digital nerve

Digital artery

Deep flex. tendon

Skin   Superficial flex. Tendon

Fig. 13-3

Positioning

The hand is pronated and rested on a flat surface or supported by an attendant.

Equipment

A standard regional anesthesia tray is prepared with the following equipment:

- Sterile towels and gauze packs

- Controlled 10-mL syringe containing local anesthetic

- $1^1/_2$-in, 25-gauge needle

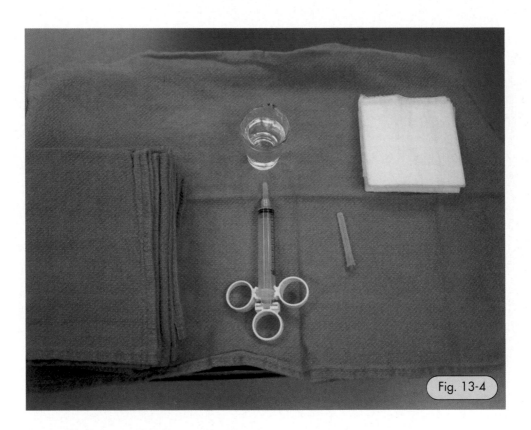

Fig. 13-4

Local Anesthetic Infiltration and Needle Insertion

Block of Volar and Dorsal Digital Nerves at the Base of the Finger

A $1^1/_2$-in, 25-gauge needle is inserted at a point on the dorsolateral aspect of the base of the finger, and a small skin wheal is raised **(Fig. 13-5)**. The needle is then directed anteriorly toward the base of the phalanx. It is then advanced until it contacts the phalanx, while the anesthesiologist observes for any protrusion from the palmar dermis directly opposite the needle path **(Fig. 13-6)**. One milliliter of solution is injected, as the needle is withdrawn 1 to 2 mm from the bone contact. An additional 1 mL is injected continuously as the needle is withdrawn back to skin level. The same procedure is repeated on each side of the base of the finger to achieve anesthesia of the entire finger **(Fig. 13-6)**.

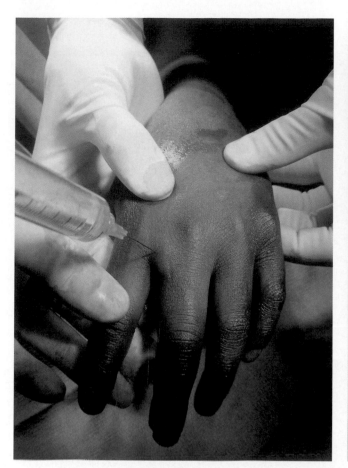

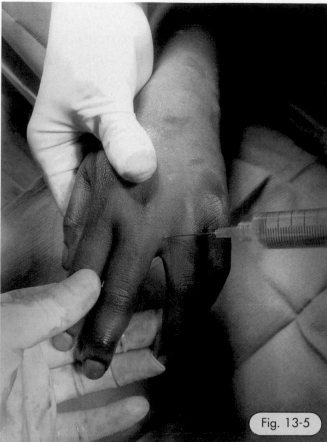

Fig. 13-5

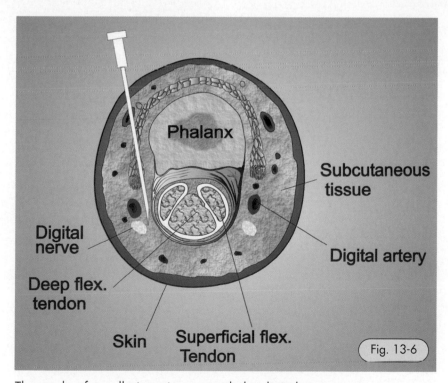

Fig. 13-6

The angle of needle insertion to reach the digital nerve.

Transthecal Digital Block

A transthecal digital block is placed by using the flexor tendon sheath for local anesthetic infusion. In this technique, with the patient's hand supinated, the flexor tendon is located. The needle should enter the skin at a 45° angle. Using a 1-in, 25- to 27-gauge needle, 2 mL of local anesthetic is injected into the flexor tendon sheath at the level of the distal palmar crease. Resistance to the injection suggests that the needle tip is against the flexor tendon. Careful withdrawal of the needle results in the free flow of medication as the potential space between the tendon and the sheath is entered. Proximal pressure can be applied to the volar surface for the duration of the injection so that the medication diffuses throughout the synovial sheath.

TIPS

▶ The advantage of transthecal approach is the ability to provide anesthesia to the entire digit with a single injection and with a reportedly higher success rate.

▶ For more extensive surgery on the finger, it may be advantageous to combine both approaches discussed in this chapter for a greater success rate and for more extensive distribution of anesthesia.

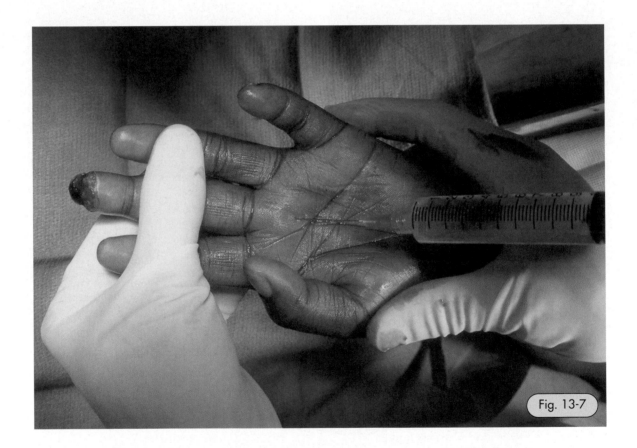

Fig. 13-7

Block Dynamics and Perioperative Management

A skin wheal at the point of needle insertion significantly reduces the discomfort during placement of the block. A digital block requires a small dose of sedative or narcotic during placement. The typical onset time for this block is 10 to 20 minutes, depending on the concentration and volume of local anesthetic used.

Choice of Local Anesthetic

The choice of the type and concentration of local anesthetic used for a digital block is based on the desired duration of blockade. The onset times and duration effect for some commonly used local anesthetic mixtures are listed in **Table 13.1**.

TABLE 13.1

Choice of Local Anesthetic for Digital Block

ANESTHETIC	ONSET (min)	DURATION OF ANESTHESIA (h)	DURATION OF ANALGESIA (h)
1.5% Mepivacaine (+ HCO$_3$)	15–20	2–3	3–5
2% Lidocaine (+ HCO$_3$)	10–20	2–5	3–8
0.5% Ropivacaine	15–30	4–8	5–12
0.75% Ropivacaine	10–15	5–10	6–24
0.5% Bupivacaine (or levobupivacaine)	15–30	5–15	6–30

Complications and How to Avoid Them

One specific complication of digital blocks is vascular insufficiency and gangrene. This catastrophe is a result of digital artery occlusion combined with collateral circulation insufficiency. A series of causative factors is often involved in producing this rare but serious condition.

TABLE 13.2
Complications of Digital Block and Preventive Techniques

Infection	• Should be very rare with the use of an aseptic technique.
Hematoma	• Avoid multiple needle insertions. • Use a 25-gauge needle (or smaller) and avoid puncturing superficial veins.
Other	• Instruct the patient on care of the insensate finger.
Gangrene of the digit(s)	• Avoid epinephrine-containing solutions for this block. • Limit the injection volume to 2 mL on each side. • The mechanical pressure effects of injecting solution into a potentially confined space should always be borne in mind, particularly in blocks at the base of the digit. • In patients with small-vessel disease, an alternative method should perhaps be sought in addition to avoiding a digital tourniquet.
Nerve injury	• Residual paresthesias can result after an inadvertent intraneuronal injection. • Systemic toxicity is rare because of the distal location of the blockade. • Do not inject when the patient complains of pain or when high pressures are met on injection.

SUGGESTED READINGS

• Brown DL, Bridenbaugh LD. The upper extremity: somatic block. In: Cousins MJ, Bridenbaugh PO, eds. *Neuronal Blockade in Clinical Anesthesia and Management of Pain*. Philadelphia, Pa: Lippincott-Raven, 1988; 345–371.

• Chiu DTW. Transthecal digital block: flexor tendon sheath used for anesthetic infusion. *J Hand Surg* 1990; 15:471–473.

• Flarity-Reed K. Methods of digital block. *J Emerg Nurs* 2002;28:351.

• Freedman RR, Mayes MD, Sabharwal SC. Digital nerve blockade in Raynaud's disease. *Circulation* 1989;80:1923.

• Kirchhoff R, Jensen PB, Nielsen NS, Boeckstyns ME. Repeated digital nerve block for pain control after tenolysis. *Scand J Plast Reconstr Surg Hand Surg* 2000;34:257.

• Morrison WG. Transthecal digital block. *Arch Emerg Med* 1993;10:35–38.

- O'Donnell J, Wilson K, Leonard PA. An avoidable complication of digital nerve block. *Emerg Med* J 2001; 18:316.
- Sarhadi NS, Shaw-Dunn J. Transthecal digital nerve block: an anatomical appraisal. *J Hand Surg* [Br] 1998; 23:490.
- Torok PJ, Flinn SD, Shin AY. Transthecal digital block at the proximal phalanx. *J Hand Surg* 2001;26:69.
- Wilhelm BJ, Blackwell SJ, Miller JH, Mancoll JS, Dardano T, Tran A, Phillips LG. Do not use epinephrine in digital blocks: myth or truth? *Plast Reconstr Surg* 2001;107:393.

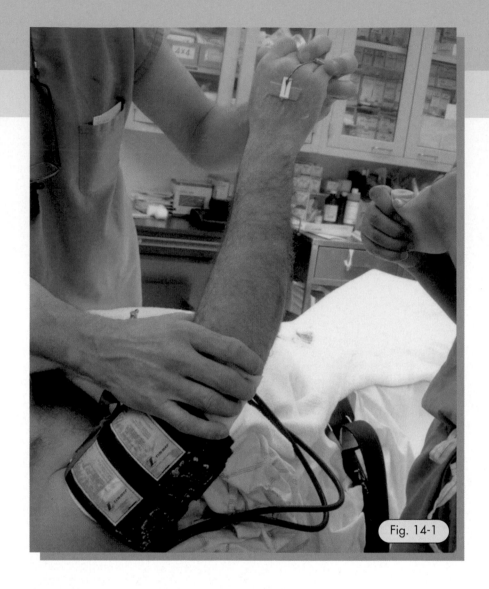

Fig. 14-1

BLOCK AT A GLANCE

- Indications: surgery on the wrist, hand, and fingers

- Local anesthetic: 12–15 mL of 2% lidocaine

- Complexity level: basic

14 INTRAVENOUS REGIONAL BLOCK OF THE UPPER EXTREMITY

GENERAL CONSIDERATIONS

Intravenous (IV) regional anesthesia was originally introduced by the German surgeon August K. G. Bier in 1908, thus the name "Bier block." Bier described complete anesthesia and motor paralysis after an IV injection of prilocaine into a previously exsanguinated limb. The resultant anesthesia is produced by direct diffusion of local anesthetic from the vessels into the nearby nerves. The technique was reintroduced into clinical practice using lidocaine as a local anesthetic in the mid-1960s. Since its reintroduction, IV regional anesthesia has become one of the most commonly used regional anesthesia techniques in the United States. This technique is best used for brief minor surgery (up to 1 hour) of the hand and forearm. Its use for longer surgical procedures is precluded by discomfort caused by the tourniquet, which limits the indications for its use. Some examples of suitable procedures include carpal tunnel release, tendon contracture release, and foreign body extraction. The main advantages of this technique are its simplicity and reliability. Its drawback is the lack of postoperative analgesia because the block quickly resolves after release of the tourniquet. In this chapter, we describe the use of IV regional anesthesia for the upper extremity; identical procedures with a larger volume of local anesthetic can be used for the lower extremity.

Regional Anesthesia Anatomy

Peripheral nerve endings of the extremities are nourished by small blood vessels. The injection of a local anesthetic solution into a venous system results in diffusion of the local anesthetic into the nerve endings with the consequent development of anesthesia. This holds true as long as the concentration of local anesthetic in the venous system remains relatively high. As will be apparent in the technique description, it is imperative that before the injection, the venous system be exsanguinated to prevent dilution of the local anesthetic.

Distribution of Anesthesia

An IV regional block results in anesthesia of the entire extremity below the level of the tourniquet. The duration of the anesthesia and analgesia is limited by the duration of the tourniquet application.

Patient Positioning

The patient is in the supine position with the arm to be blocked elevated to achieve passive exsanguination **(Fig. 14-1)**. This is a crucial step, and care should be taken to allow 1 to 2 minutes for passive return of blood to the dependent levels. Before beginning the block procedure, an IV line is started on the side opposite the one to be blocked.

Equipment

A standard regional anesthesia tray is prepared with the following equipment:

- 22-gauge IV catheter

- Flexible extension tubing

- 5-in Esmarch bandage

- Double-cuff tourniquet

- 20-mL syringe with local anesthetic

- Pressure source

- Double-cuff tourniquet with in-line valves

Local Anesthetic Infiltration and Needle Insertion

A tourniquet should be placed on the proximal arm of the extremity to be blocked **(Fig. 14-2)**. We use a double cuff to increase the reliability of the technique and help reduce tourniquet pressure pain. The arm should

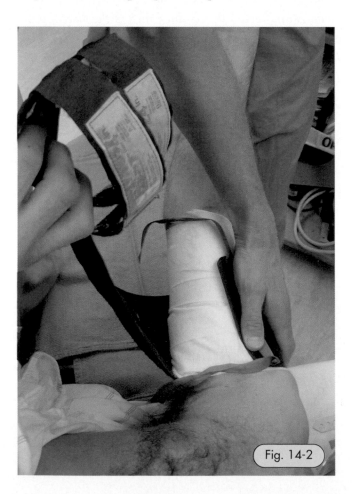

Fig. 14-2

be generously wrapped with a soft cloth at the tourniquet site to prevent discomfort on application of the tourniquet and skin bruising where the tourniquet may pinch the unprotected skin **(Fig. 14-2)**. The tourniquet should be well-secured and fastened to prevent inadvertent slipping or opening with consequent loss of anesthesia and/or systemic toxicity due to access of the injected local anesthetic to the central circulation.

Prior to proceeding, it is of utmost importance to check the functionality of the tourniquet by briefly inflating both tourniquet cuffs and squeezing the inflated cuffs and observing that there are no leaks.

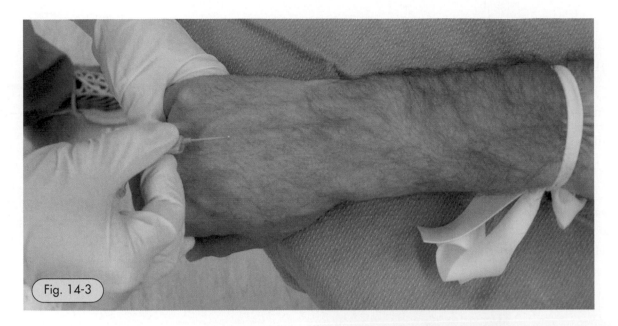

Fig. 14-3

A small IV catheter (e.g., 22-gauge) is introduced into the dorsum of the patient's hand of the arm to be anesthetized **(Fig. 14-3)**. The catheter should be firmly secured in place to prevent dislodgment during exsanguination with the Esmarch tourniquet or during the injection procedure. The arm is then elevated at least for 1 minute to allow passive exsanguination, which occurs as the large veins are emptied into the more proximal circulation **(Fig. 14-4)**. Then, a 5-in Esmarch tourniquet is applied systematically from the fingertips to the distal cuff **(Fig. 14-4)**. Proper methodical application of the tourniquet requires some skill, as well as an assistant to hold the arm correctly in the upright position. The tourniquet should be always slightly stretched before applying the next turn-wrap around the extremity.

TIP

▶ Proper methodical application of the tourniquet and completeness of the exsanguination as blood is squeezed from the vascular beds into the proximal circulation are the most important factors for ensuring a high success rate with this technique.

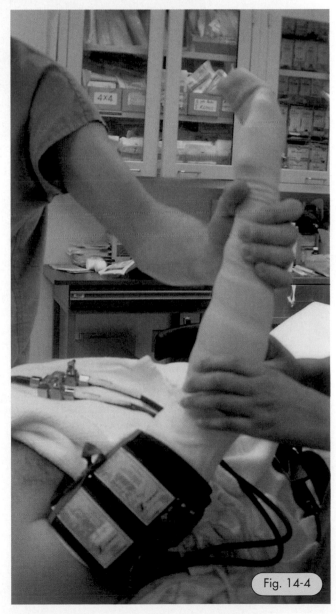

Fig. 14-4

Once the tourniquet is applied, the following maneuvers are undertaken to complete exsanguination of the extremity **(Fig. 14-5)**:

1. Inflate the *distal* cuff.

2. Inflate the *proximal* cuff.

3. Deflate the *distal* cuff.

The cuffs should be inflated to a pressure of 100 mm Hg above the systolic blood pressure or at least to 300 mm Hg. The tourniquet is then unwrapped, and the extremity is checked for color (pale skin) and arterial occlusion (absence of a radial pulse).

TIPS

▶ Inadequate occlusion of arterial blood flow by the tourniquet can result in venostasis and venous engorgement of the extremity, and occasionally this makes it difficult to operate.

▶ The extremity is then lowered, and the local anesthetic is slowly injected through a previously inserted IV catheter.

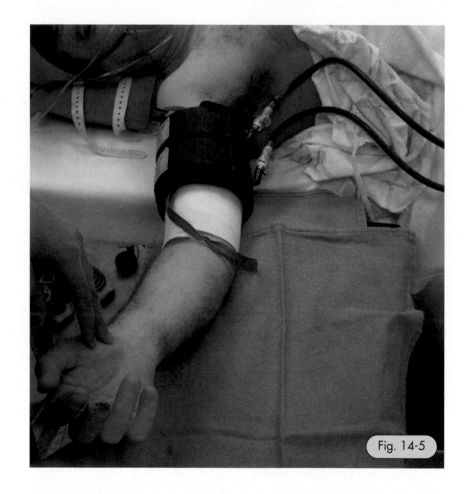

Fig. 14-5

Once the absence of arterial pulsation and the functionality of the tourniquet are confirmed, the local anesthetic is slowly injected (over 5–10 seconds) through the catheter **(Fig. 14-6)**.

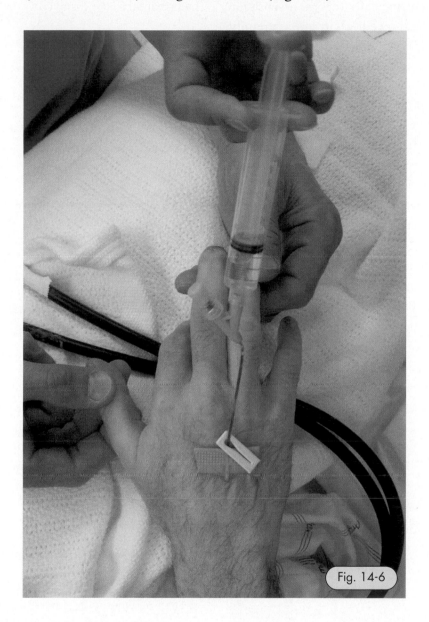

Fig. 14-6

Choice of Local Anesthetic

Lidocaine is the most commonly used drug for IV regional anesthesia. Many authors recommend a large volume of a dilute solution of local anesthetic (e.g., 50 mL of 0.5% lidocaine). We prefer a smaller volume of a concentrated drug (e.g., 12 to 15 mL of 2% lidocaine) because the dilution and drawing of the drug in multiple syringes is time-consuming and not necessary. In addition, smaller volumes are easier to inject and simpler to prepare.

Several other local anesthetic solutions and additives are reported to result in a slight prolongation of analgesia, such as 0.25% bupivacaine, 0.2% ropivacaine, meperidine, tramadol, ketorolac, and clonidine. However, it is our opinion that the marginal potential improvements in analgesia obtained with these medications or their adjuvants do not justify the compromise in safety and increase in complexity or side effects of this otherwise safe, straightforward technique.

Block Dynamics and Perioperative Management

The onset of anesthesia with this technique is within 5 minutes. The patient typically reports a sensation described as "pins and needles" in the extremity. However, this sign is almost always missed in our practice because we routinely administer small doses of midazolam (2 to 4 mg IV) to ensure the patient's comfort during the procedure. Most patients invariably report pressure at the site of the tourniquet after 30 to 45 minutes, sometimes even earlier. When the discomfort becomes troublesome and requires significant additional sedation and analgesics, the distal cuff over the anesthetized extremity is inflated and the proximal cuff is deflated. This provides immediate relief of discomfort caused by pressure from the proximal cuff. This maneuver provides an additional 15 to 30 minutes of comfort. When tourniquet pain is first reported by the patient, the surgeon should be consulted for information on the expected time required to complete the surgery. The proximal tourniquet should not be released prematurely. The proper procedure for changing the tourniquet from the proximal to the distal cuff is as follows **(Fig. 14-7)**:

1. Inflate the *distal* cuff.

2. Check the pressure in the distal cuff by squeezing the cuff and documenting the oscillations on the manometer.

3. Deflate the *proximal* cuff.

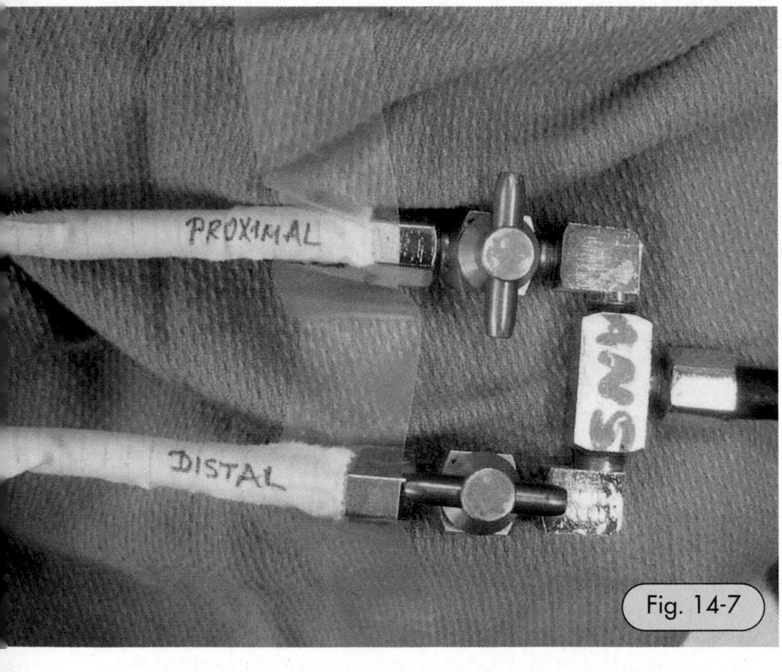

> **TIP**
>
> ▶ It is important to properly label the proximal and distal cuffs and their respective valves to avoid deflation of the wrong cuff and the abrupt loss of anesthesia that would ensue, or the risk of local anesthetic toxicity **(Fig. 14-7)**.

Deflating the tourniquet correctly at the end of surgery is important to avoid the risk of local anesthetic toxicity when the procedure is completed within 45 minutes after the injection of local anesthetic. A two-stage deflation is suggested whereby the cuff is deflated for 10 seconds and reinflated for 1 minute before the final release. This practice allows for a more gradual washout of local anesthetic.

> **TIP**
>
> ▶ Release of the tourniquet results in a rapid resolution of anesthesia and analgesia. The surgeon should be instructed to infiltrate local anesthetic into the wound before release of the tourniquet to prevent sudden oncoming pain. When this is not possible, judicious doses of analgesic should be administered preemptively in anticipation of postoperative pain.

Fig. 14-7

Complications and How to Avoid Them

Complications associated with IV regional blocks are few and are mostly limited to systemic toxicity from the local anesthetic that is related to problems with the tourniquet.

TABLE 14.1
Complications of IV Regional Block and Techniques To Prevent Them

Systemic toxicity of local anesthetic	• The risk comes mainly from inadequate tourniquet application or equipment failure at the beginning of the procedure. • Every precaution should be taken to ensure that the tourniquet is reliable and the pressure is maintained. • Gradually release the tourniquet in steps to prevent a massive washout of local anesthetic into the systemic circulation. • After the surgical procedure is completed, within 20 minutes after injection of local anesthetic, gradually release the tourniquet in several steps, with 2-minute intervals between deflations.
Hematoma	• Use a small-gauge intravenous (IV) catheter. • If superficial veins are punctured during an unsuccessful attempt at placement of the IV catheter, apply firm pressure on the puncture site for 2–3 min. Failure to do so will invariably lead to venous bleeding during application of the tourniquet.
Engorgement of the extremity	• In order to avoid venostasis, ensure that the tourniquet is fully functional and that the arterial pulse is absent. • This scenario may be more common in patients with arteriosclerosis; the calcifications in the arterial walls may prevent effective function of the tourniquet; consequently, the arterial blood continues to enter the distal extremity while the venous blood is unable to escape, resulting in engorgement of the extremity and occasionally ecchymotic hemorrhage in the subcutaneous tissue.
Ecchymoses and subcutaneous hemorrhage	• The above principle applies. • Ensure that adequate padding is used over the arm where the tourniquet is to be applied.

SUGGESTED READINGS

• Bannister M. Bier's block. *Anaesthesia* 1997;52:713.

• Blyth MJ, Kinninmonth AW, Asante DK. Bier's block: a change of injection site. *J Trauma* 1995;39:726.

• Brown EM, McGriff JT, Malinowski RW. Intravenous regional anaesthesia (Bier block): review of 20 years' experience. *Can J Anaesth* 1989;36:307.

• Casale R, Glynn C, Buonocore M. The role of ischaemia in the analgesia which follows Bier's block technique. *Pain* 1992;50:169.

• de May JC. Bier's block. Anaesthesia 1997;52:713.

• Farrell RG, Swanson SL, Walter JR. Safe and effective IV regional anesthesia for use in the emergency department. *Ann Emerg Med* 1985;14:288.

• Hadžić A, Vloka JD, Kuroda MM, Koorn R, Birnbach DJ. The practice of peripheral nerve blocks in the United States: a national survey. *Reg Anesth Pain Med* 1998;23:241–246.

• Hilgenhurst G. The Bier block after 80 years: a historical review. *Reg Anesth* 1990;15:2.

• Holmes CM. Intravenous regional neural blockade. In: Cousins MJ, Bridenbaugh PO, eds. *Neuronal Blockade in Clinical Anesthesia and Management of Pain*. Philadelphia, Pa: Lippincott-Raven, 1988;395–409.

• Hunt SJ, Cartwright PD. Bier's block—under pressure? *Anaesthesia* 1997;52:188.

• Moore DC. Bupivacaine toxicity and Bier block: the drug, the technique, or the anesthetist. *Anesthesiology* 1984;61:782.

• Tramer MR, Glynn CJ. Magnesium Bier's block for treatment of chronic limb pain: a randomised, double-blind, cross-over study. *Pain* 2002;99:235.

• Wilson JK, Lyon GD. Bier block tourniquet pressure. *Anesth Analg* 1989;68:823.

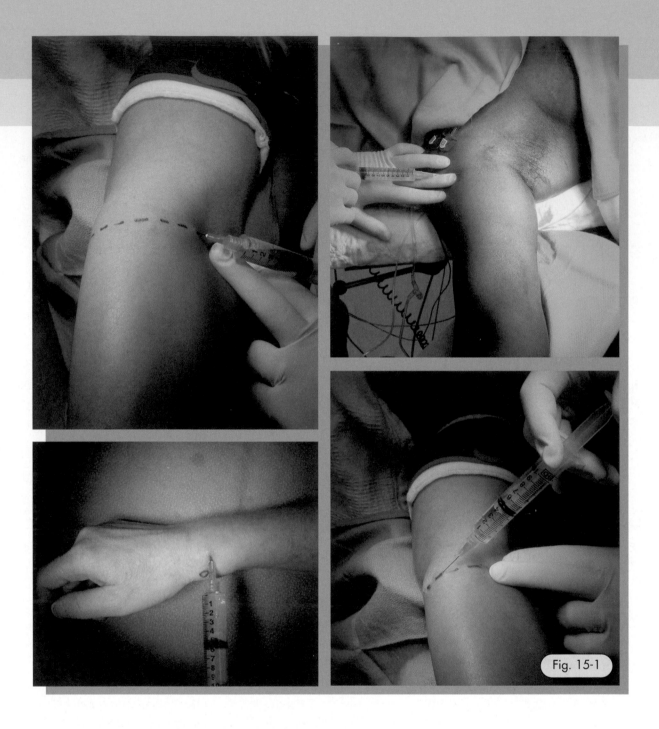

Fig. 15-1

BLOCK AT A GLANCE

- Indications: mostly used as a supplement to major blocks of the upper extremity

- Local anesthetic: 5 to 10 mL

- Complexity level: basic

15 CUTANEOUS
NERVE BLOCKS OF THE UPPER EXTREMITY

GENERAL CONSIDERATIONS

Cutaneous nerve blocks of the upper extremity are used mainly for supplementing brachial plexus blocks. These blocks are simple to learn and perform, are essentially devoid of complications, and can be useful as complements to major conduction blocks of the upper extremity. Their judicious use can help prevent tourniquet pain or salvage an incomplete brachial plexus block. The techniques discussed in this chapter focus primarily on the blocks that are most useful clinically: blocks of the intercostobrachial, medial, and lateral cutaneous nerves of the forearm and the superficial radial nerve.

Regional Anesthesia Anatomy

Cutaneous nerve blockade is achieved by the injection of local anesthetic into the subcutaneous layers above the muscle fascia. The subcutaneous tissue contains a variable amount of fat, superficial nerves, and vessels. Deeper, there is a tough, membranous layer, the deep fascia of the lower extremity, which encloses the muscles of the arm and forearm. Numerous superficial nerves and vessels penetrate the deep fascia.

The cutaneous innervation of the upper extremity originates from the superficial cervical plexus, the brachial plexus, and the intercostal nerves **(Table 15.1, Fig. 15-2, and Fig. 15-3)**. Only a few cutaneous nerves of the upper extremity exist as individual nerves. These originate directly from the spinal nerves (intercosto-

brachial [T2 and T3] and occasionally the cutaneous nerve of the arm [C8 and T1]). These nerves are not anesthetized with a brachial plexus block and need to be specifically blocked when skin anesthesia of their respective territories is desired. Most of the cutaneous nerves of the upper extremity emanate from the cords or individual nerves of the brachial plexus. These nerves are anesthetized with a successful brachial plexus block. The radial nerve (posterior cord) provides the majority of the cutaneous innervation (posterior cutaneous nerve of the arm, posterior cutaneous nerve of the forearm). The medial and ulnar nerves provide only small cutaneous branches to the hand.

TABLE 15.1
Origin of the Cutaneous Nerves of the Upper Extremity

SUPERFICIAL CERVICAL PLEXUS	BRACHIAL PLEXUS	INTERCOSTAL NERVES
Supraclavicular nerves	Superior lateral cutaneous nerve of arm	Intercostobrachial nerve (T2 and occasionally T3)
	Posterior cutaneous nerve of the arm	Medial cutaneous nerve of the arm (C8 and T1)
	Posterior cutaneous nerve of the forearm	
	Medial cutaneous nerve of the forearm	
	Lateral cutaneous nerve of the forearm (musculocutaneous nerve)	
	Superficial radial nerve	
	Dorsal cutaneous of the ulnar nerve	
	Palmar cutaneous branch of the median (R2) nerve	

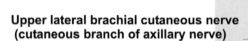

Upper lateral brachial cutaneous nerve (cutaneous branch of axillary nerve)

Intercostobrachial nerve

Cutaneous branches of radial nerve

Lower lateral brachial cutaneous nerve

Posterior antebrachial cutaneous nerve

Posterior antebrachial cutaneous nerve

Lateral antebrachial cutaneous nerve, posterior branch

Radial nerve, superficial branch

Posterior brachial cutaneous nerve, (cutaneous branch of radial nerve)

Medial antebrachial cutaneous nerve, ulnar (posterior) branches

Dorsal (cutaneous) branch of ulnar nerve

Fig. 15-2

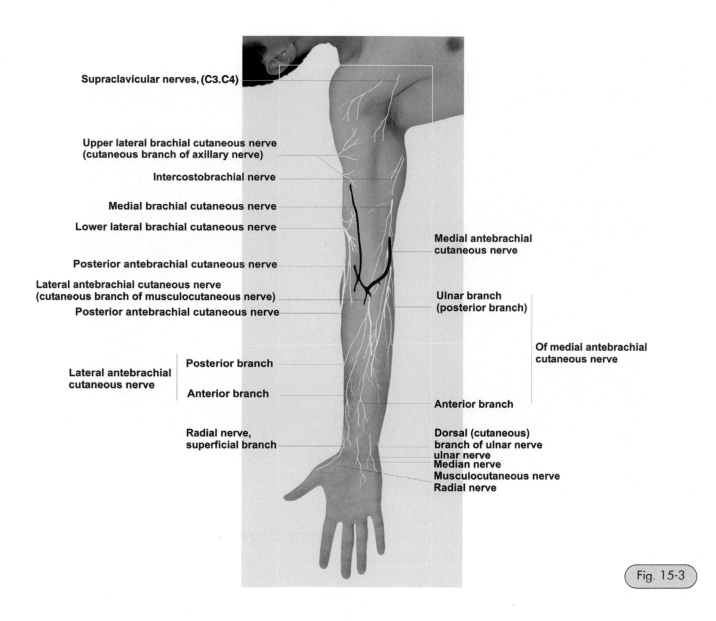

Supraclavicular nerves, (C3.C4)

Upper lateral brachial cutaneous nerve
(cutaneous branch of axillary nerve)

Intercostobrachial nerve

Medial brachial cutaneous nerve

Lower lateral brachial cutaneous nerve

Posterior antebrachial cutaneous nerve

Lateral antebrachial cutaneous nerve
(cutaneous branch of musculocutaneous nerve)

Posterior antebrachial cutaneous nerve

Lateral antebrachial
cutaneous nerve

Posterior branch

Anterior branch

Radial nerve,
superficial branch

Medial antebrachial
cutaneous nerve

Ulnar branch
(posterior branch)

Of medial antebrachial
cutaneous nerve

Anterior branch

Dorsal (cutaneous)
branch of ulnar nerve
ulnar nerve
Median nerve
Musculocutaneous nerve
Radial nerve

Fig. 15-3

INTERCOSTOBRACHIAL NERVE BLOCK

Anatomy

The intercostobrachial nerve is the lateral cutaneous branch of the ventral primary ramus of T2. It provides innervation to the axilla and the skin of the medial aspect of the arm. The intercostobrachial nerve communicates with the medial cutaneous nerve of the arm. Both nerves are anesthetized by subcutaneous infiltration of the skin of the medial aspect of the arm.

Indications

Blocks of these nerves are often combined with an infraclavicular or axillary block to achieve more complete anesthesia of the upper arm.

Technique

A $1^1/_2$-in, 25-gauge needle is inserted at the level of the axillary fossa **(Fig. 15-4)**. The entire width of the medial aspect of the arm is infiltrated with local anesthetic to raise a subcutaneous "wheal" of anesthesia.

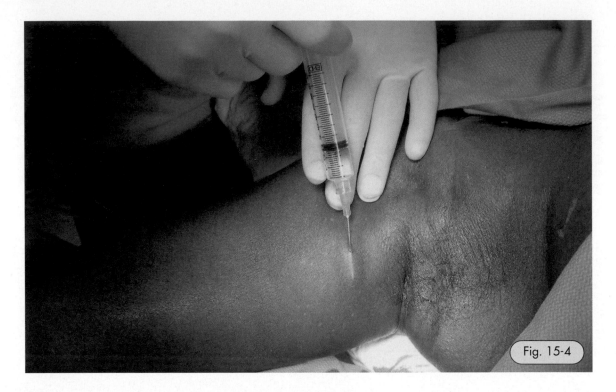

Fig. 15-4

Medial Cutaneous Nerve of the Forearm Block

Anatomy

The medial cutaneous nerve of the forearm originates within the medial cord. This nerve supplies branches to the skin of the medial side of the forearm **(Fig. 15-5)**.

Indications

The medial antebrachial cutaneous nerve is blocked by infiltration of local anesthetic into the subcuta-

neous tissue on the anteromedial and dorsomedial surfaces of the forearm just below the elbow crease. Along with blockade of the lateral antebrachial cutaneous nerve, anesthesia for the insertion of an arteriovenous graft on the forearm can be achieved.

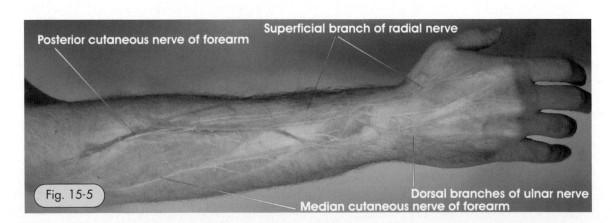

Posterior cutaneous nerve of forearm

Superficial branch of radial nerve

Fig. 15-5

Dorsal branches of ulnar nerve

Median cutaneous nerve of forearm

Technique

A $1^{1}/_{2}$-in, 25-gauge needle is used to infiltrate local anesthetic subcutaneously over the entire medial aspect of the arm just below the elbow crease **(Fig. 15-6)**.

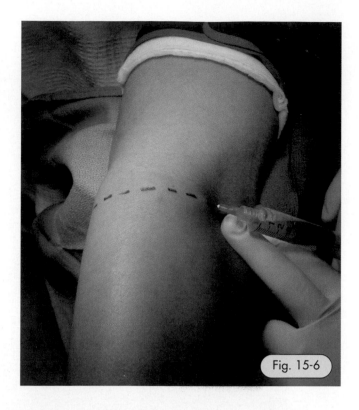

Fig. 15-6

Lateral Cutaneous Nerve of the Forearm Block

Anatomy

The lateral cutaneous nerve of the forearm is a cutaneous extension of the musculocutaneous nerve, which originates from C4 through C7 and separates from the brachial plexus through the lateral cord. The musculocutaneous nerve runs through the bodies of the coracobrachials and biceps muscles, emerges between the biceps and brachioradialis muscles, and pierces the deep brachial fascia just above the elbow crease lateral to the biceps tendon **(Fig. 15-7)**. As soon as the nerve emerges above the fascia, it becomes the lateral antebrachial cutaneous nerve and descends on the anterolateral surface of the forearm. The musculocutaneous nerve supplies branches to the anterolateral and posterior surfaces of the forearm. Its distal branches reach the lateral surface of the wrist.

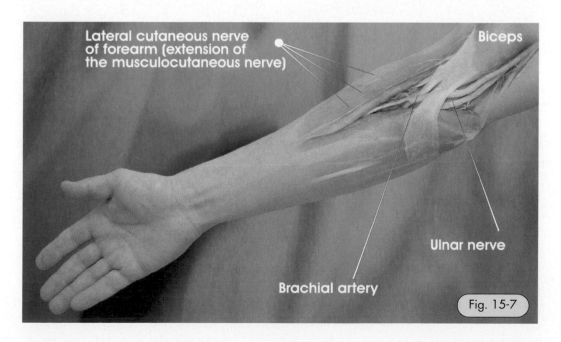

Lateral cutaneous nerve of forearm (extension of the musculocutaneous nerve)

Biceps

Ulnar nerve

Brachial artery

Fig. 15-7

Indications

Blockade of the lateral cutaneous and medial cutaneous nerves of the forearm results in anesthesia of the anterior and lateral surfaces of the forearm. This block is suitable for the insertion of arteriovenous grafts, a procedure used in patients with chronic renal failure.

Technique

The nerve can be blocked at the level of the arm (musculocutaneous block; see "Axillary Block" for a description) or when it emerges at the elbow level. To block the lateral cutaneous nerve of the forearm at the *level of the elbow*, the patient is placed in the supine position with the arm extended 90°. After aseptic skin preparation, a 50-mm, 25-gauge needle is introduced just below the elbow crease **(Fig. 15-8)**. A subcutaneous infiltration of local anesthetic is made lateral to the biceps muscle tendon.

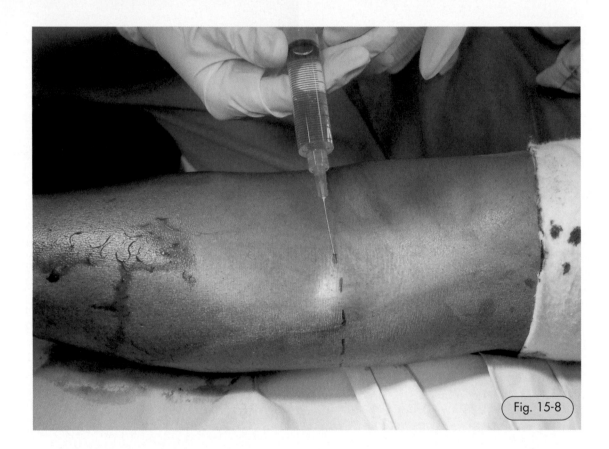

Fig. 15-8

Choice of Local Anesthetic

The choice of local anesthetic is primarily based on the desired duration of the blockade. Because these blocks do not result in motor blockade, longer-acting local anesthetic are most commonly chosen (e.g., 0.2% to 0.5% ropivacaine or 0.25% bupivacaine).

Complications and How to Avoid Them

Complications from cutaneous nerve blocks are few, they are discussed in **Table 15.2**.

TABLE 15.2

Complications of Cutaneous Blocks and Preventive Techniques

Systemic toxicity of local anesthetic	• The risk is small and may be of concern mostly when used in conjunction with other high-dose major conduction blocks.
Hematoma	• Avoid multiple needle insertions. • Avoid inserting the needle through superficial veins.
Nerve injury	• Usually manifested as transient paresthesias or dysesthesias and results from inadvertent intraneuronal injection. • Injections should not be made when high pressures are felt on injection or when the patient reports pain in the distribution of the nerve.

SUGGESTED READINGS

• Agur AMR, Lee MJ. *Grant's Atlas of Anatomy*. Baltimore, Md: Lippincott Williams & Wilkins, 1999.

• Jankovic D, Wells C. *Regional Nerve Blocks*. 2nd ed. Wissenchafts-Verlag Berlin, Blackwell Scientific Publications, 2001.

• Pernkopf E. *Atlas of Topographical and Applied Human Anatomy*. Vol II: Thorax, Abdomen and Extremities. 2nd ed. Munich, Germany: U&S Saunders, 1980.

• Raj PP. *Textbook of Regional Anesthesia*. London, England: Churchill Livingstone, 2002.

• Viscomi CM, Reese J, Rathmell JP. Medial and lateral antebrachial cutaneous nerve blocks: an easily learned regional anesthetic for forearm arteriovenous fistula surgery. *Reg Anesth* 1996;21:2–5.

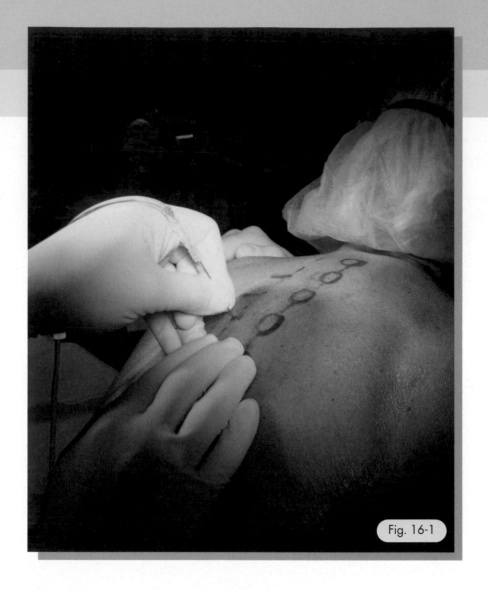

Fig. 16-1

BLOCK AT A GLANCE

- Indications: Breast surgery, pain management after thoracic surgery or rib fractures

- Landmarks: spinal process at the desired thoracic dermatomal level

- Needle insertion: 2.5 cm lateral to the midline

- Target: needle insertion 1 cm past the transverse process

- Local anesthetic: 3 to 5 mL per level

- Complexity level: advanced

GENERAL CONSIDERATIONS

A thoracic paravertebral block is a technique of injecting local anesthetic in the vicinity of the thoracic spinal nerves emerging from the intervertebral foramen with the resultant ipsilateral somatic and sympathetic nerve blockade. The resultant anesthesia or analgesia is conceptually similar to a "unilateral" epidural anesthesia. Higher or lower levels can be chosen to accomplish a unilateral, bandlike, segmental blockade at the desired levels without significant hemodynamic changes. This technique is one of the easiest and most time-efficient to perform but more challenging to teach because it requires stereotactic needle maneuvering. A certain "mechanical" mind or sense of geometry is necessary for mastering it. In our practice this block is performed most commonly for surgery in patients undergoing breast (mastectomy and cosmetic breast surgery) and thoracic surgery. A catheter can also be inserted for continuous infusion of local anesthetic.

Anatomy

The thoracic paravertebral space is a wedge-shaped area that lies on either side of the vertebral column **(Fig. 16-2)**. Its walls are formed by the parietal pleura anterolaterally; the vertebral body, intervertebral disk, and intervertebral foramen medially; and the superior costotransverse process posteriorly. The spinal nerves in the paravertebral space are organized in small bundles submerged in the fat of the area. At this location, they are not enveloped by a thick fascial sheath. Therefore, they are relatively easily anesthetized by the injection of local anesthetic. The thoracic paravertebral space is continuous, with the intercostal space laterally, epidural space medially, and contralateral paravertebral space via the prevertebral fascia. The mechanism of action of a paravertebral blockade includes direct penetration of local anesthetic into the spinal nerve, lateral extension along with the intercostal nerve, and medial extension through the intervertebral foramina.

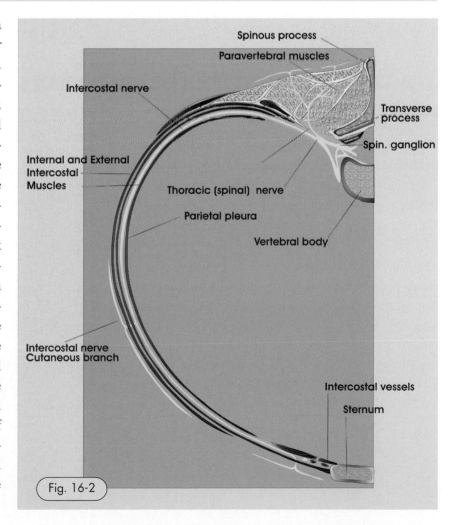

Fig. 16-2

Distribution of Anesthesia

Thoracic paravertebral blockade results in ipsilateral anesthesia. The location of the resulting dermatomal distribution of anesthesia or analgesia is a function of the level blocked and the volume of local anesthetic injected **(Fig. 16-3)**.

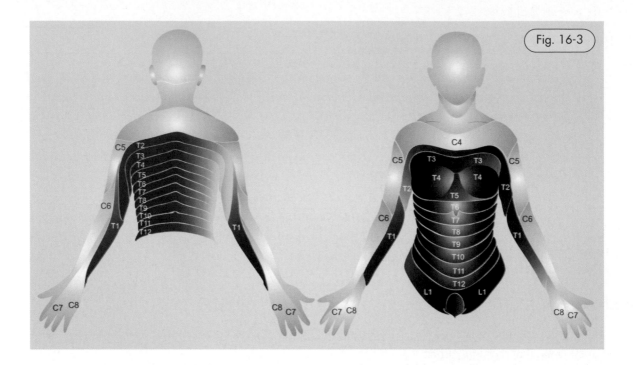

Fig. 16-3

SINGLE-INJECTION THORACIC PARAVERTEBRAL BLOCK

Patient Positioning

The patient is positioned in the sitting or lateral decubitus position and supported by an attendant **(Fig. 16-4)**. The back should assume kyphosis, similar to the position required for neuraxial anesthesia. The patient's feet rest on a stool to allow greater patient comfort and a greater degree of kyphosis. This increases the distance between the adjacent transverse processes and facilitates advancement of the needle beyond contact with the transverse process.

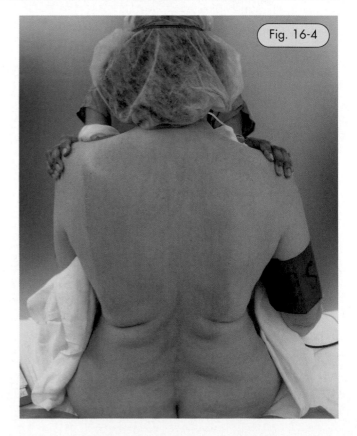

Fig. 16-4

Equipment

A standard regional anesthesia tray is prepared with the following equipment **(Fig. 16-5)**:

- Sterile towels and gauze packs

- 20-mL syringes containing local anesthetic

- Sterile gloves and marking pen

- 1½-in, 25-gauge needle for skin infiltration

- 10-cm, 22-gauge, Quincke- or Tuohy-tip spinal needle

TIP

▶ The use of needles with markings to indicate the depth of insertions is suggested for greater precision.

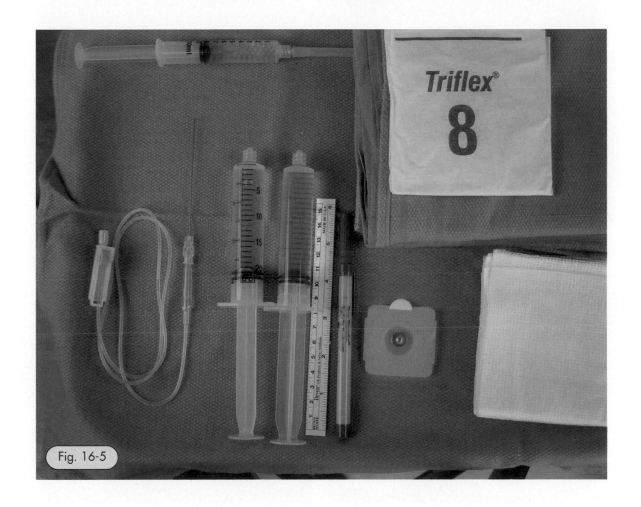

Fig. 16-5

Anatomic Landmarks

The following surface anatomy landmarks are used to identify spinal levels and estimate the position of the transverse processes (**Fig. 16-6 and 16-7**):

1. Spinous processes (midline)

2. Tips of scapulae (corresponds to T7)

3. Paramedial line 2.5 cm lateral to the midline

TIPS

▶ It should be noted that labeling the position of each individual transverse process at the level to be blocked is at best a rough estimation.

▶ It is more practical to outline the midline instead and simply draw the line 2.5 cm laterally to it. All injections will be along this line. Once two first transverse processes are identified, the rest follow the same cranial-caudal spacing.

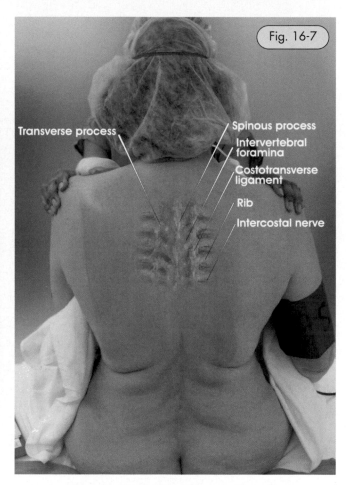

Fig. 16-6

Fig. 16-7

Transverse process

Spinous process

Intervertebral foramina

Costotransverse ligament

Rib

Intercostal nerve

The location of the important anatomic structures: (1) spinous processes, (2) transverse process, (3) intervertebral foramina, (4) costo-transverse ligament, (5) rib, and (6) intercostal nerve.

Local Anesthetic Skin Infiltration

After cleaning the skin with an antiseptic solution, 6 to 10 mL of dilute local anesthetic is infiltrated subcutaneously along the line where the injections will be made **(Fig. 16-8)**. The injection should be carried out slowly to avoid pain on injection. New needle reinsertions should be made through previously anesthetized skin.

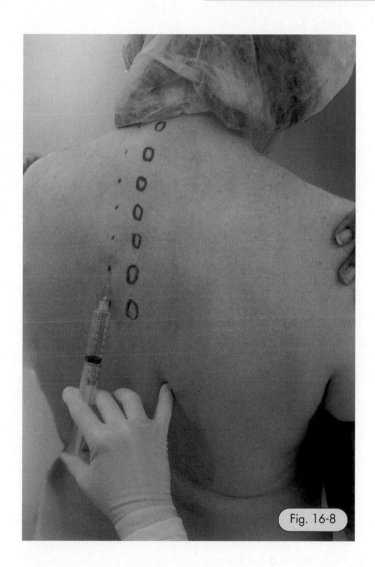

Fig. 16-8

Needle Insertion

The needle is inserted perpendicularly to the skin while paying constant attention to the depth of needle insertion and the medial-lateral needle orientation. The utmost care should be taken to avoid directing the needle medially (risking epidural or spinal injection). After the transverse process is contacted, the needle is withdrawn to skin level and redirected superiorly or inferiorly to "walk off" the transverse process **(Fig. 16-9)**. The ultimate goal is to insert the needle to a depth of 1 cm past the transverse process **(Fig. 16-10)**. A certain "give" occasionally can be felt as the needle passes through the costotransverse ligament; however, this is nonspecific and should not be relied on.

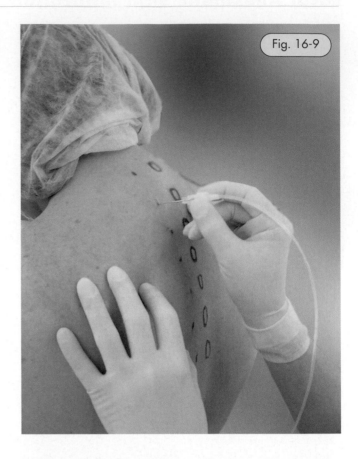

Fig. 16-9

TIP

▶ The block procedure essentially consists of 3 maneuvers **(Fig. 16-10)**:

1. Contact the transverse process of individual vertebrae and note the depth at which the process was contacted (usually 2 to 4 cm), *(needle 1.)*

2. Withdraw the needle to skin level and reinsert it at a 10° caudal or cephalad angulation.

3. Walk off the transverse process 1 cm deeper to the transverse process and inject 4 to 5 mL of local anesthetic, *(needle 2.)*

The needle can be redirected to walk off the superior or inferior aspect of the transverse process. At levels of T7 and below, walking off the inferior aspect of the transverse process is recommended to reduce the risk of intrapleural placement of the needle **(Fig. 16-11)**. Proper handling of the needle is important both for accuracy and safety. Once the transverse process is contacted, the needle should be regripped so that the gripping fingers allow only a 1-cm deeper insertion.

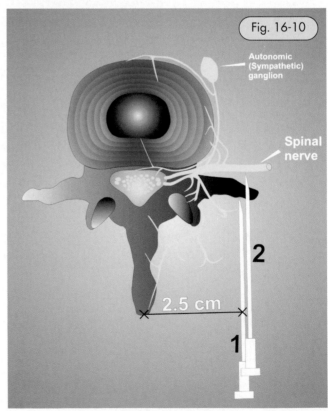

Fig. 16-10

Autonomic (Sympathetic) ganglion

Spinal nerve

2

2.5 cm

1

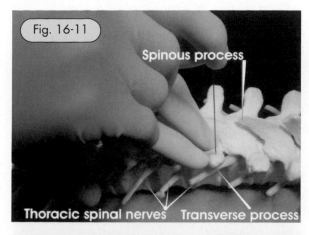

Spinous process

Thoracic spinal nerves   Transverse process

Fig. 16-11

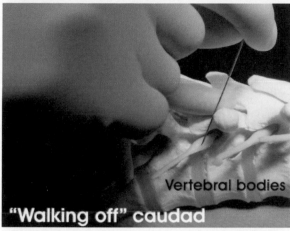

Vertebral bodies

"Walking off" caudad

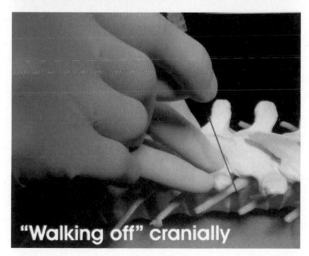

"Walking off" cranially

► While some authors suggest using a loss-of-resistance technique to identify the paravertebral space, such a change in resistance is subtle and nonspecific at best. For this reason, we do not pay attention to the loss of resistance but carefully measure the skin–transverse process distance and simply advance the needle 1 cm past the transverse process.

► Never redirect the needle medially because of the risk of intraforaminal needle passage and consequent spinal cord injury.

► Use common sense in advancing the needle. The depth at which the transverse processes are contacted varies with a patient's body habitus and the level at which the block is performed. The deepest levels are at the high thoracic (T1 and T2) and low lumbar levels (L4 and T5) where the transverse process is contacted at a depth of 6 to 8 cm in average-sized patients. The shallowest depth is at the midthoracic levels (T5 and T10) where the transverse processes are contacted at 2 to 4 cm in an average-sized patients.

► Never disconnect the needle from the tubing or the syringe containing local anesthetic while the needle is inserted. Instead, use a stopcock to switch from syringe to syringe during injection.

Choice of Local Anesthetic

It is almost always beneficial to achieve longer-acting anesthesia or analgesia in a thoracic paravertebral blockade by using a longer-acting local anesthetic. Unless lower lumbar levels (L2 through L5) are scheduled to be blocked, paravertebral blocks do not result in motor blockade of an extremity and do not impair the patient's ability to ambulate or take care of themselves. In addition, relatively small volumes injected at several levels do not present a concern for local anesthetic toxicity.

Some commonly used local anesthetic solutions and their dynamics with this block are listed in **Table 16.1.**

TABLE 16.1
Choice of Local Anesthetic for Paravertebral Block

ANESTHETIC	ONSET (min)	DURATION OF ANESTHESIA (h)	DURATION OF ANALGESIA (h)
1.5% Mepivacaine (+ HCO$_3$ plus epinephrine)	10–20	2–3	3–4
2% Lidocaine (HCO$_3$ + epinephrine)	10–15	2–3	3–4
0.5% Ropivacaine	15–25	3–5	8–12
0.75% Ropivacaine	10–15	4–6	12–18
0.5% Bupivacaine (+ epinephrine)	15–25	4–6	12–18
0.5% 1-bupivacaine (+ epinephrine)	15–25	4–6	12–18

TIP

▶ In patients undergoing multiple-level blockade, consider using alkalinized 3-chloroprocaine for skin infiltration to decrease the total dose of the more toxic long-acting local anesthetic. Chloroprocaine is rapidly metabolized by plasma cholinesterase on absorption.

Block Dynamics and Perioperative Management

Placement of a paravertebral block is associated with moderate patient discomfort. Adequate sedation (midazolam 2 to 4 mg) is necessary to facilitate placement of the block. We routinely administer alfentanil 250 to 750 μg just before beginning the block procedure. However, excessive sedation should be avoided because positioning becomes difficult when patients cannot keep their balance in a sitting position. The blockade depends on dispersion of the anesthetic within the space to reach the individual roots at the level of the injection. The first sign of the blockade is the loss of pinprick sensation at the dermatomal distribution of the root being blocked. The higher the concentration and volume of local anesthetic used, the faster the onset.

CONTINUOUS THORACIC PARAVERTEBRAL BLOCK

Continuous thoracic paravertebral blockade is an advanced regional anesthesia technique, and adequate experience with the single-injection technique is necessary. The continuous thoracic paravertebral block technique is more suitable for analgesia than for surgical anesthesia. The resultant blockade can be thought of as a unilateral continuous thoracic epidural, except that there are no significant hemodynamic changes. The technique is somewhat similar to the single-injection technique, except that the needle should be properly angled to allow insertion of the catheter. This technique provides excellent analgesia and is devoid of significant hemodynamic effects in patients following mastectomy and unilateral chest surgery.

Patient Positioning

The patient is positioned in the supine or lateral decubitus position **(Fig. 16-12)**. In our practice, this block is used mostly with patients undergoing various thoracic procedures. For practical reasons, most catheters are placed postoperatively, just before the patient emerges from general anesthesia. Because these patients are typically already positioned in the lateral decubitus position, this practice precludes the need for special patient positioning or premedication for the block placement. In addition, the risk of pneumothorax is nonexistent because the patients already have a chest tube inserted. However, the ability to clearly visualize spinous processes is crucial.

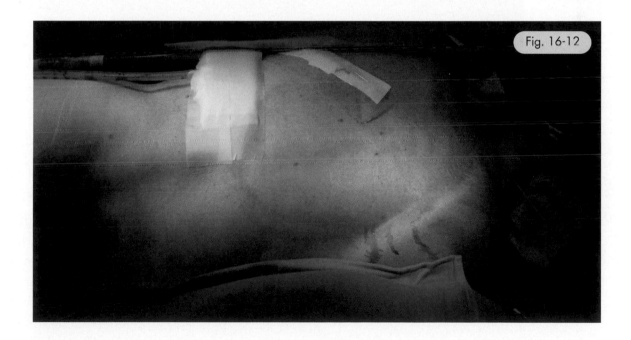

Fig. 16-12

Equipment

A standard regional anesthesia tray is prepared with the following equipment:

- Sterile towels and gauze packs

- 20-mL syringe containing local anesthetic

- Sterile gloves and marking pen

- $1^1/_2$-in, 25-gauge needle for skin infiltration

- 5-cm, insulated stimulating needle (Tuohy-style or Quincke tip)

- Catheter

Landmarks

The landmarks for a continuous paravertebral block are identical to those for the single-injection technique **(see Fig. 16-3)**:

1. Midline (spinous processes)

2. Paramedial line (2.5 cm lateral to the spinous processes)

TIP

▶ For continuous paravertebral blockade, the catheter is ideally inserted one to two segmental levels below the thoracotomy incision line.

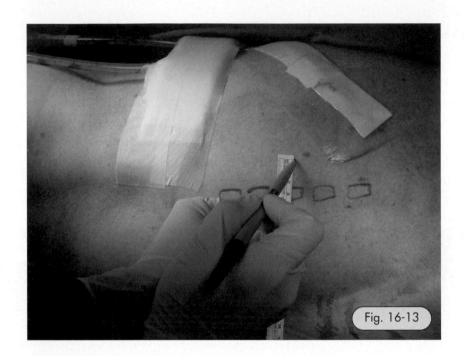

Fig. 16-13

Local Anesthetic Infiltration and Needle Insertion

The subcutaneous tissues and paravertebral muscles are infiltrated with local anethetic to decrease the discomfort at the site of needle insertion. The needle is attached to a syringe containing local anethetic via an extension tubing and advanced in a saggital, slightly cephalad plane to contact the transverse process **(Fig. 16-14)**. Once the transverse process is contacted, the needle is withdrawn back to skin level and reinserted cephalad at a 10° to 15° angle to walk off 1 cm past the transverse process and enter the paravertebral space. As the paravertebral space is entered, a certain "give" is sometimes perceived, but it should not be relied on as the target. Once the paravertebral space is entered, the initial bolus of local anesthetic (5 to 6 mL) is injected through the needle. The catheter is inserted about 5 cm beyond the needle tip **(Fig. 16-15)**. The catheter is then secured using a solution of benzoin and an occlusive dressing and clearly labeled "paravertebral nerve block catheter" **(Fig. 16-16)**. The catheter should be carefully checked for air, cerebrospinal fluid, and blood before administering a local anesthetic or starting a continuous infusion.

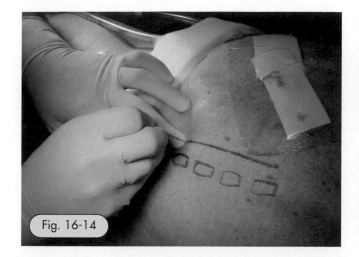

Fig. 16-14

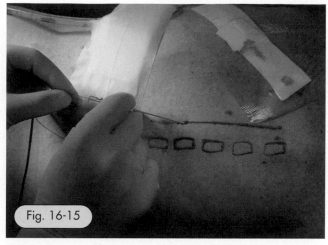

Fig. 16-15

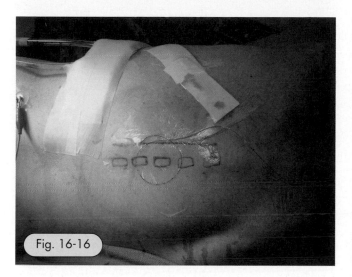

Fig. 16-16

TIPS

► Care must be exercised to prevent medial orientation of the needle (risk of intraepidural or spinal placement).

► If it is deemed that the needle is inserted too laterally (inability to advance due to needle-rib contact), the needle should be *reinserted* medially rather than oriented medially (to avoid a risk of spinal cord injury).

► A distinct "give" is often felt as the needle passes through the costovertebral ligament. However, advancing the needle geometrically 1 cm past the transverse process is more accurate.

Management of the Continuous Infusion

Continuous infusion is initiated after an initial bolus of dilute local anesthetic is administered through the catheter. The bolus injection consists of a small volume of 0.5% ropivacaine or bupivacaine (e.g., 8 mL). For continuous infusion, 0.2% ropivacaine or 0.25% bupivacaine (levobupivacaine) is also suitable. Local anesthetic is infused at 10 mL/hr or 6 mL/h when a patient-controlled analgesia (PCA) dose (4 mL every 30 minutes) is planned.

TIPS

► Breakthrough pain in patients undergoing continuous infusion is always managed by administering a bolus of local anesthetic. Increasing the rate of infusion alone is rarely adequate.

► When the bolus injection through the catheter fails to result in blockade after 30 minutes, the catheter should be considered dislodged and should be removed.

► Every patient receiving a paravertebral block infusion should be prescribed an immediately available alternative pain management protocol because incomplete analgesia and catheter dislodgment can occur. For inpatients, this is probably best done using backup intravenous PCA.

Complications and How to Avoid Them

TABLE 16.2
Complications of Thoracic Paravertebral Block and Preventive Techniques

Infection	• A strict aseptic technique should be used.
Hematoma	• Avoid multiple needle insertions in patients undergoing anticoagulation therapy.
Local anesthetic toxicity	• Rare.
	• Large volumes of long-acting anesthetic should be reconsidered in older and frail patients.
	• Consider using chloroprocaine for skin infiltration to decrease the total dose of the more toxic, long-acting local anesthetic.
Nerve injury	• Local anesthetic should never be injected when a patient complains of severe pain or exhibits a withdrawal reaction on injection.
Total spinal anesthesia	• Avoid medial angulation of the needle, which can result in an inadvertent epidural or subarachnoid needle placement.
	• Aspirate before injection (to detect blood and cerebrospinal fluid).
Quadriceps muscle weakness	• Can occur when the levels are not accurately determined and the levels below L1 are blocked (femoral nerve; L2 through L4).
Paravertebral muscle pain	• Paravertebral muscle pain, resembling a muscle spasm, is occasionally seen, particularly in young, muscular men and when a larger-gauge, Tuohy-tip needle is used.
	• Injection of local anesthetic into the paravertebral muscle before needle insertion and the use of a smaller-gauge (e.g., 22 gauge) Quincke-tip needle is suggested to avoid this side effect.

SUGGESTED READINGS

Paravertebral Block

• Conacher ID, Kokri M. Postoperative paravertebral blocks for thoracic surgery: a radiological appraisal. Br J Anaesth 1987;59:155.

• Coveney E, Weltz CR, Greengrass R, Iglehart JD, Leight GS, Steele SM, Lyerly HK. Use of paravertebral block anesthesia in the surgical management of breast cancer: experience in 156 cases. Ann Surg 1998;227:496–501.

• Greengrass RA, Klein SM, D'Ercole FJ, Gleason DG, Shimer CL, Steele SM. Lumbar plexus and sciatic nerve block for knee arthroplasty: comparison of ropivacaine and bupivacaine. Can J Anaesth 1998;45:1094–1096.

• Hadžić A, Vloka JD, Kuroda MM, Koorn R, Birnbach DJ. The practice of peripheral nerve blocks in the United States: a national survey. Reg Anesth Pain Med 1998;23:241–246.

• Karmakar MK. Thoracic paravertebral block. Anesthesiology 2001;95:771–780.

• Klein SM, Bergh A, Steele SM, Georgiade GS, Greengrass RA. Thoracic paravertebral block for breast surgery. Anesth Analg 2000;90:1402–1405.

- Kopacz DJ, Thompson GE. Neural blockade of the thorax and abdomen. In: Cousins MJ, Bridenbaugh PO, eds. *Neuronal Blockade in Clinical Anesthesia and Management of Pain.* Philadelphia, Pa: Lippincott-Raven, 1988;451–485.
- Pusch F, Wildling E, Klimscha W, Weinstable C. Sonographic measurement of needle insertion depth in paravertebral blocks in women. *Br J Anaesth* 2002;85:841-843.
- Richardson J, Sabanathan S. Thoracic paravertebral analgesia. *Acta Anaesthesiol Scand* 1995;39:1005–1015.
- Terheggen MA, Wille F, Borel Rinkes IH, Ionescu TI, Knape JT. Paravertebral blockade for minor breast surgery. *Anesth Analg* 2002;94:355–359.
- Wheeler LJ. Peripheral nerve stimulation end-point for thoracic paravertebral block. *Br J Anaesth* 2001;86:598.

Continuous Paravertebral Block

- Buckenmaier CC III, Steele SM, Nielsen KC, Martin AH, Klein SM. Bilateral continuous paravertebral catheters for reduction mammoplasty. *Acta Anaesthesiol Scand* 2002;46:1042–1045.
- Catala E, Casas JI, Unzueta MC, Diaz X, Aliaga L, Landeira JM. Continuous infusion is superior to bolus doses with thoracic paravertebral blocks after thoracotomies. *J Cardiothorac Vasc Anesth* 1996;10:586–588.
- Cheung SL, Booker PD, Franks R, Pozzi M. Serum concentrations of bupivacaine during prolonged continuous paravertebral infusion in young infants. *Br J Anaesth* 1997;79:9–13.
- Eng J, Sabanathan S. Continuous paravertebral block for postthoracotomy analgesia in children. *J Pediatr Surg* 1992;27:556–557.
- Johnson LR, Rocco AG, Ferrante FM. Continuous subpleural-paravertebral block in acute thoracic herpes zoster. *Anesth Analg* 1988;67:1105–1108.
- Ganapathy S, Murkin JM, Boyd DW, Dobkowski W, Morgan J. Continuous percutaneous paravertebral block for minimally invasive cardiac surgery. *J Cardiothorac Vasc Anesth* 1999;13:594-596.
- Hultman JL, Schuleman S, Sharp T, Gilbert TJ. Continuous thoracic paravertebral block. *J Cardiothorac Anesth* 1989;3:54.
- Karmakar MK, Booker PD, Franks R. Bilateral continuous paravertebral block used for postoperative analgesia in an infant having bilateral thoracotomy. *Paediatr Anaesth* 1997;7:469–471.
- Richardson J, Sabanathan S, Jones J, Shah RD, Cheema S, Mearns AJ. A prospective, randomized comparison of preoperative and continuous balanced epidural or paravertebral bupivacaine on post-thoracotomy pain, pulmonary function and stress responses. *Br J Anaesth* 1999;83:387–392.
- Terheggen MA, Wille F, Borel Rinkes IH, Ionescu TI, Knape JT. Paravertebral blockade for minor breast surgery. *Anesth Analg* 2002;94:355–359.

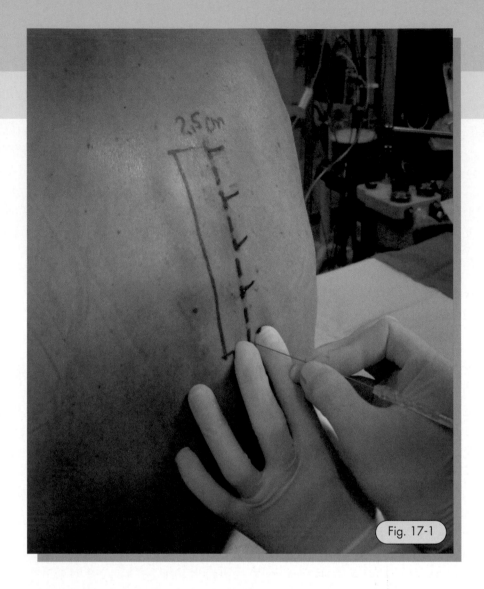

Fig. 17-1

BLOCK AT A GLANCE

- Indications: Inguinal hernia surgery, lateral abdominal wall surgery

- Landmarks: spinal processes T9 through L5 (the number and location of levels is chosen for each indication), transverse process

- Needle insertion: 2 cm lateral to the midline

- Target: needle insertion 1 cm past the transverse process

- Local anesthetic: 5 mL per level

- Complexity level: advanced

17 THORACOLUMBAR
PARAVERTEBRAL BLOCK

GENERAL CONSIDERATIONS

A paravertebral block is an advanced nerve block technique. Although in principle the procedure is similar to that for a thoracic prevertebral block, its anatomy and indications are sufficiently distinct to deserve separate consideration. It is paradoxical that this technique is one of the easiest and most time-efficient to perform, yet it is one of the most difficult to teach. It involves stereotactic needle maneuvering, and a certain mechanical ability or sense of geometry is helpful in mastering it. A paravertebral block is a selective block of the nerve roots at the chosen levels, and the resultant anesthesia or analgesia is conceptually similar to a "unilateral" epidural anesthesia. Higher or lower levels can be chosen to accomplish a bandlike segmental blockade at the desired levels. However, a paravertebral block does not result in a hemodynamically significant sympathetic blockade; therefore, hypotension is not commonly seen. This block is used most commonly in our practice for surgical patients undergoing inguinal herniorrhaphy. For this indication, it is important to avoid blockade of the L2 level (femoral nerve), which affects the ability to ambulate. The technique is also well-suited for pain management after hip surgery (T12 through L5).

Anatomy

The walls of the paravertebral space in this region are formed by the parietal pleura or iliopsoas muscle anterolaterally; the vertebral body, intervertebral disk, and intervertebral foramen medially; and the superior costotransverse process posteriorly (higher levels). The spinal nerves in the paravertebral space are submerged in the paravertebral adipose tissue.

The paravertebral space is continuous with the epidural space medially and the contralateral paravertebral space via the prevertebral fascia. The mechanism of action of a paravertebral blockade at this level includes direct penetration of the local anesthetic into the spinal nerve and medial extension through the intervertebral foramina.

Distribution of Anesthesia

A thoracolumbar paravertebral block results in ipsilateral dermatomal anesthesia **(Fig. 17-2)**. The location of the resulting dermatomal distribution of anesthesia or analgesia is the function of the level blocked and the volume of local anesthetic injected.

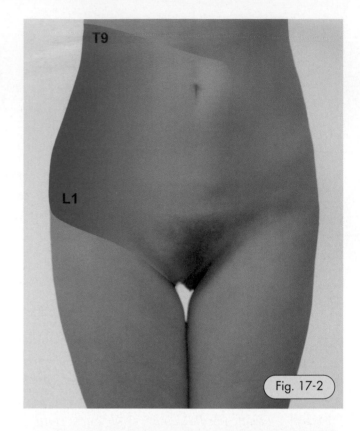

Fig. 17-2

Patient Positioning

The patient is positioned in the sitting or lateral decubitus position and supported by an attendant **(Fig. 17-3)**. The back should assume kyphosis, similar to the position required for neuraxial anesthesia. The patient's feet should rest on a stool to allow for greater comfort and a greater degree of kyphosis. This increases the distance between the adjacent transverse processes and facilitates advancement of the needle beyond contact with the transverse process.

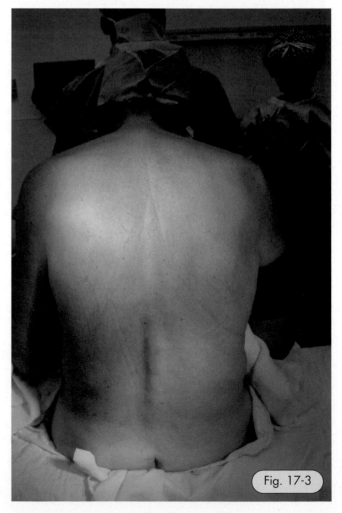

Fig. 17-3

Equipment

A standard regional anesthesia tray is prepared with the following equipment **(Fig. 17-4)**:

- Sterile towels and gauze packs

- 20-mL syringes containing local anesthetic

- Sterile gloves, marking pen

- $1^1/_2$-in, 25- gauge needle for skin infiltration

- 10-cm, long 22-gauge, Quincke or Tuohy-tip spinal needle

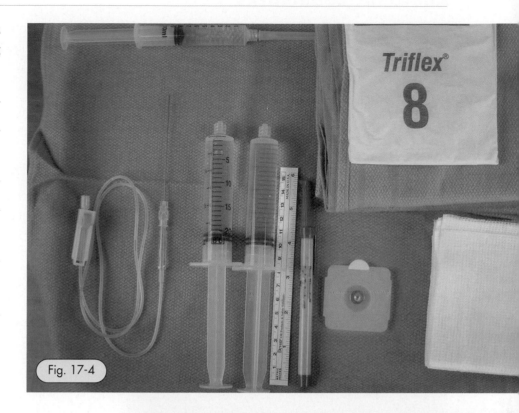

Fig. 17-4

Surface Landmarks

The following bony surface anatomy landmarks are helpful in identifying spinal levels and in estimating the position of the transverse processes **(Fig. 17-5)**:

1. Iliac crest (corresponds to L3-4 or L2-3)

2. Spinous processes (midline)

3. Tips of scapulae (corresponds to T7)

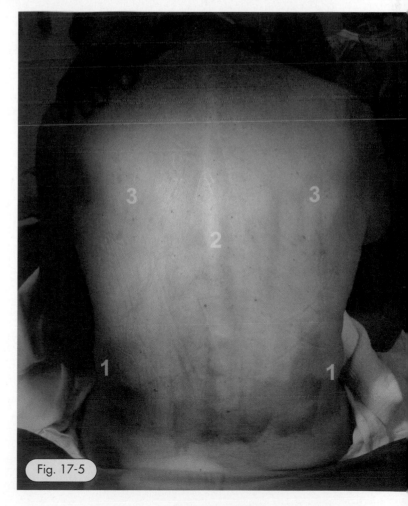

Fig. 17-5

Anatomic Landmarks

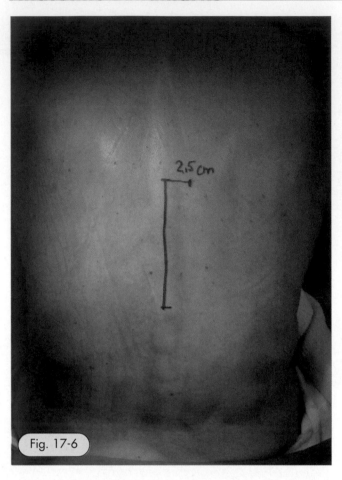

Fig. 17-6

Before attempting the block, all relevant landmarks should be outlined with a pen **(Fig. 17-6)**. These include:

1. Midline

2. 2.5 cm lateral to the midline

TIPS

▶ It should be noted that labeling the position of each individual transverse process at the level to be blocked is at best a rough estimation.

▶ Instead it is more practical to outline the midline instead and simply draw the line 2.5 cm lateral to it. All injections will be along this line. Once the first two transverse processes are identified, the rest will follow the same cranial-caudal spacing.

▶ When lower lumbar levels are involved, keep in mind that the needle should be inserted closer to 2-cm lateral to the midline because the transverse processes of the lower lumbar vertebrae are shorter and smaller than at the higher lumbar or thoracic levels.

Local Anesthetic Skin Infiltration

After cleaning the skin with an antiseptic solution, 5 to 10 mL of dilute local anesthetic is infiltrated subcutaneously along the line where the injections will be made. The injection should be carried out slowly to avoid pain on injection; new needle re-insertions should be made through previously anesthetized skin.

Hand Position

The fingers of the palpating hand should straddle the paramedial line and fix the skin to avoid medial-lateral skin movement **(Fig. 17-7)**. This hand is moved in the cranial-caudal position only during block placement. The needle is inserted perpendicular to the skin, paying constant attention to the depth of insertion and the medial-lateral orientation. The entire block procedure consists of 3 maneuvers **(Fig. 17-8)**:

1. Contact the transverse process of the individual vertebrae and note the depth at which the process was contacted **(Fig. 17-8A)**.

2. Withdraw the needle to skin level and reinsert it at a 10° superior or inferior angle.

3. "Walk off" the transverse process 1 cm deeper to the transverse process and inject 4 to 5 mL of local anesthetic **(Fig. 17-8B)**.

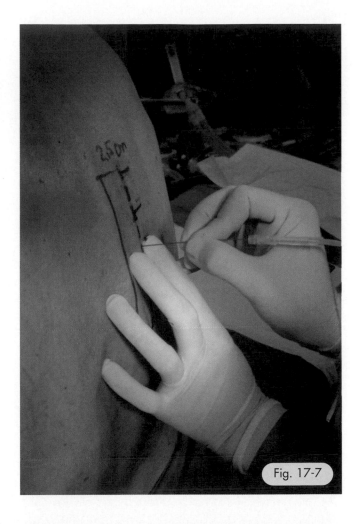

Fig. 17-7

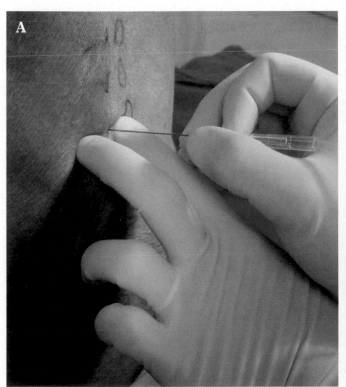

A

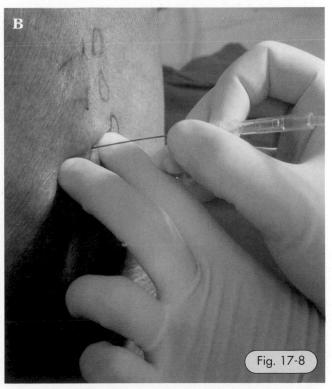

B

Fig. 17-8

An example of caudal needle redirection after contacting the transverse process.

Some authors suggest using a loss-of-resistance technique to identify the paravertebral space. However, such a change in resistance, even when present, is very subtle and nonspecific at best. For this reason, we do not pay attention to the loss of resistance but carefully measure the skin–transverse process distance and simply advance the needle 1 cm past the process. A certain "give" may occasionally be felt as the needle passes through the costotransverse ligament; however, this is obviously not the case at the lumbar level.

Proper handling of the needle is important for both accuracy and safety. Once the transverse process is contacted, the needle should be regripped so that the fingers allow insertion of the needle 1 cm beyond the transverse process.

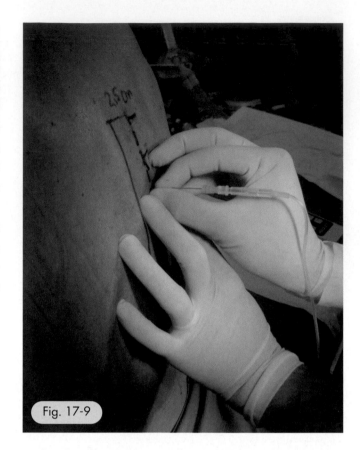

Fig. 17-9

TIPS

▶ The needle should not be directed medially because of the risk of intra-foraminal needle passage and consequent spinal cord injury.

▶ Use common sense in advancing the needle. The depth at which the transverse processes are contacted varies with the patient's body habitus and the level at which the block is performed. The deepest levels are at the high thoracic (T1 and T2) and low lumbar levels (L4 and L5) where the transverse process is contacted at a depth of 6 to 8 cm in average-sized patients. The shallowest depth is at the mid-thoracic levels (T5 to T10) where the transverse processes are contacted at 2 to 4 cm in average-sized patients.

▶ Never disconnect the tubing from the needle (e.g., for a syringe change) during the block procedure when performing blocks at the thoracic levels. In cases where the needle tip is inadvertently placed in the chest cavity, a pneumothorax should not occur as long as the needle opening is sealed (no communication between the chest cavity and the air outside).

▶ Needles with depth markings are particularly well-suited for this block.

Choice of Local Anesthetic

Unless lower lumbar levels (L2 through L5) are blocked, paravertebral blocks do not result in motor block of an extremity and do not impair the patient's ability to ambulate. In addition, relatively small volumes injected at several levels do not present a concern for local anesthetic toxicity. For these reasons, it is almost always beneficial to achieve longer-acting blockade by using longer-acting local anesthetic. Some commonly used local anesthetic solutions and their dynamics with this block are listed in **Table 17.1.**

TABLE 17.1
Choice of Local Anesthetic for Paravertebral Block

ANESTHETIC	ONSET (min)	DURATION OF ANESTHESIA (h)	DURATION OF ANALGESIA (h)
1.5% Mepivacaine (HCO$_3$ + epinephrine)	10–20	2–3	3–4
2% Lidocaine (HCO$_3$ + epinephrine)	10–15	2–3	3–4
0.5% Ropivacaine	15–25	3–5	8–12
0.75% Ropivacaine	10–15	4–6	12–18
0.5% Bupivacaine (+ epinephrine)	15–25	4–6	12–18
0.5% Levobupivacaine (+ epinephrine)	15–25	4–6	12–18

TIP

▶ In patients undergoing a multiple-level blockade, consider using alkalinized 3-chloroprocaine for skin infiltration to decrease the total dose of the more toxic long-acting local anesthetic. Chloroprocaine is an ester-linked local anesthetic and is rapidly metabolized by plasma cholinesterase on absorption.

Block Dynamics and Perioperative Management

The onset time for this block is slightly longer than for many other block techniques (15 to 25 minutes). The blockade depends on anesthetic dispersion within the space to reach the individual roots at the level of the injection. The first sign of blockade is the loss of pinprick sensation at the dermatomal distribution of the root being blocked. The higher the concentration of local anesthetic used, the sooner the onset can be expected.

TABLE 17.2
Complications of Thoracic Lumbar Paravertebral Block and Preventive Techniques

Infection	• A strict aseptic technique should be used.
Hematoma	• Avoid multiple needle insertions.
Local anesthetic toxicity	• Large volumes of long-acting anesthetic should be reconsidered in older and frail patients. • Consider using chloroprocaine for skin infiltration to decrease the total dose of the more toxic, long-acting local anesthetic.
Nerve injury	• Local anesthetic should never be injected when the patient complains of severe pain or exhibits a withdrawal reaction on injection.
Total spinal anesthesia	• Can result due to inadvertent subarachnoid injection or longitudinal spread of local anesthetic within dural sleeves. • Avoid medial angulation of the needle, which may result in an inadvertent epidural or subarachnoid needle placement. • Aspirate before injection (to check for blood and cerebrospinal fluid) and avoid forceful injections.
Quadriceps muscle weakness	• This may occur when the levels are not accurately determined and the levels below L1 are blocked (femoral nerve, L2 through L4). When unsure, use shorter acting local anesthetic for the estimated L1 level.
Paravertebral muscle pain	• Paravertebral muscle pain, resembling a muscle spasm, is occasionally seen, particularly in young, muscular men and when a larger-gauge Tuohy needle is used. • Injection of local anesthetic into the paravertebral muscle before needle insertion and the use of a smaller-gauge (e.g., 22-gauge) Quincke-tip needle is suggested to avoid this side effect.

SUGGESTED READINGS

- Karmakar MK. Paravertebral somatic nerve block for outpatient inguinal herniorrhaphy. *Reg Anesth Pain Med* 1999;24:96–97.

- Karmakar MK, Gin T, Ho AM. Ipsilateral thoraco-lumbar anaesthesia and paravertebral spread after low thoracic paravertebral injection. *Br J Anaesth* 2001; 87:312–316.

- Klein SM, Greengrass RA, Weltz C, Warner DS. Paravertebral somatic nerve block for outpatient inguinal herniorrhaphy: an expanded case report of 22 patients. *Reg Anesth Pain Med* 1998;23:306–310.

- Klein SM, Pietrobon R, Nielsen KC, Steele SM, Warner DS, Moylan JA, Eubanks WS, Greengrass RAL. Paravertebral somatic nerve block compared with peripheral nerve blocks for outpatient inguinal herniorrhaphy. *Reg Anesth Pain Med* 2002;27:476–480.

- Kopacz DJ, Thompson GE. Neural blockade of the thorax and abdomen. In: Cousins MJ, Bridenbaugh PO, eds. *Neuronal Blockade in Clinical Anesthesia and Management of Pain.* Philadelphia, Pa: Lippincott-Raven, 1988;451–485.

- Lonnqvist PA, Hildingsson U. The caudal boundary of the thoracic paravertebral space: a study in human cadavers. *Anaesthesia* 1992;47:1051–1052.

- Naja Z, Lonnqvist PA. Somatic paravertebral nerve blockade: incidence of failed block and complications. *Anaesthesia* 2001;56:1184–1188.

- Naja Z, Ziade MF, Lonnqvist PA. Bilateral paravertebral somatic nerve block for ventral hernia repair. *Eur J Anaesthesiol* 2002;19:197–202.

- Pusch F, Wildling E, Klimscha W, Weinstable C. Sonographic measurement of needle insertion depth in paravertebral blocks in women. *Br J Anaesth* 2002; 85:841–843.

- Richardson J, Sabanathan S. Thoracic paravertebral analgesia. *Acta Anaesthesiol Scand* 1995;39:1005-1015.

- Richardson J, Vowden P, Sabanathan S. Bilateral paravertebral analgesia for major abdominal vascular surgery: a preliminary report. *Anaesthesia* 1995; 50:995–998.

- Wassef MR, Randazzo T, Ward W. The paravertebral nerve root block for inguinal herniorrhaphy—a comparison with the field block approach. *Reg Anesth Pain Med* 1998;23:451–456.

- Wheeler LJ. Peripheral nerve stimulation end-point for thoracic paravertebral block. *Br J Anaesth* 2001;86:598.

- Wood GJ, Lloyd JW, Bullingham RE, Britton BJ, Finch DR. Postoperative analgesia for day-case herniorrhaphy patients: a comparison of cryoanalgesia, paravertebral blockade and oral analgesia. *Anaesthesia* 1981; 36:603–610.

- Wyatt SS, Price RA. Complications of paravertebral block. *Br J Anaesth* 2000;84:424.

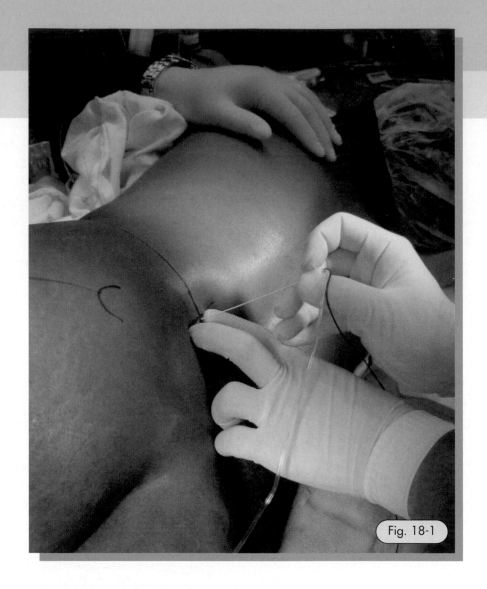

Fig. 18-1

BLOCK AT A GLANCE

- Indications: hip, anterior thigh, and knee surgery

- Landmarks: iliac crest, spinous processes (midline)

- Nerve stimulation: twitch of the quadriceps muscle at 0.5 to 1.0 mA current

- Local anesthetic: 25 to 35 mL

GENERAL CONSIDERATIONS

The lumbar plexus block is an advanced nerve block technique. It has significant clinical applicability and, for this reason, is used commonly in our practice. However, this block has a relatively higher potential for complications and should be practiced only after appropriate training. Because of placement of the needle in the deep muscle beds, the potential for systemic toxicity is greater than with many other techniques. In addition, the proximity of the lumbar nerve roots and epidural space carries a risk of an epidural spread. For these reasons, care should be taken when selecting the type, volume, and concentration of local anesthetic, particularly in elderly and frail patients. In addition, because of the depth of the needle placement, this block is best avoided in very obese patients. A lumbar plexus block provides anesthesia or analgesia to the entire distribution of the lumbar plexus, including the anterolateral and medial thigh, the knee, and the saphenous nerve below the knee. When combined with a sciatic nerve block, anesthesia of the entire leg can be achieved.

Regional Anesthesia Anatomy

The lumbar plexus consists of five nerves on each side, the first of which emerges between the first and second lumbar vertebrae and the last one between the last lumbar vertebra and the base of the sacrum **(Fig. 18-2)**. As soon as the L2 through L4 roots of the lumbar plexus split off their spinal nerves and emerge from the intervertebral foramina, they become embedded in the psoas major muscle. This is because the psoas is attached to the lateral surfaces and transverse processes of the lumbar vertebrae. Within the muscle, these roots then split into anterior and posterior divisions, which then reunite to form the individual branches (nerves) of the plexus.

The major branches of the lumbar plexus are the genitofemoral nerve, lateral femoral cutaneous nerve, femoral nerve, and obturator nerves. The femoral nerve is formed by the posterior divisions of L2 through L4 and descends from the plexus laterally to the psoas muscle. The anterior divisions of the same roots join to form the other major branch of the lumbar plexus, the obturator nerve.

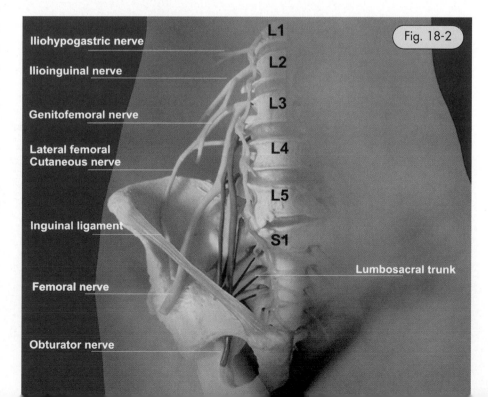

Fig. 18-2

Iliohypogastric nerve
Ilioinguinal nerve
Genitofemoral nerve
Lateral femoral Cutaneous nerve
Inguinal ligament
Femoral nerve
Obturator nerve

L1
L2
L3
L4
L5
S1

Lumbosacral trunk

Distribution of Anesthesia

The femoral nerve supplies motor fibers to the quadriceps muscle (knee extension), the skin of the anteromedial thigh, and the medial aspect of the leg below the knee and foot **(Fig. 18-3)**. The obturator nerve sends motor branches to the adductors of the hip and a highly variable cutaneous area on the medial thigh or knee joint. The lateral femoral cutaneous and genitofemoral nerves are purely cutaneous nerves.

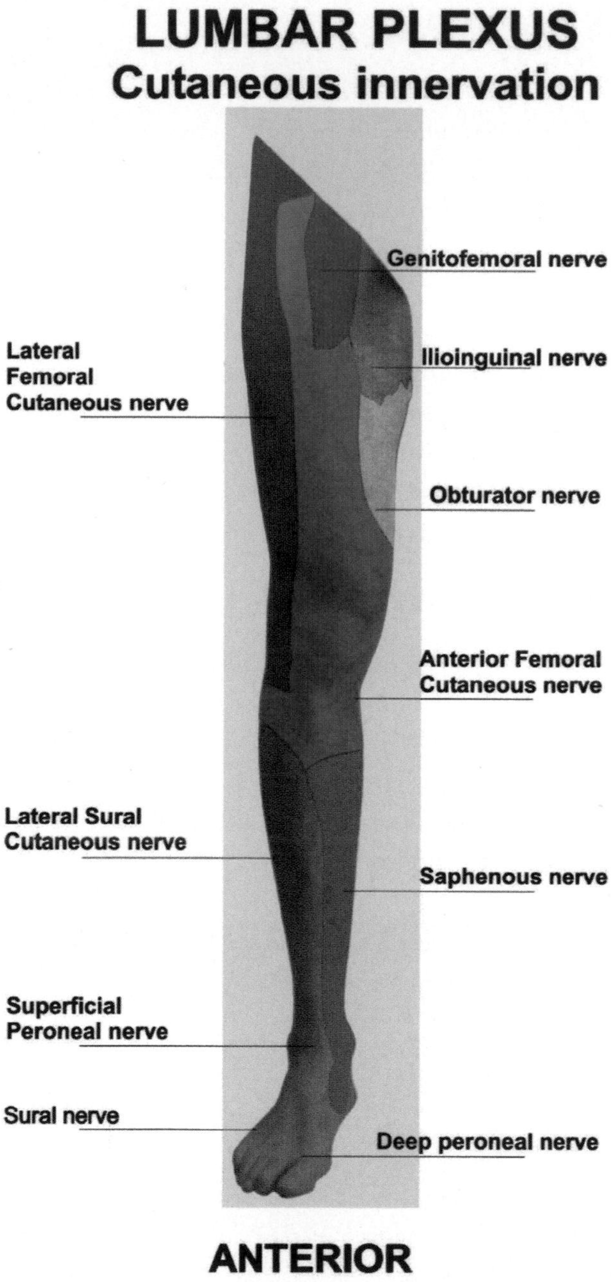

LUMBAR PLEXUS
Cutaneous innervation

Genitofemoral nerve

Lateral Femoral Cutaneous nerve

Ilioinguinal nerve

Obturator nerve

Anterior Femoral Cutaneous nerve

Lateral Sural Cutaneous nerve

Saphenous nerve

Superficial Peroneal nerve

Sural nerve

Deep peroneal nerve

ANTERIOR

Fig. 18-3

The cutaneous innervation of the lumbar plexus.

SINGLE-INJECTION LUMBAR PLEXUS BLOCK

Patient Positioning

The patient is in the lateral decubitus position with a slight forward tilt (**Fig. 18-4**). The foot on the side to be blocked should be positioned over the dependent leg so that twitches of the patella can be seen easily. It is equally important that the anesthesiologist assume a position from which the anterior thigh can be seen so that contractions of the quadriceps muscle are visible.

TIP

▶A slightly forward pelvic tilt in the patient position allows for a more ergonomic position for the anesthesiologist.

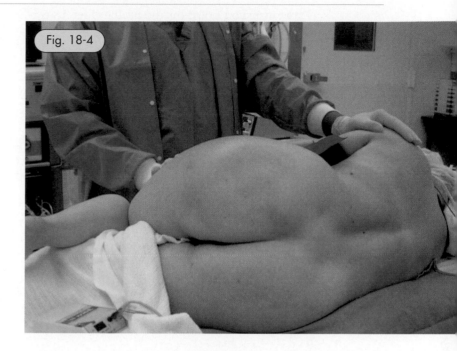

Fig. 18-4

Equipment

A standard regional anesthesia tray is prepared with the following equipment (**Fig. 18-5**):

- Sterile towels and gauze packs

- 20-mL syringes containing local anesthetic

- Sterile gloves, marking pen, and surface electrode

- $1^{1}/_{2}$-in, 25-gauge needle for skin infiltration

- 10-cm, short-bevel, insulated stimulating needle

- Peripheral nerve stimulator

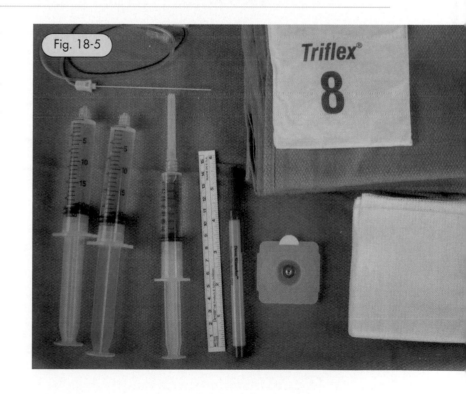

Fig. 18-5

Surface Landmarks

There are only two surface anatomy landmarks that are important in determining the insertion point for the needle **(Fig. 18-6)**:

1. Iliac crest

2. Spinous processes (midline)

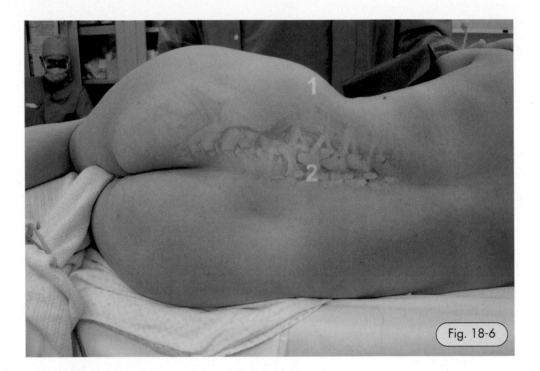

Fig. 18-6

TIPS

▶ The gluteal crease tends to sag to a dependent position. It should never be assumed that it coincides with the midline.

▶ Always use spinous processes to accurately determine the midline.

▶ Position the patient carefully to avoid spinal rotation.

Anatomic Landmarks

Landmarks for the lumbar plexus block include **(Fig. 18-7)**:

1. Iliac crest

2. Midline (spinous processes)

3. Needle insertion 4 cm lateral to the intersection of landmarks 1 and 2

TIPS

▶ Palpation of the iliac crest is best accomplished by placing the palpating hand over the ridge of the pelvic bone and pressing firmly against it **(Fig. 18-8)**.

▶ To better estimate the location of the iliac crest, the thickness of the adipose tissue over the iliac crest should be considered.

▶ Pelvic proportions greatly vary among people; thus a visual "reality check" is always performed. If the estimated iliac crest line appears to be almost at the level of the midtorso or touching the rib cage (too cranial), make an appropriate adjustment to avoid too cranial insertion of the needle.

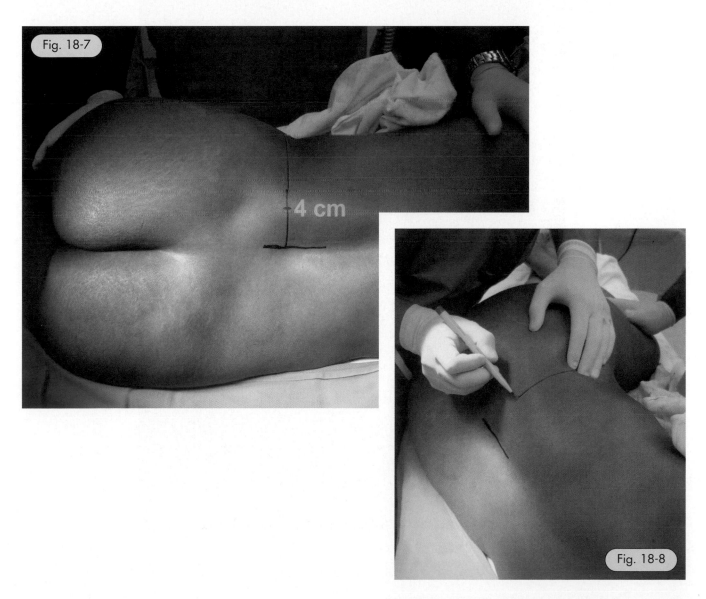

Fig. 18-7

Fig. 18-8

Local Anesthetic Infiltration and Needle Insertion

Local Anesthetic Skin Infiltration

After a cleaning with an antiseptic solution, the skin is anesthetized by infiltrating local anesthetic subcutaneously at the determined needle insertion site **(Fig. 18-9)**.

> **TIP**
>
> ▶ Because the needle can be inserted at any point on the line 4 cm lateral and parallel to the midline, local infiltration should be done along this line rather than at a single projected needle insertion point. This allows for needle reinsertion at another point (if necessary) without a need for additional skin infilration.

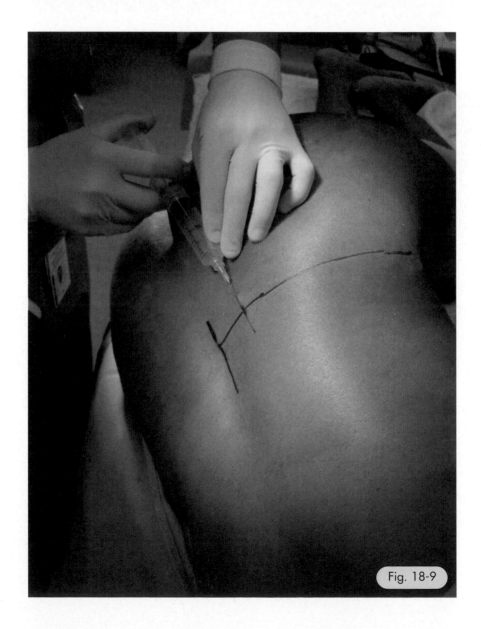

Fig. 18-9

Needle Insertion

The fingers of the palpating hand are firmly pressed against the paravertebral muscles to stabilize the landmark and decrease the skin-nerve distance

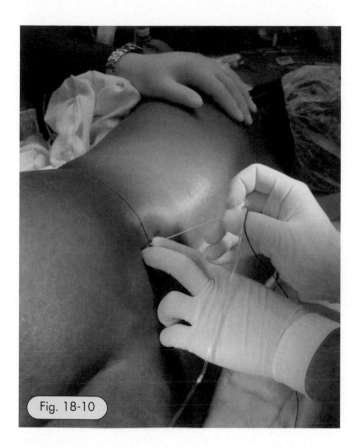

Fig. 18-10

(**Fig. 18-10**). The palpating hand should not be moved during the entire block placement procedure so that precise redirections of the angle of needle insertion can be made, if necessary. The needle is inserted at an angle perpendicular to the skin. The nerve stimulator should be set initially to deliver a current of 1.5 mA. As the needle is advanced, local twitches of the paravertebral muscles are first obtained at a depth of a few centimeters. The needle is then advanced further until twitches of the quadriceps muscle are obtained (usually at a depth of 6 to 8 cm) (**Fig. 18-11**). After these twitches are observed, the current should be lowered to produce stimulation between 0.5 and 1.0 mA. At this point, 25 to 35 mL of local anesthetic is slowly injected with frequent aspirations to rule out inadvertent intravascular placement of the needle.

GOAL

- *Visible or palpable twitches of the quadriceps muscle at 0.5 to 1.0 mA.*

TIPS

▶ A successful lumbar plexus blockade depends on dispersion of the local anesthetic in the fascial plane (psoas muscle) where the roots of the plexus are situated. Thus, the goal of nerve stimulation is to identify this plane by eliciting stimulation of one of the roots.

▶ Stimulation at currents less than 0.5 mA should not be sought when using this technique. Dural sleeves thickly envelop the roots of the lumbar plexus. Motor stimulation with a low current may indicate placement of the needle inside a dural sleeve. An injection inside this sheath can result in tracking of local anesthetic toward the epidural or subarachnoid space, resulting in consequent epidural or spinal anesthesia.

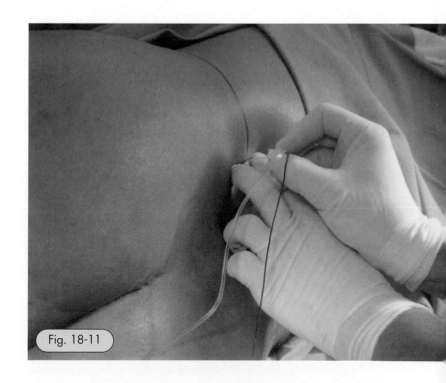

Fig. 18-11

Failure to Obtain a Quadriceps Twitch on the First Needle Pass

When insertion of the needle does not result in quadriceps muscle stimulation, the following maneuvers should be followed:

1. Withdraw the needle to skin level, redirect it 5° to 10° cranially, and repeat the procedure.

2. Withdraw the needle to skin level, redirect it 5° to 10° caudally, and repeat the procedure.

3. Withdraw the needle to skin level, redirect it 5° to 10° medially, and repeat the procedure.

4. Withdraw the needle to skin level, reinsert it 2 cm caudally or cranially, and repeat the procedure.

Interpreting Responses to Nerve Stimulation

TABLE 18.1

Some Common Responses to Nerve Stimulation and the Course of Action to Take to Obtain the Proper Response

RESPONSE OBTAINED	INTERPRETATION	PROBLEM	ACTION
Local twitch of the paraspinal muscles	Direct stimulation of the paraspinal muscles	Too shallow a placement of the needle	Continue advancing the needle
Needle contacts bone at a 4- to 6-cm depth; no twitches are seen	Needle advancement is stopped by the transverse process	Indicates proper needle placement, but requires redirection of the needle	Withdraw the needle to skin level and redirect it 5° cranially or caudally
Twitches of the hamstring muscles are seen; needle is inserted 6–8 cm	This is the result of stimulation of the roots of the sciatic plexus (sciatic nerve)	Needle inserted too caudally	Withdraw the needle and reinsert it 3–5 cm cranially
Flexion of the thigh at a depth of >6–8 cm	This subtle and often missed response is caused by direct stimulation of the psoas muscle	Needle inserted too deep (missed the lumbar plexus roots); further advancement may place the needle intraperitoneally	Stop advancing the needle; withdraw the needle and reinsert it using the protocol outlined in the technique description
The needle is placed deep (10 cm), but twitches were not elicited and bone is not contacted	Needle missed the transverse process and roots of the lumbar plexus	Too deep placement of needle	Withdraw the needle and reinsert it using the protocol outlined in the technique description

Choice of Local Anesthetic

A lumbar plexus blockade requires a relatively large volume of local anesthetic to achieve anesthesia of the entire plexus. The choice of the type and concentration of local anesthetic should be based on whether the block is planned for surgical anesthesia or pain management **(Table 18.2)**. Because of the highly vascular nature of the area, there is a relatively high potential for inadvertent intravascular injection or rapid absorption from the deep muscle beds.

TABLE 18.2
Choice of Local Anesthetic for Lumbar Plexus Block

ANESTHETIC	ONSET (min)	DURATION OF ANESTHESIA (h)	DURATION OF ANALGESIA (h)
3% 2-Chloroprocaine (HCO_3 + epinephrine)	10–15	1.5	2
1.5% Mepivacaine (+ HCO_3)	10–15	2	2–4
1.5% Mepivacaine (HCO_3 + epinephrine)	10–15	2.5–3	2–5
2% Lidocaine (+ HCO_3)	10–20	2.5–3	2–5
2% Lidocaine (HCO_3 + epinephrine)	10–20	5–6	5–8
0.5% Ropivacaine	15–20	4–6	6–10

TIPS

▶ Always assess the risk/benefit ratio of using large volumes and concentrations of long-acting local anesthetic for a lumbar plexus blockade.

▶ A lumbar plexus block carries a higher risk of local anesthetic toxicity than many other nerve block techniques because of its deep location and the close proximity of muscles. For this reason, we tend to avoid high concentrations and large volumes of long-acting local anesthetic with this block.

▶ Smaller volumes and concentrations can be used successfully for analgesia (e.g., 20 mL); however, for surgical anesthesia, 30 mL is usually necessary to achieve a dense blockade of the entire lumbar plexus.

▶ Consider using a less toxic local anesthetic (e.g., alkalinized 3% chloroprocaine) for skin infiltration to avoid a large cumulative dose of local anesthetic.

Block Dynamics and Perioperative Management

A lumbar plexus block can be associated with significant patient discomfort during nerve localization because the needle passes through multiple muscle planes. Adequate sedation and analgesia are necessary to ensure a still, cooperative patient. Typically, we use midazolam 4 to 6 mg after the patient is positioned, and alfentanil 500 to 1000 µg just before needle insertion. A typical onset time for this block is 15 to 25 minutes, depending on the type, concentration, and volume of local anesthetic and the level at which the needle is placed. For example, although an almost immediate onset of anesthesia in the anterior thigh and knee can be achieved with an injection at the L3 level, additional time is required for a local anesthetic to block the lateral thigh (L1) or obturator nerve (L5). The first sign of the onset of blockade is usually a loss of sensation in the saphenous nerve territory (medial skin below the knee).

TIP

▶ Inadequate skin anesthesia despite the apparent timely onset of the blockade can occur. It can take up to 30 minutes for full sensory-motor anesthesia to develop. Local infiltration by the surgeon at the site of the incision is often all that is needed to allow the surgery to proceed.

CONTINUOUS LUMBAR PLEXUS BLOCK

A continuous lumbar plexus blockade is an advanced regional anesthesia technique, and adequate experience with the single-injection technique is a prerequisite to ensure its efficacy and safety. Otherwise, the technique is quite similar to the single-injection procedure, except that a Tuohy-style needle is preferred. The needle opening should be directed cephalad to facilitate threading of the catheter. This technique can be used for postoperative pain management in patients undergoing hip, femur, and knee surgery.

Patient Positioning

As for the single-injection technique, the patient is positioned in the lateral decubitus position with the side to be blocked up and at a slightly forward pelvic tilt **(Fig. 18-12)**. An assistant helps to maintain flexion of the spine, as in positioning a patient for an epidural or spinal block in the lateral position.

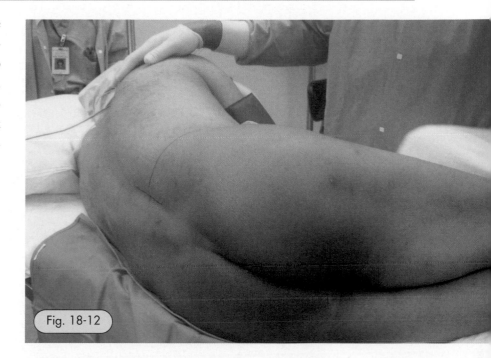

Fig. 18-12

Equipment

A standard regional anesthesia tray is prepared with the following equipment **(Fig. 18-13)**:

- Sterile towels and gauze packs

- 20-mL syringes containing local anesthetic

- Sterile gloves, marking pen, and surface electrode

- $1^1/_2$-in, 25-gauge needle for skin infiltration

- 10-cm, insulated stimulating needle (preferably with a Tuohy-style tip)

- Catheter

- Peripheral nerve stimulator

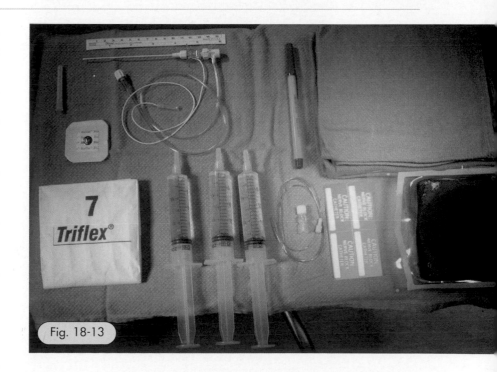

Fig. 18-13

Landmarks

The landmarks for a continuous lumbar plexus block are the same as for the single-injection technique **(Fig. 18-14)**:

1. Iliac crest

2. Midline (spinous processes)

3. Needle insertion site 4 cm lateral to the midline and above the iliac crest line

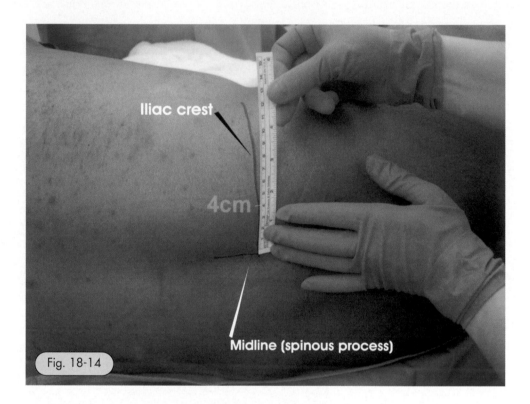

Fig. 18-14

Local Anesthetic Infiltration and Needle Insertion

The skin and subcutaneous tissues are anesthetized with local anethetic. The needle is attached to the nerve stimulator (1.5 mA, 2 Hz, 100–300 μs) and to a syringe containing local anesthetic, via flexible tubing. The palpating hand should be firmly pressed and anchored against the paraspinal muscles to facilitate needle insertion and redirection of the needle when necessary **(Fig. 18-15)**. A 10-cm, Tuohy-style continuous block needle is inserted at a perpendicular angle and advanced until the quadriceps twitch response is obtained at 0.5 to 1.0 mA current. At this point, the initial volume of local anesthetic is injected (e.g., 15 to 25 mL) and the catheter is inserted approximately 8 to 10 cm beyond the needle tip. The needle is then withdrawn back to skin level while the catheter is simultaneously advanced. This method prevents inadvertent removal of the catheter. Before administering local anesthetic, the catheter is checked for inadvertent intravascular and intrathecal placement by performing an aspiration test.

▶ It is useful to inject some local anesthetic intramuscularly to prevent pain on advancement of a larger-gauge or blunt-tipped needle used for a continuous block.

▶ The opening of the needle tip should be oriented cephalad before threading the catheter.

▶The skin in the lumbar area may be highly movable, thus, insertion of the catheter to a depth of 8 to10 cm is necessary to help prevent its removal during patient repositioning, and so on.

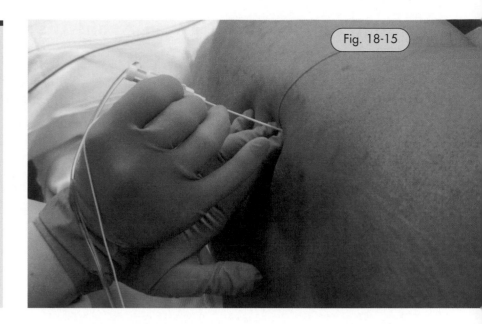

Fig. 18-15

Continuous Infusion

Continuous infusion is always initiated after an initial bolus of dilute local anesthetic through the catheter. For this purpose, we routinely use 0.2% ropivacaine 15 to 20 mL. Diluted bupivacaine or levobupivacaine is also suitable but can result in additional motor blockade. The infusion is maintained at 10 mL/h or 5 mL/h when a patient-controlled analgesia (PCA) dose (5 mL every 30 minutes) is planned.

▶Breakthrough pain in patients receiving a continuous infusion is always managed by administering a bolus of local anesthetic (**Fig. 18-16**). Simply increasing the rate of infusion is rarely adequate. For patients on the ward, a higher concentration of a shorter-acting local anesthetic (e.g., 1% mepivacaine) is useful to both manage the pain and test the position of the catheter.

▶When the bolus injection through the catheter fails to result in a blockade after 30 minutes, the catheter should be considered dislodged and should be removed.

▶ Every patient receiving a lumbar plexus block infusion should be prescribed an alternative pain management protocol because incomplete analgesia and catheter dislodgment can occur. For inpatients, this is probably best done using backup intravenous PCA.

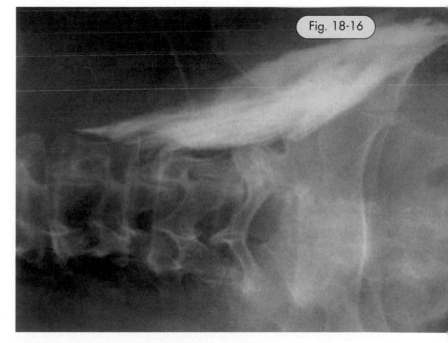

Fig. 18-16

Figure 18.16 shows the dispersion of 20 mL of a contrast solution within the psoas sheath.

Complications and How to Avoid Them

The lumbar plexus block carries a potential for serious complications, but is an advanced technique with a significant clinical applicability. Some general and specific instructions on possible complications and methods for avoiding them are discussed in **Table 18.3**.

TABLE 18.3
Complications of Lumbar Plexus Block and Preventive Techniques

Infection	• A strict aseptic technique is used.
Hematoma	• Avoid multiple needle insertions. • Continuous lumbar plexus blocks are best avoided in patients receiving anticoagulant therapy. • The use of antiplatelet therapy is not a contraindication for this block in the absence of spontaneous bleeding.
Vascular puncture	• Vascular puncture is not common with this technique. • Deep needle insertion should be avoided (vena cava, aorta).
Local anesthetic toxicity	• Higher volume of local anesthetic result in more solid, complete, and faster blockade; however, it carries a higher risk of toxicity. • Large volumes of long-acting anesthetic should be avoided in older and frail patients. • Careful, frequent aspiration should be performed during the injection. • Avoid fast, forceful injection of local anesthetic.
Nerve injury	• The risk of nerve injury after lumbar plexus is low. • Local anesthetic should never be injected when the patient complains of pain on injection or abnormally high pressure is noted. • When stimulation is obtained with current intensity of <0.5 mA, the needle should be pulled back to obtain the same response with a current of 0.5 to 10 mA before injecting local anesthetic to avoid injection into the dural sleeves and the consequent epidural or spinal spread.
Hemodynamic consequences	• Lumbar plexus blockade results in unilateral sympathectomy; as such, significant hypotension is rare in the absence of epidural spread of local anesthetic. • Spread of the local anesthetic to the epidural space may result in significant hypotension and occurs in as many as 15% of patients. • Every patient receiving a lumbar plexus block should be monitored to the same extent as patients receiving epidural anesthesia.

SUGGESTED READINGS

- Brown DL, Bridenbaugh LD. The upper extremity: somatic block. In: Cousins MJ, Bridenbaugh PO, eds. *Neuronal Blockade in Clinical Anesthesia and Management of Pain*. Philadelphia, Pa: Lippincott-Raven, 1988; 345–371.

- Capdevila X, Macaire P, Dadure C, Choquet O, Biboulet P, Ryckwaert Y, D'Athis F. Continuous psoas compartment block for postoperative analgesia after total hip arthroplasty: new landmarks, technical guidelines, and clinical evaluation. *Anesth Analg* 2002;94:1606–1613.

- Chelly JE, Casati A, Fanelli G. *Continuous Peripheral Nerve Block Techniques: An Illustrated Guide*. London, England: Mosby International; 2001.

- Farny J, Drolet P, Girard M. Anatomy of the posterior approach to the lumbar plexus block. *Can J Anaesth* 1994;41:480–485.

- Farny J, Girard M, Drolet P. Posterior approach to the lumbar plexus combined with a sciatic nerve block using lidocaine. *Can J Anaesth* 1994;1:486–491.

- Hanna MH, Peat SJ, D'Costa F. Lumbar plexus block: an anatomical study. *Anaesthesia* 1993;48:675.

- Kirchmair L, Entner T, Wissel J, Moriggl B, Kapral S, Mitterschiffthaler G. A study of the paravertebral anatomy for ultrasound-guided posterior lumbar plexus block. *Anesth Analg* 2001;93:477.

- Lang S. Posterior lumbar plexus block. *Can J Anaesth* 1994;41:1238.

- Mansour NY, Bennetts FE. An observational study of combined continuous lumbar plexus and single-shot sciatic nerve blocks for post-knee surgery analgesia. *Reg Anesth* 1996;21:287.

- Pandin PC, Vandesteene A, d'Hollander AA. Lumbar plexus posterior approach: a catheter placement description using electrical nerve stimulation. *Anesth Analg* 2002;95:1428.

- Stevens RD, Van Gessel E, Flory N, Fournier R, Gamulin Z. Lumbar plexus block reduces pain and blood loss associated with total hip arthroplasty. *Anesthesiology* 2000;93:115.

- Vaghadia H, Kapnoudhis P, Jenkins LC, Taylor D. Continuous lumbosacral block using a Tuohy needle and catheter technique. *Can J Anaesth* 1992;39:75.

- Vloka JD, Hadžić A. Obturator and genitofemoral nerve blocks. *Tech Reg Anesth Pain Management* 1999:3;28–32.

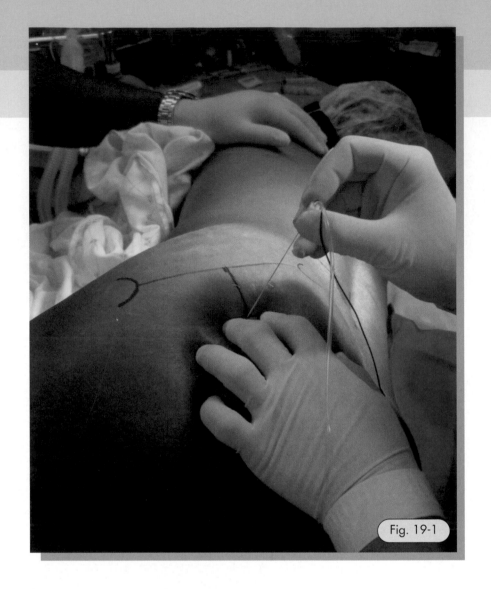

Fig. 19-1

BLOCK AT A GLANCE

- Indications: surgery on the knee, tibia, ankle, and foot

- Landmarks: greater trochanter, superior posterior iliac spine, midline between the two

- Nerve stimulation: twitch of the hamstring, calf, foot, or toes at 0.2 to 0.5 mA current

- Local anesthetic: 20 mL

- Complexity level: intermediate

GENERAL CONSIDERATIONS

The posterior approach to a sciatic blockade has wide clinical applicability for surgery and pain management of the lower extremity. Consequently, a sciatic block is one of the techniques most commonly used in our practice. In contrast to common belief, this block is relatively easy to perform. It is associated with a high success rate when properly performed. It is particularly well-suited for surgery on the knee, calf, Achilles tendon, ankle, and foot. It provides complete anesthesia of the leg below the knee with the exception of the medial strip of skin, which is innervated by the saphenous nerve. When combined with a femoral nerve or lumbar plexus block, anesthesia of almost the entire leg is achieved.

Anatomy

The sciatic nerve is formed from the L4 through S3 roots. These roots of the sacral plexus form on the anterior surface of the lateral sacrum and are assembled into the sciatic nerve on the anterior surface of the piriformis muscle. The sciatic nerve is the largest nerve in the body and measures nearly 2 cm in breadth at its commencement. It exits the pelvis through the greater sciatic foramen below the piriformis and descends between the greater trochanter of the femur and the tuberosity of the ischium **(Fig. 19-2)**. It then runs along the back of the thigh to about its lower one-third, where it diverges into two large branches, the tibial and the common peroneal nerves. The course of the nerve can be estimated by drawing a line on the back of the thigh beginning from the apex of the popliteal fossa to the midpoint of the line joining the ischial tuberosity to the apex of the greater trochanter. The sciatic nerve also gives off numerous articular (hip, knee) and muscular branches.

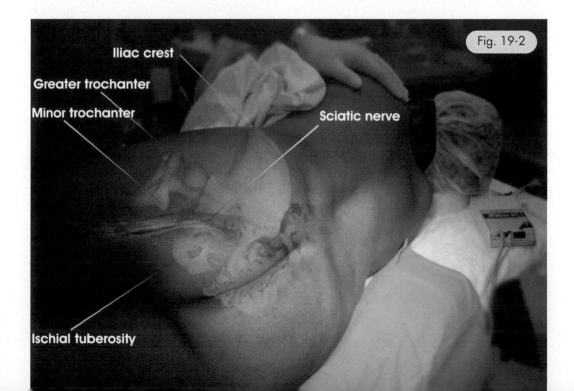

Fig. 19-2

Iliac crest

Greater trochanter

Minor trochanter

Sciatic nerve

Ischial tuberosity

In the upper part of its course, the sciatic nerve is situated deep in the major gluteal muscle and initially rests on the posterior surface of the ischium. It crosses the external rotators and the obturator internus gemelli muscle and then passes on to the quadratus femoris, by which it is separated from the obturator externus and the hip joint. On its medial side, the sciatic nerve is accompanied by the posterior cutaneous nerve of the thigh and the inferior gluteal artery. More distally, it lies on the adductor magnus. It is crossed obliquely by the long head of the biceps femoris. The articular branches of the sciatic nerve arise from the upper part of the nerve and supply the hip joint by perforating the posterior part of its capsule; they are sometimes derived directly from the sacral plexus. The muscular branches of the sciatic nerve are distributed to the biceps femoris, semitendinosus, and semimembranosus muscles and to the ischial head of the adductor magnus; the branches of the latter two arise by a common trunk. The nerve to the short head of the biceps femoris comes from the common peroneal division, and the other muscular branches from the tibial division of the sciatic nerve.

TIPS

▶ There are variations in the course of the sciatic nerve through the gluteal region. In about 15% of the population, the piriformis muscle divides the nerve. The common peroneal component passes through or above the muscle, and only the tibial component passes below it.

▶ The components of the sciatic nerve diverge at a variable distance from the knee joint. By and large, most nerves diverge at 7–10 cm above the popliteal fossa crease.

Distribution of Anesthesia

A sciatic nerve blockade results in anesthesia of the skin of the posterior aspect of the thigh, hamstring, and biceps muscles, part of hip and knee joint, and the entire leg below the knee with the exception of the skin of the medial aspect of the lower leg **(Fig. 19-3)**. Depending on the level of surgery, the addition of a saphenous or femoral nerve block may be required.

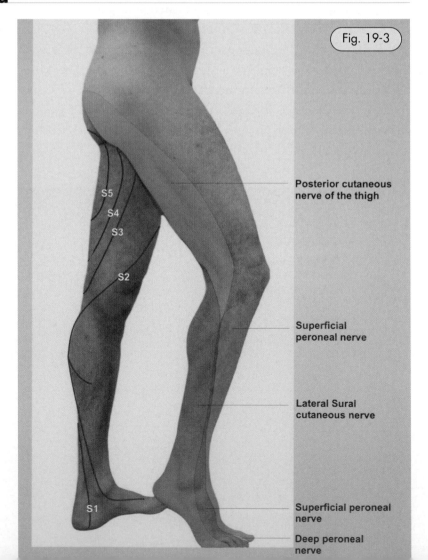

Fig. 19-3

S5
S4
S3
S2
S1

Posterior cutaneous nerve of the thigh

Superficial peroneal nerve

Lateral Sural cutaneous nerve

Superficial peroneal nerve

Deep peroneal nerve

Patient Positioning

The patient is in the lateral decubitus position tilted slightly forward **(Fig. 19-4)**. The foot on the side to be blocked should be positioned over the dependent leg so that twitches of the foot or toes can be easily observed.

TIP

▶ It should be noted that the skin over the gluteal area is highly movable. Therefore, it is important that the patient remains in the same position in which the landmarks are outlined. A small forward or backward tilt can result in a significant shift of the landmarks due to sagging of the skin and subcutaneous tissue, leading to difficulty in localizing the sciatic nerve.

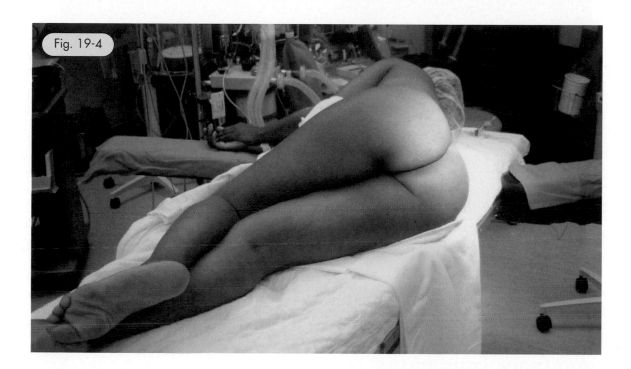

Fig. 19-4

Equipment

A standard regional anesthesia tray is prepared with the following equipment:

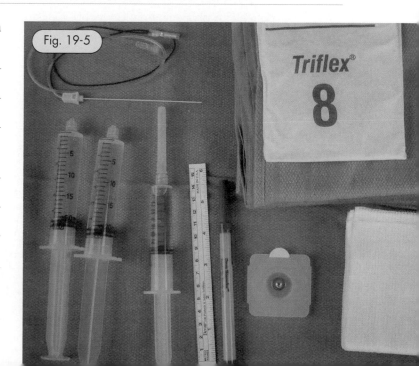

Fig. 19-5

Triflex®

8

- Sterile towels and gauze packs

- 20-mL syringes containing a local anesthetic

- Sterile gloves, marking pen, and surface electrode

- $1\frac{1}{2}$-in, 25-gauge needle for skin infiltration

- 10-cm, short-bevel, insulated stimulating needle

- Peripheral nerve stimulator

Surface Landmarks

The only two surface anatomy landmarks that are important in determining the insertion point for the needle are **(Fig. 19-6)**:

1. Greater trochanter

2. Posterior superior iliac spine.

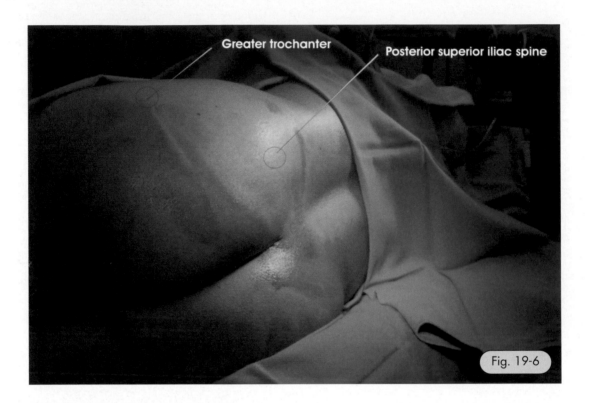

Greater trochanter

Posterior superior iliac spine

Fig. 19-6

Anatomic Landmarks

Landmarks for the posterior approach to a sciatic blockade are easily identified in most patients. A proper palpation technique is of utmost importance because the adipose tissue over the gluteal area may obscure these bony prominences. The landmarks are outlined with a marking pen **(Fig. 19-9)**:

1. Greater trochanter

2. Posterior superior iliac spine

3. Needle insertion point 4 cm distal to the midpoint between landmarks 1 and 2

A line between the greater trochanter and the posterior superior iliac spine is drawn and divided in half. A line passing through the midpoint of this line and perpendicular to it is extended 4 cm caudal and marked as the needle insertion point.

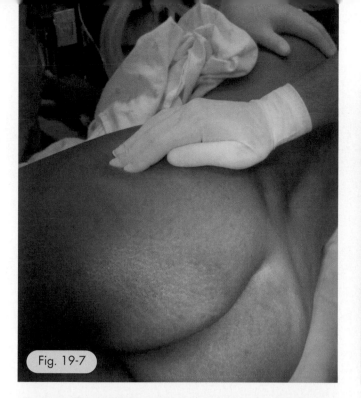

Fig. 19-7

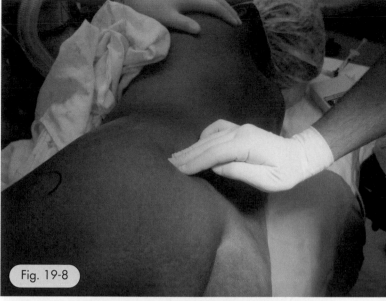

Fig. 19-8

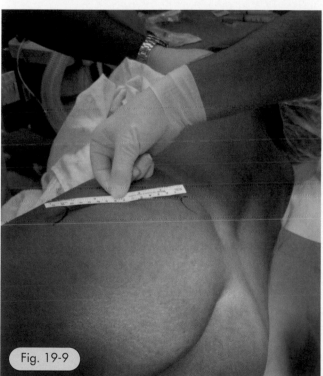

Fig. 19-9

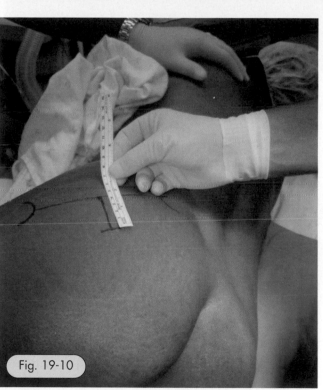

Fig. 19-10

TIPS

▶ Palpating the greater trochanter **(Fig. 19-7)**: it is important that the structure of the greater trochanter be approached from its posterior aspect.

▶Palpating the posterior superior iliac spine: the palpating hand is rolled back until the fingers meet the posterior superior iliac spine **(Fig. 19-8)**. This land-

mark should be labeled on the side facing the great trochanter.

▶ Palpating and labeling of the "inner" aspects of the greater trochanter and the posterior superior iliac spine results in a shorter line connecting the two **(Fig. 19-9)** and a more precise approximation of the position of the sciatic nerve.

Local Anesthetic Skin Infiltration

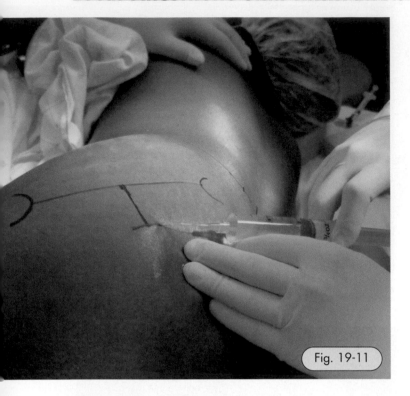

Fig. 19-11

After cleaning the area with an antiseptic solution, local anesthetic is infiltrated subcutaneously at the determined needle insertion site **(Fig. 19-11)**. The anesthesiologist performing the block should assume an ergonomic position to allow precise needle maneuvering and monitoring of the responses to nerve stimulation.

TIP

▶ The height of the bed should be raised to allow a comfortable and stable position for the patient during block placement and for observation of the muscle twitches occurring during nerve stimulation.

Needle Insertion

The fingers of the palpating hand should be firmly pressed on the gluteus muscle to decrease the skin-nerve distance **(Fig. 19-12)**. Also, the skin between the index and middle fingers should be stretched to allow greater precision during block placement. The palpating hand should not be moved during the entire procedure. Even small movements of the palpating hand can change the position of the needle insertion site because of the highly movable skin and soft tissues in the gluteal region. The needle is introduced perpendicular to the spherical skin plane. The nerve stimulator should be initially set to deliver 1.5 mA current (2 Hz, 100–300 μs) to allow detection of twitches of the gluteal muscles and stimulation of the sciatic nerve.

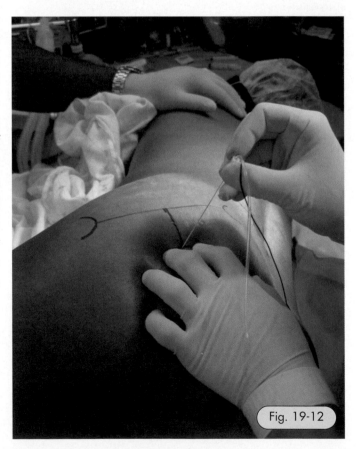

Fig. 19-12

Needle Advancement

As the needle is advanced, twitches of the gluteal muscles are observed first **(Fig. 19-13)**. These twitches merely indicate that the needle position is still too shallow. Once the gluteal twitches disappear, brisk response of the sciatic nerve to stimulation is observed (hamstring, calf, foot, or toe twitches). After an initial stimulation of the sciatic nerve is obtained, the stimulating current is gradually decreased until twitches are still seen or felt at 0.2 to 0.5 mA. This typically occurs at a depth of 5 to 8 cm. After obtaining negative results from an aspiration test for blood, 15 to 20 mL of local anesthetic is slowly injected. Any resistance to the injection of local anesthetic should prompt withdrawal of the needle by 1 mm. Injection should then be reattempted. Persistent resistance to injection should prompt complete needle withdrawal and flushing to ensure the patency of the needle before reattempting the procedure.

TIP

▶ The choice of medication, as well as the dose and mode of administration, should take into consideration the individual patient's characteristics, response to drugs, and overall medical status.

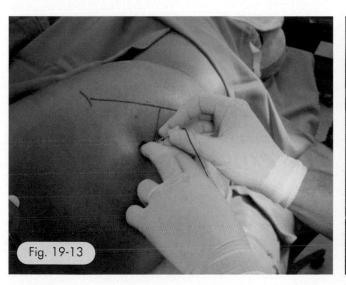

Fig. 19-13

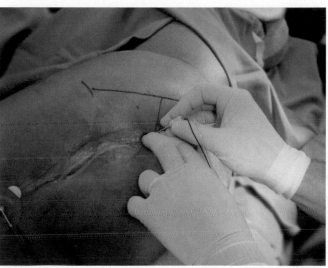

This figure shows the proper needle insertion and hands stabilization during posterior sciatic nerve block. The figure to the right illustrates the relationship of the needle insertion site to the course of the sciatic nerve. The sciatic nerve shown is digitally superimposed from an image taken during sciatic nerve dissection in a human cadaver. Note the sizeable width of the sciatic nerve and its thick epineural sheath.

GOAL

Visible or palpable twitches of the hamstrings, calf muscles, foot, or toes at 0.2 to 0.5 mA current. Twitches of the hamstring are equally acceptable because this approach blocks the nerve proximal to the separation of the neuronal branches to the hamstring muscle.

Interpreting Responses to Nerve Stimulation

Some common responses to nerve stimulation and the course of action to take to obtain the proper response are listed in **Table 19.1.**

TABLE 19.1
Some Common Responses to Nerve Stimulation

RESPONSE OBTAINED	INTERPRETATION	PROBLEM	ACTION
Local twitch of the gluteus muscle	Direct stimulation of the gluteus muscle	Too shallow (superficial) placement of the needle	Continue advancing the needle
Needle contacts bone but local twitch of the gluteus muscle is not elicited	Needle is inserted close to the attachment of the gluteus muscle to the iliac bone	Too superior placement of the needle	Stop the procedure, recheck the patient's position, and reassess the landmarks
Needle encounters bone; sciatic twitches not elicited	Needle missed the plane of the sciatic nerve and is stopped by the hip joint or ischial bone	The needle is inserted to laterally (hip joint) or medially (ischial bone)	Withdraw the needle and redirect it slightly medially or laterally (5º–10º) **(Fig. 19-14)**
Hamstring twitch	Stimulation of the main trunk of the sciatic nerve	None. These branches are within the sciatic nerve sheath at this level	Accept and inject local anesthetic
Needle is placed deep (10 cm); twitches not elicited; bone is not contacted	Needle has passed through the sciatic notch	Too inferior placement of the needle	Withdraw the needle and redirect it slightly superiorly

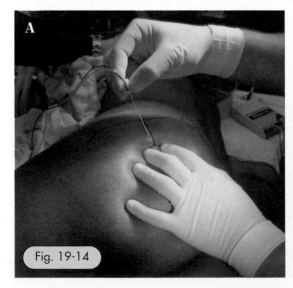

Fig. 19-14

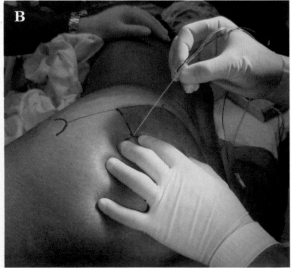

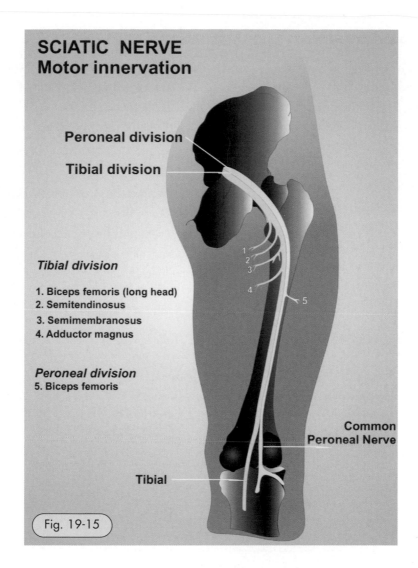

SCIATIC NERVE
Motor innervation

Peroneal division

Tibial division

Tibial division

1. Biceps femoris (long head)
2. Semitendinosus
3. Semimembranosus
4. Adductor magnus

Peroneal division
5. Biceps femoris

Common
Peroneal Nerve

Tibial

Fig. 19-15

TIPS

▶ Stimulation at a current intensity of less than 0.5 mA may not be possible in some patients. This is occasionally (but not frequently) the case in elderly patients and in patients with long-standing diabetes mellitus, peripheral neuropathy, sepsis, or severe peripheral vascular disease. In these cases, stimulating currents up to 1.0 mA should be accepted as long as the motor response is specific and clearly seen or felt.

▶ Because the level of the blockade with this approach to sciatic block is above the departure of these branches, twitches in any of the hamstring muscles can be accepted as a reliable sign of localization of the sciatic nerve (**Fig. 19-15**).

Choice of Local Anesthetic

A sciatic block requires a relatively low volume of local anesthetic to achieve anesthesia of the entire trunk of the nerve. The choice of the type and concentration of local anesthetic should be based on whether the block is planned for surgical anesthesia or pain management (**Table 19.2**). Because the duration of a sciatic blockade is longer than that of any other peripheral nerve block, we tend to use a shorter-acting local anesthetic more commonly. However, when prolonged pain relief is desired, a longer-acting local anesthetic may be more appropriate. Because very long duration of blockade can be achieved with epinephrine-containing local anesthetics, we rarely add epinephrine to local anesthetics for sciatic nerve blockade. Too long a duration of dense sciatic nerve anesthesia may increase risk of nerve injury because of the possibility of stretching or sitting on the anesthetized nerve.

> **TIP**
>
> ▶ Avoid the use of epinephrine during sciatic nerve blockade because of the peculiar blood supply to the sciatic nerve, the possibility of additional ischemia due to stretching or sitting on the anesthetized nerve, and the long duration of blockade.

TABLE 19.2
Choice of Local Anesthetic for Sciatic Nerve Block

ANESTHETIC	ONSET (min)	DURATION OF ANESTHESIA (h)	DURATION OF ANALGESIA (h)
3% 2-Chloroprocaine (+ HCO₃)	10–15	2	2.5
1.5% Mepivacaine (+ HCO₃)	10–15	4–5	5–8
2% Lidocaine (+ HCO₃)	10–20	5–6	5–8
0.5% Ropivacaine	15–20	6–12	6–24
0.75% Ropivacaine	10–15	8–12	8–24
0.5 Bupivacaine (or levobupivacaine)	15–30	8–16	10–48

Block Dynamics and Perioperative Management

This technique is associated with moderate patient discomfort because the needle passes through the gluteus muscles. Adequate sedation and analgesia are very important to ensure that the patient is still and tranquil. We typically use midazolam 2 to 4 mg after the patient is positioned, and alfentanil 500 to 750 μg just before the needle is inserted. A typical onset time for this block is 10 in 25 minutes, depending on the type, concentration, and volume of local anesthetic used. The first signs of onset of the blockade are usually a report by the patient that the foot "feels different" or inability to wiggle the toes.

> **TIP**
>
> ▶Inadequate skin anesthesia despite an apparently timely onset of the blockade can occur. It can take up to 30 minutes for full sensory-motor anesthesia to develop. However, local infiltration by the surgeon at the site of the incision is often all that is needed to allow the surgery to proceed until the block fully sets in.

CONTINUOUS SCIATIC NERVE BLOCK

A continuous sciatic nerve block is an advanced regional anesthesia technique, and experience with the single-injection technique is recommended to ensure its efficacy and safety. The procedure is quite similar to the single-injection procedure; however, a slight angulation of the needle caudally is necessary to facilitate threading of the catheter. Securing and maintaining the catheter is easy and convenient. This technique can be used for surgery and postoperative pain management in patients undergoing a wide variety of lower leg, foot, and ankle surgeries. In our practice, perhaps the single most important indication for use of this block is for amputation of the lower extremity.

Patient Positioning

Proper patient positioning at the outset and maintenance of this position during continuous sciatic nerve blockade is crucial for precise catheter placement. A slightly forward pelvic tilt prevents "sagging" of the soft tissues in the gluteal area and significantly facilitates block placement **(Fig. 19-16)**.

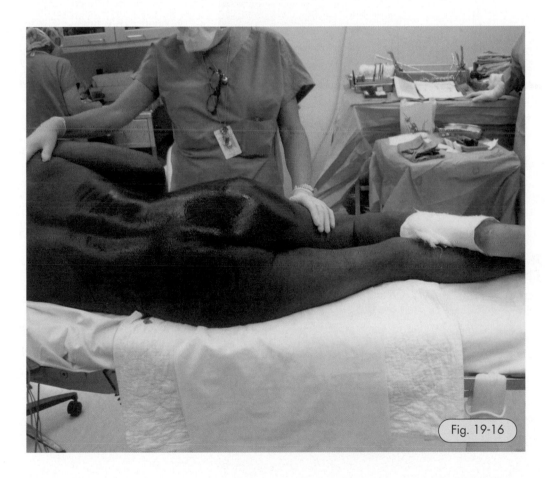

Fig. 19-16

Equipment

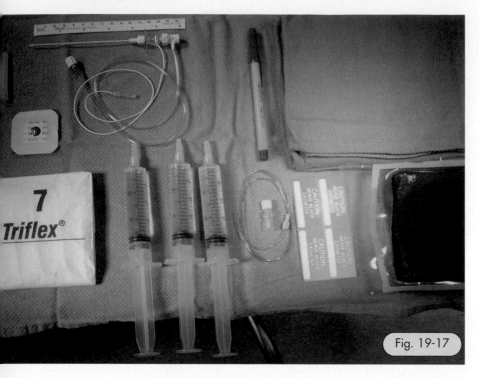

Fig. 19-17

A standard regional anesthesia tray is prepared with the following equipment **(Fig. 19-17)**:

- Sterile towels and gauze packs

- 20-mL syringes containing a local anesthetic

- Sterile gloves, marking pen, and surface electrode

- $1^1/_2$-in, 25-gauge needle for skin infiltration

- 10-cm, insulated stimulating needle (preferably with a Tuohy-style tip)

- Catheter

- Peripheral nerve stimulator

Landmarks

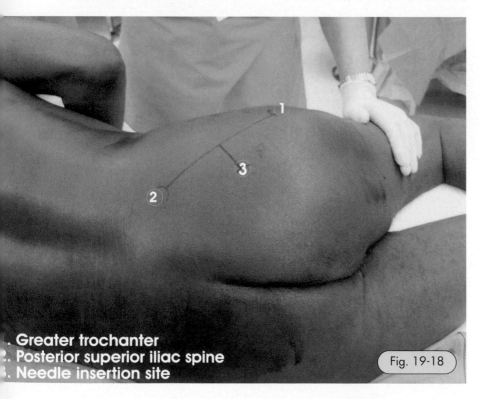

1. Greater trochanter
2. Posterior superior iliac spine
3. Needle insertion site

Fig. 19-18

The landmarks for a continuous sciatic block are the same as those in the single-injection technique **(Fig. 19-18)**:

1. Greater trochanter

2. Posterior-superior iliac spine

3. Needle insertion site 4 cm caudal to the midpoint of the line between landmarks 1 and 2.

Local Anesthetic Infiltration and Needle Insertion

The continuous sciatic block technique is similar to the single-injection technique. With the patient in the lateral decubitus position and tilted slightly forward, the landmarks are identified and marked with the pen. After a thorough cleaning of the area with an antiseptic solution, the skin at the needle insertion site is infiltrated with local anesthetic **(Fig. 19-19)**. The palpating hand is positioned and fixed around the site of needle insertion to shorten the skin nerve distance.

A 10-cm continuous block needle is connected to the nerve stimulator and inserted perpendicularly to the skin. The opening of the needle should face distally (pointing toward the patient's foot) to facilitate catheter insertion. The initial intensity of the stimulating current should be 1.0 to 1.5 mA.

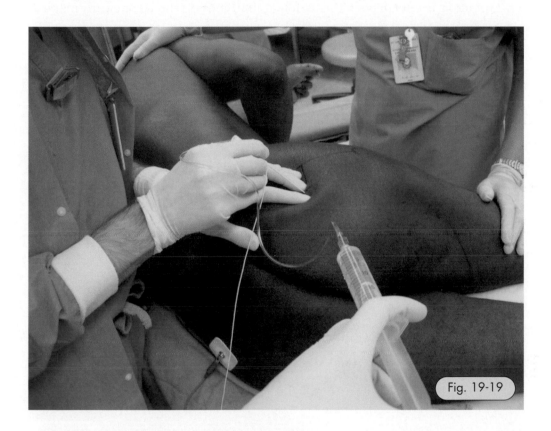

Fig. 19-19

TIP

▶It is useful to inject some local anesthetic intramuscularly to prevent pain during advancement of the larger-gauge and blunt-tipped needles typically used for this block.

As the needle is advanced, twitches of the glutcus muscle are observed first. Deeper needle advancement results in stimulation of the sciatic nerve. The principles of nerve stimulation and needle redirection are identical to those for the single-injection technique. After obtaining the appropriate twitches, the needle is manipulated until the desired response (twitches of the hamstrings muscles or foot) is seen or felt using a current of 0.2 to 0.5 mA. At this point, a bolus of local anesthetic (20 mL) is injected after obtaining negative results from an aspiration test for blood. This is followed by insertion of the catheter about 5 to 10 cm beyond the needle tip. The needle is then withdrawn back to skin level, and the catheter advanced simultaneously to prevent inadvertent removal of the catheter **(Fig. 19-20)**. An aspiration test for blood should be used to check the catheter for accidental intravascular placement before local anesthetic is administered.

Several techniques for securing the catheter to the skin have been proposed. A benzoin skin preparation, followed by application of a clear dressing and a cloth tape, is a simple, efficacious method **(Fig. 19-21)**. The infusion port should be clearly marked "continuous sciatic block."

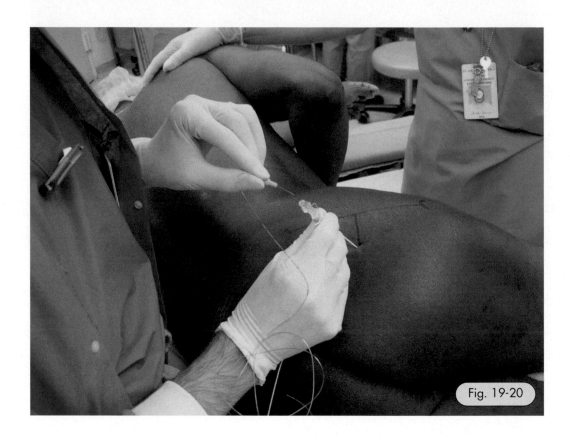

Fig. 19-20

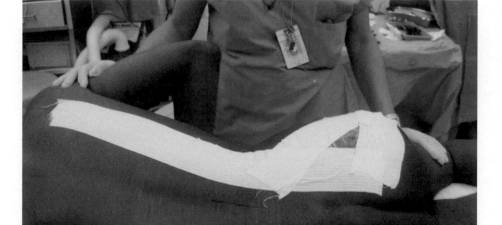

Fig. 19-21

Continuous Infusion

Continuous infusion is always initiated after administration of an initial bolus of dilute local anesthetic through the catheter **(Fig. 19-22)**. For this purpose, we routinely use 0.2% ropivacaine 15 to 20 mL. Diluted bupivacaine or levobupivacaine is also suitable, but can result in more pronounced motor blockade. The infusion is maintained at 10 or 5 mL/h when a patient-controlled analgesic (PCA) dose (5 mL/h) is planned.

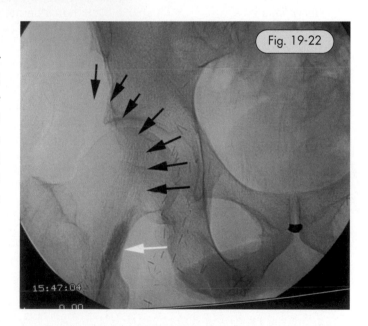

Fig. 19-22

The course of the sciatic catheter (black arrows) and the dispersion of 2 mL of contrast solution (white arrow) injected through the catheter.

Complications and How to Avoid Them

Some general and specific instructions on possible complications and methods used to avoid them are listed in **Table 19.3.**

TABLE 19.3
Complications of Sciatic Nerve Block and Preventive Techniques

Infection	• A strict aseptic technique is used.
Hematoma	• Avoid multiple needle insertions, particularly in patients undergoing anticoagulant therapy.
Vascular puncture	• Vascular puncture is not common with this technique. • Deep needle insertion should be avoided (pelvic vessels).
Local anesthetic toxicity	• Avoid using large volumes and doses of local anesthetic because of the proximity of the muscle beds and the potential for rapid absorption.
Nerve injury	• A sciatic block has a unique predisposition for mechanical and pressure injury. • Nerve stimulation and slow needle advancement should be employed. • Local anesthetic should never be injected when the patient complains of pain or abnormally high pressure on injection is noted. • When stimulation is obtained with a current intensity of <0.2 mA, the needle should be pulled back to obtain the same response with a current intensity of >0.2 mA before injecting local anesthetic. • Advance the needle slowly when twitches of the gluteus muscle cease to avoid impaling the sciatic nerve on the rapidly advancing needle.
Other	• Instruct the patient and nursing staff on the care of the insensate extremity. • Explain the need for frequent body repositioning to avoid stretching and prolonged ischemia (sitting) on the anesthetized sciatic nerve.

SUGGESTED READINGS

Single-Injection Nerve Block, Posterior Approach

• Bailey SL, Parkinson SK, Little WL, Simmerman SR. Sciatic nerve block: a comparison of single versus double injection technique. *Reg Anesth* 1994;19:9–13.

• Bridenbaugh PO, Wedel DJ. The lower extremity: somatic blockade. In: Cousins MJ, Bridenbaugh PO, eds. *Neuronal Blockade in Clinical Anesthesia and Management of Pain.* 3rd ed. Philadelphia, Pa: Lippincott-Raven, 1998;375–394.

• Dalens B, Tanguy A, Vanneuville G. Sciatic nerve blocks in children: comparison of the posterior, anterior, and lateral approaches in 180 pediatric patients. *Anesth Analg* 1990;70:131–137.

• Farny J, Girard M, Drolet P. Posterior approach to the lumbar plexus combined with a sciatic nerve block using lidocaine. *Can J Anaesth* 1994;41:486–491.

• Hadžić A, Vloka JD, Kuroda MM, Koorn R, Birnbach DJ. The practice of peripheral nerve blocks in the United States: a national survey. *Reg Anesth Pain Med* 1998;23:241–246.

- Kilpatrick AW, Coventry DM, Todd JG. A comparison of two approaches to sciatic nerve block. *Anaesthesia* 1992;47:155–157.
- Mansour NY, Bennetts FE. An observational study of combined continuous lumbar plexus and single-shot sciatic nerve blocks for post-knee surgery analgesia. *Reg Anesth* 1996;21:287–291.
- Smith BE, Siggins D. Low volume high concentration block of the sciatic nerve. *Anesthesia* 1988;43:8–11.

Continuous Sciatic Nerve Block, Posterior Approach

- Bridenbaugh PO, Wedel DJ. The lower extremity: somatic blockade. In: Cousins MJ, Bridenbaugh PO, eds. *Neuronal Blockade in Clinical Anesthesia and Management of Pain.* 3rd ed. Philadelphia, Pa: Lippincott-Raven, 1998,375–394.
- Chelly JE, Casati A, Fanelli G. *Continuous Peripheral Nerve Block Techniques: An Illustrated Guide.* London, England: Mosby International, 2001.
- di Benedetto P, Casati A, Bertini L. Continuous subgluteus sciatic nerve block after orthopedic foot and ankle surgery: comparison of two infusion techniques. *Reg Anesth Pain Med* 2002;27:168–172.
- di Benedetto P, Casati A, Bertini L, Fanelli G, Chelly JE. Postoperative analgesia with continuous sciatic nerve block after foot surgery: a prospective, randomized comparison between the popliteal and subgluteal approaches. *Anesth Analg* 2002;94:996–1000.
- Klein SM, Greengrass RA, Grant SA, Higgins LD, Nielsen KC, Steele SM. Ambulatory surgery for multiligament knee reconstruction with continuous dual catheter peripheral nerve blockade. *Can J Anaesth* 2001;48:375–378.
- Souron V, Eyrolle L, Rosencher N. The Mansour's sacral plexus block: an effective technique for continuous block. *Reg Anesth Pain Med* 2000;25:208–209.
- Sutherland ID. Continuous sciatic nerve infusion: expanded case report describing a new approach. *Reg Anesth Pain Med* 1998;23:496–501

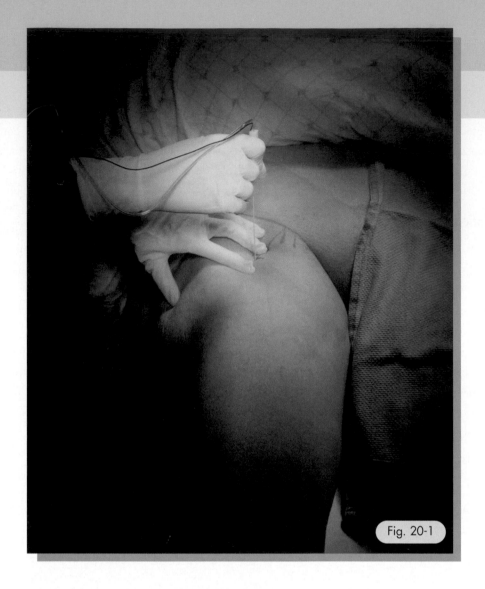

Fig. 20-1

BLOCK AT A GLANCE

- Indications: surgery on the knee, tibia, fibula, ankle, and foot

- Landmarks: femoral crease, femoral artery

- Needle: 15 cm

- Nerve stimulation: twitch of the foot or toes at 0.2 to 0.5 mA current

- Local anesthetic: 20 ml

- Complexity level: advanced

SCIATIC
NERVE BLOCK: ANTERIOR APPROACH

GENERAL CONSIDERATIONS

The anterior approach to a sciatic block is an advanced nerve block technique. This block is well-suited for surgery on the leg below the knee, particularly on the ankle and foot. It provides complete anesthesia of the leg below the knee with the exception of the medial strip of skin, which is innervated by the saphenous nerve. Combined with a femoral nerve block, this procedure results in anesthesia of the entire knee and the leg below. It should be noted that the anterior approach is less applicable compared to the posterior approach. The sciatic nerve is blocked more distally, and a higher level of skill is required to achieve reliable anesthesia. Consequently, we reserve the use of this block for patients that cannot be repositioned into the lateral position needed for the posterior approach. This technique is not suitable for catheter insertion because of the deep location and perpendicular angle of insertion required to reach the sciatic nerve.

Anatomy

The sciatic nerve is formed from the L4 through S3 roots **(Fig. 20-2)**. The roots of the lumbosacral plexus form on the anterior surface of the sacrum and are assembled into the sciatic nerve on the anterior surface of the piriformis muscle. The course of the nerve can be estimated by drawing a line on the back of the thigh from the apex of the popliteal fossa to the midpoint of a line joining the ischial tuberosity to the apex of the greater trochanter. The nerve exits the pelvis through the greater sciatic notch and gives off numerous articular (hip, knee) and muscular branches. Once in the upper thigh, it continues its descent behind the lesser trochanter and becomes completely covered by the femur. The only part of the nerve that is accessible to blockade through an anterior approach is a short segment slightly above and below the lesser trochanter. The muscular branches of the sciatic nerve are distributed to the biceps femoris, semitendinosus, and semimembranosus and to the ischial head of the adductor magnus; the branches of the latter two arise by a common trunk. The nerve to the short head of the biceps femoris comes from the common peroneal division, and the other muscular branches from the tibial division of the sciatic nerve. At the level of the block, the nerve is partly hidden by the femur (minor trochanter).

▶ There are variations in the course of the sciatic nerve through the gluteal region. In about 15% of the population, the piriformis muscle divides the nerve. The common peroneal component passes through the muscle or above it, and only the tibial component passes below the muscle.

▶ The components of the sciatic nerve diverge at a variable distance from the knee joint; most sciatic nerves diverge at or more than 7 cm from the popliteal fossa crease.

▶ Because the level of the blockade with this approach to sciatic block is often below the exit of these branches, twitches of the hamstring muscles can *not* be accepted as a reliable sign of localization of the sciatic nerve as long as the motor response is specific and clearly seen or felt.

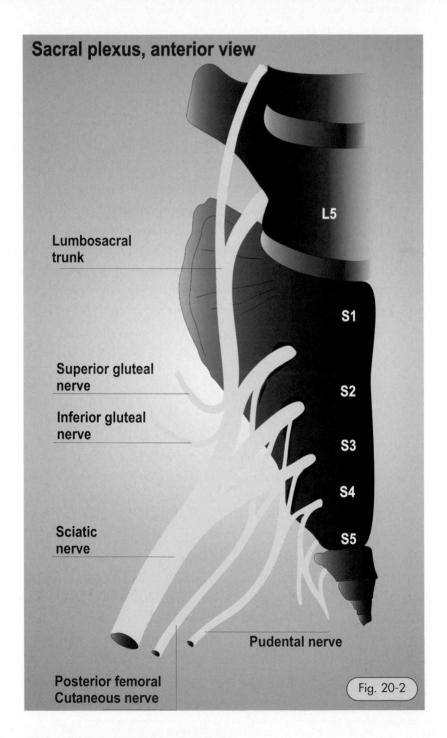

Sacral plexus, anterior view

Lumbosacral trunk

Superior gluteal nerve

Inferior gluteal nerve

Sciatic nerve

Posterior femoral Cutaneous nerve

Pudental nerve

L5

S1

S2

S3

S4

S5

Fig. 20-2

Distribution of Anesthesia

A sciatic nerve block through the anterior approach results in anesthesia of the hamstring muscles below the blockade and the entire leg below the knee (including the ankle and foot) except for a strip of skin over the medial aspect **(Fig. 20-3)**. The saphenous nerve, a superficial cutaneous branch of the femoral nerve, innervates this medial area of skin below the knee. The posterior cutaneous nerve of the thigh or articular branches of the hip are not anesthetized with this technique. Therefore, the anterior approach to a sciatic block can be chosen for selected patients for knee or below-knee surgery. A proximal thigh tourniquet should be avoided with this technique because of the risk of prolonged ischemia of the sciatic nerve.

The shaded areas indicate the cutaneous distribution of anesthesia with the anterior approach to a sciatic nerve block. A distal two-thirds of the hamstring muscles are also anesthetized with this technique (not shown in the illustration).

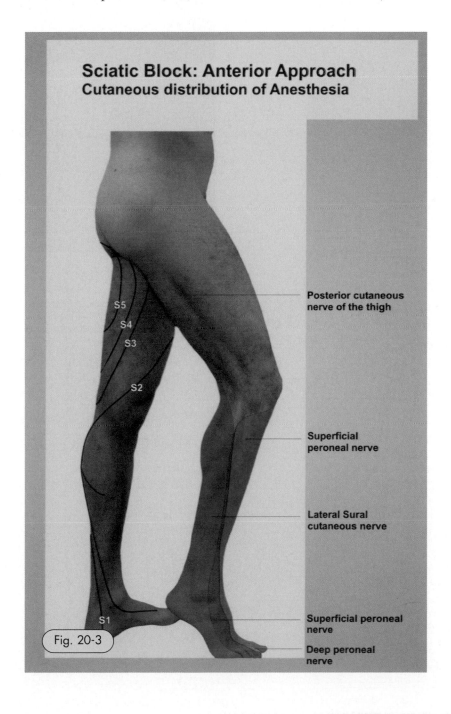

Sciatic Block: Anterior Approach
Cutaneous distribution of Anesthesia

Posterior cutaneous nerve of the thigh

Superficial peroneal nerve

Lateral Sural cutaneous nerve

Superficial peroneal nerve

Deep peroneal nerve

Fig. 20-3

Patient Positioning

The patient is in the supine position with both legs fully extended **(Fig. 20-4)**.

> **TIP**
>
> ▶ Placing a pillow underneath the patient's hips can be useful to optimize access to the groin and landmarks for the block.

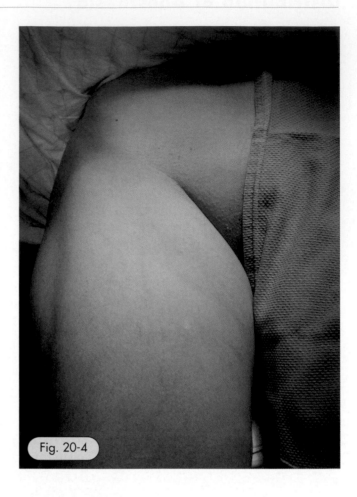

Fig. 20-4

Equipment

A standard regional anesthesia tray is prepared with the following equipment:

- Sterile towels and gauze packs

- 20-mL syringes containing local anesthetic

- Sterile gloves, marking pen, and surface electrode

- 1$\frac{1}{2}$-in, 25-gauge needle for skin infiltration

- 15-cm, short-bevel, insulated stimulating needle

- Peripheral nerve stimulator

> **TIP**
>
> ▶ Although it sometimes may appear that a 150-mm needle is too long (e.g., in a slim adult) more often than not, shorter needles (e.g., 100 mm) are unable to reach the sciatic nerve and may result in unnecessary unsuccessful attempts.

Surface Landmarks

The only surface anatomy landmark that is important in determining the insertion point for the needle is the femoral crease line.

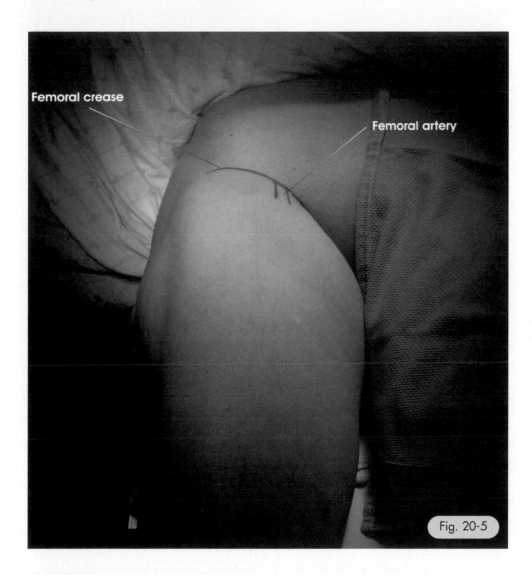

Femoral crease

Femoral artery

Fig. 20-5

TIP

▶ Note that the description of this technique differs from common descriptions of the anterior approach to a sciatic block. This technique does not rely on identification of the inguinal ligament, which can be difficult to estimate in obese patients. Instead, this much simplified technique relies on the femoral crease, which is easily recognized in all patients even without palpation.

Anatomic Landmarks

The following landmarks should routinely be outlined using a marking pen:

1. Femoral crease

2. Femoral artery pulse

3. Needle insertion point is marked 4 to 5 cm distally on a line passing through the pulse of the femoral artery and perpendicularly to the femoral crease **(Fig. 20-6)**.

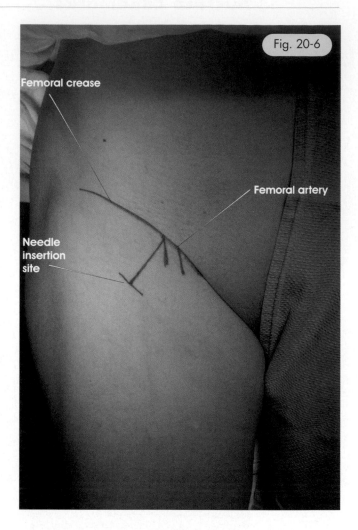

Fig. 20-6

Femoral crease

Femoral artery

Needle insertion site

TIPS

▶ Avoid pushing the soft tissues laterally or medially during palpation of the femoral artery. The skin and subcutaneous tissue in this area are highly movable, and lateral or medial displacement of the tissues may skew the femoral artery landmark.

▶ The femoral crease is easily identifiable in all patients. Retraction of the adipose tissue of the lower abdomen is useful in exposing the femoral crease, facilitating palpation of the femoral artery, and block placement in obese patients.

Local Anesthetic Skin Infiltration

After cleaning the area with an antiseptic solution, local anesthetic is infiltrated subcutaneously at the determined needle insertion site. The anesthesiologist performing the block should stand on the side of the patient to be blocked to be able to monitor the patient and the responses to nerve stimulation.

Needle Insertion and Advancement

The fingers of the palpating hand should be firmly pressed against the quadriceps muscle to decrease the skin-nerve distance **(Fig. 20-7)**. The needle is introduced at an angle perpendicular to the skin plane. The nerve stimulator should be initially set to deliver a 1.5 mA current. The twitch of the foot or toes typically occurs at a depth of 10 to 12 cm. After obtaining nega-

tive results from an aspiration test for blood, 20 mL of local anesthetic is slowly injected. Any resistance to the injection of local anesthetic should prompt cessation of the injection attempt; this should then be reattempted. Persistent resistance to injection should prompt complete needle withdrawal and flushing before reintroduction of the needle.

TIP

▶ Because the needle transverses muscle planes, it is occasionally obstructed by muscle fibers. However, when resistance to injection is met, it is never correct to assume that the needle is obstructed. The proper action is to withdraw the needle and check its patency by flushing before reinserting it.

GOAL

Visible or palpable twitches of the calf muscles, foot, or toes at 0.2 to 0.5 mA current.

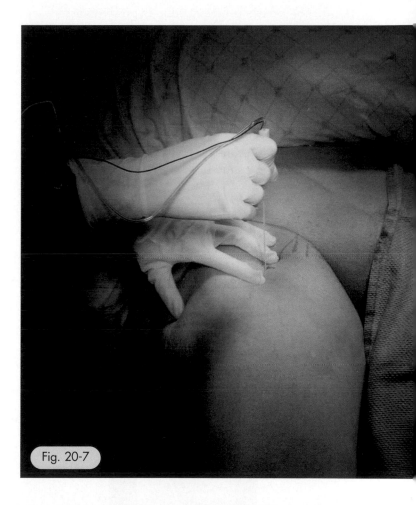

Fig. 20-7

TIPS

▶ Local twitches of the quadriceps muscle are often elicited during needle advancement. The needle should be advanced past these twitches.

▶ Although there is a concern about femoral nerve injury with further needle advancement, this concern is theoretical. At this level, the femoral nerve is divided into smaller terminal branches that are movable and are unlikely to be penetrated by a slowly advancing, short-beveled needle.

▶ Resting the heel on the bed surface may prevent the foot from twitching even when the sciatic nerve is stimulated. This can be prevented by placing the ankle on a footrest or by having an assistant continuously palpate the calf or Achilles tendon.

▶ Because branches to the hamstring muscle may leave the main trunk of the sciatic nerve at the level of needle insertion, twitches of the hamstring should not be accepted as a reliable sign of sciatic nerve localization **(Fig. 20.8)**.

► Bone contact is frequently encountered during needle advancement, indicating that the needle has contacted the femur (usually the lesser trochanter) **(Fig. 20-9)**. When the needle is stopped by bone, the algorithm below should be followed:

1. The needle is withdrawn 2 to 3 cm.
2. The foot is rotated inward (internal rotation) **(Fig. 20-10)**.
3. The needle is advanced to bypass the lesser trochanter. The internal rotation of the leg swings the lesser trochanter downward and away from the path of the needle and often allows passage of the needle toward the sciatic nerve.
4. When steps 1 through 3 fail to facilitate passage of the needle, the needle is withdrawn back to the skin and reinserted at a slightly medial angulation **(Fig. 20-11)**. Steps 1 through 3 are then repeated.

► Failure to pass the needle or achieve nerve stimulation should prompt its withdrawal, and the following actions should be taken:

1. Ensure that the nerve stimulator is functional, properly connected to the patient and to the needle, and set to deliver a current of desired intensity.
2. Reassess the landmarks.
3. Insert the needle 1 cm medially to the original insertion site.

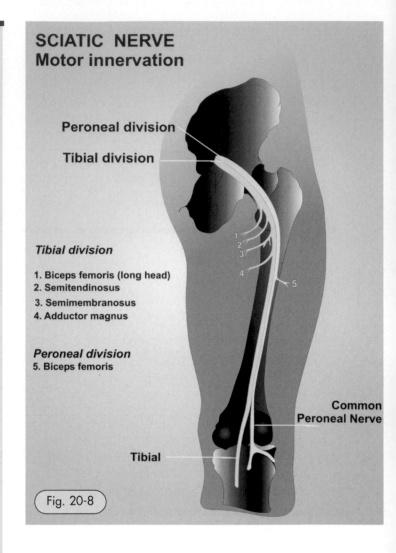

SCIATIC NERVE
Motor innervation

Peroneal division

Tibial division

Tibial division

1. Biceps femoris (long head)
2. Semitendinosus
3. Semimembranosus
4. Adductor magnus

Peroneal division
5. Biceps femoris

Common Peroneal Nerve

Tibial

Fig. 20-8

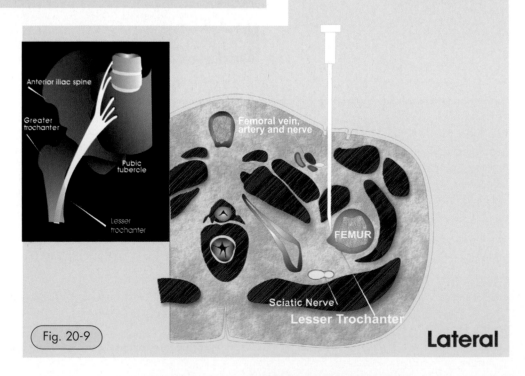

ANTERIOR

Anterior iliac spine

Greater trochanter

Pubic tubercle

Lesser trochanter

Femoral vein, artery and nerve

FEMUR

Sciatic Nerve

Lesser Trochanter

Fig. 20-9

Lateral

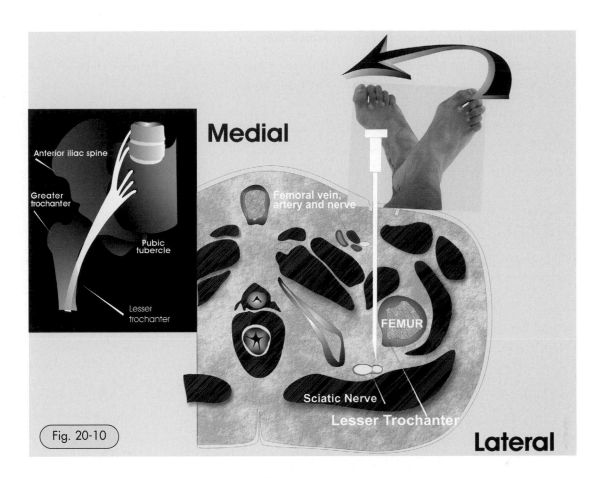

Fig. 20-10

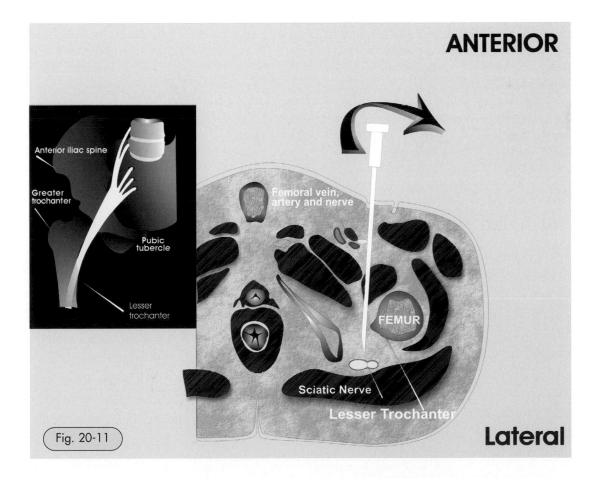

Fig. 20-11

Interpreting Responses to Nerve Stimulation

Some common responses to nerve stimulation and the course of action to take to obtain the proper response are given in **Table 20.1.**

TABLE 20.1

Some Common Responses to Nerve Stimulation and the Course of Action to Take to Obtain the Proper Response

RESPONSE OBTAINED	INTERPRETATION	PROBLEM	ACTION
Twitch of the quadriceps muscle (patella twitch)	Common; stimulation of the branches of the femoral nerve	Too shallow a (superficial) placement of the needle	Continue advancing the needle
Local twitch at the femoral crease area	Direct stimulation of the iliopsoas or pectineus muscles	Too superior insertion of the needle	Stop the procedure and reassess the landmarks
Hamstring twitch	The needle may be stimulating branch(es) of the sciatic nerve to the hamstring muscle; direct stimulation of the hamstring with higher current is also possible	Unreliable	Withdraw needle and redirect it slightly medially or laterally (5°–10°)
The needle is placed deep (12–15 cm) but twitches were not elicited and bone is not contacted	The needle is likely too medial		Withdraw needle and redirect it slightly laterally
Twitches of the calf, foot, or toes	Stimulation of the sciatic nerve	None	Accept and inject local anesthetic

Choice of Local Anesthetic

A sciatic blockade requires a relatively low volume of local anesthetic to achieve anesthesia of the entire trunk of the nerve. The choice of the type and concentration of local anesthetic should be based on whether the block is planned for surgical anesthesia or pain management **(Table 20.2)**. Because the duration of a sciatic blockade is longer than that of any other peripheral nerve block, we tend to use a shorter-acting local anesthetic more commonly. However, when prolonged pain relief is desired, a longer-acting local anesthetic may be more appropriate.

TIP

▶ We suggest that the use of epinephrine for the anterior approach to a sciatic nerve block be avoided because of the risk of nerve ischemia due to the combined effects of the vasoconstrictive action of epinephrine, nerve stretching, and application of a tourniquet.

TABLE 20.2
Choice of Local Anesthetic for Sciatic Nerve Block

ANESTHETIC	ONSET (min)	DURATION OF ANESTHESIA (h)	DURATION OF ANALGESIA (h)
3% 2-Chloroprocaine (+ HCO3)	10–15	2	2.5
1.5% Mepivacaine (+ HCO3)	10–15	4–5	5–8
2% Lidocaine (+ HCO3)	10–20	5–6	5–8
0.5% Ropivacaine	15–20	6–12	6–24
0.75% Ropivacaine	10–15	8–12	8–24
0.5 Bupivacaine (or levobupivacaine)	15–30	8–16	10–48

Block Dynamics and Perioperative Management

An anterior approach to a sciatic block can be associated with significant patient discomfort because the needle must transverse multiple muscle planes on its way to the sciatic nerve. The administration of midazolam 2 to 6 mg after the patient is positioned and alfentanil 500 to 1000 mg just before infiltration of local anesthetic are usually sufficient for most patients. The need for this premedication is also suggested by the fact that most of our indications for this block are in patients with lower-extremity trauma, making patient positioning and leg manipulation even more uncomfortable. A typical onset time for this block is 10 to 25 minutes, depending on the type, concentration, and volume of local anesthetic used. Usually, the first sign of blockade onset is a report by the patient that the foot "feels different" or inability to wiggle the toes.

TIP

▶ Inadequate skin anesthesia despite an apparently timely onset of the blockade can occur. With some blocks, it can take up to 30 minutes for full sensory-motor anesthesia to develop. Local infiltration by the surgeon at the site of the incision is often all that is needed to allow the surgery to proceed.

Complications and How to Avoid Them

Some general and specific instructions on possible complications and methods that can be used to avoid them are presented in **Table 20.3**.

TABLE 20.3
Complications of Anterior Approach to Sciatic Nerve Block and Preventive Techniques

Infection	• A strict aseptic technique should always be used.
Hematoma	• Avoid multiple needle insertions. • This technique should be avoided in patients receiving anticoagulant therapy.
Vascular puncture	• Vascular puncture is not common with this technique; when it occurs, it is usually because of too medial a placement of the needle (femoral artery and vein).
Local anesthetic toxicity	• Systemic toxicity after sciatic blockade is not common; however, it is important to avoid injecting large volumes and doses of local anesthetic because of the proximity of the muscle beds and the potential for rapid absorption.
Nerve injury	• A sciatic block is uniquely sensitive to mechanical and pressure injury. • Nerve stimulation and slow needle advancement should be employed. • Local anesthetic should never be injected when a patient complains of pain. • Never forcefully inject local anesthetic when an abnormally high pressure on injection is noted. • It is never correct to assume that the needle is obstructed with tissue debris when resistance to injection is met; the needle should be taken out and checked for the patency (flush) before reinsertion and another attempt is made to inject. • When stimulation is obtained with current intensity of <0.2 mA, the needle should be pulled back to obtain the same response with a current intensity of 0.2–0.5 mA before injecting local anesthetic.
Tourniquet	• Avoid the use of a tourniquet when possible. • Injection of the local anesthetic within the sciatic nerve sheath, epinephrine, and a tourniquet over the site of injection can all combine to cause ischemia of the sciatic nerve.
Other	• Instruct the patient and nursing staff on care of the insensate extremity. • Explain to the patient that frequent body repositioning is needed to avoid stretching and prolonged ischemia (sitting) of the anesthetized sciatic nerve. • Advise the use of heel padding during prolonged bed rest or sleep.

SUGGESTED READINGS

- Chelly JE, Delaunay L. A new anterior approach to the sciatic nerve block. *Anesthesiology* 1999; 91:1655–1660.
- Magora F, Pessachovitch B, Shoham I. Sciatic nerve block by the anterior approach for operations on the lower extremity. *Br J Anaesth* 1974;46:121–123.
- Mansour NY. Anterior approach revisited and another new sciatic nerve block in the supine position. *Reg Anesth* 1993;18:265–266.
- McNicol LR. Anterior approach to sciatic nerve block in children: loss of resistance or nerve stimulator for identifying the neurovascular compartment. *Anesth Analg* 1987;66:1199–1200.
- McNicol LR. Sciatic nerve block for children: sciatic nerve block by the anterior approach for postoperative pain relief. *Anaesthesia* 1985;40:410–414.
- Van Elstraete AC, Poey C, Lebrun T, Pastureau F. New landmarks for the anterior approach to the sciatic nerve block: imaging and clinical study. *Anesth Analg* 2002;95:214–218.
- Vloka JD, Hadžić A, April E, Thys DM. Anterior approach to the sciatic nerve block: the effects of leg rotation. *Anesth Analg* 2001;92:460–462.

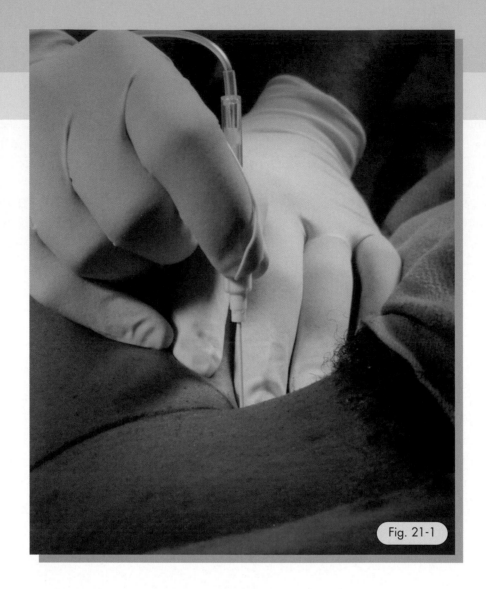

Fig. 21-1

BLOCK AT A GLANCE

- Indications: anterior thigh and knee surgery

- Landmarks: femoral (inguinal) crease, femoral artery pulse

- Needle: 5 cm

- Nerve stimulation: twitch of the patella (quadriceps) at 0.2 to 0.5 mA current

- Local anesthetic volume: 20 mL

- Complexity level: basic

21 FEMORAL
NERVE BLOCK

GENERAL CONSIDERATIONS

A femoral nerve block is a basic nerve block technique that is easy to master, carries a low risk of complications, and has significant clinical applicability for surgical anesthesia and postoperative pain management. This block is well-suited for surgery on the anterior thigh, knee, quadriceps tendon repair, and postoperative pain management after femur and knee surgery. When combined with a block of the sciatic nerve, anesthesia of almost the entire lower extremity from the midthigh level can be achieved. The success rate of this block for surgery is high, nearing 95%.

Anatomy

The femoral nerve is the largest branch of the lumbar plexus. It arises from the second, third, and fourth lumbar nerves. The nerve descends through the fibers of the psoas muscle, emerging from the psoas at the lower part of its border, and runs downward between the psoas and the iliacus. Eventually, the femoral nerve passes underneath the inguinal ligament into the thigh, where it assumes a more flattened shape **(Fig. 21-2)**. As it passes beneath the inguinal ligament, it is positioned immediately lateral and slightly deeper than the femoral artery.

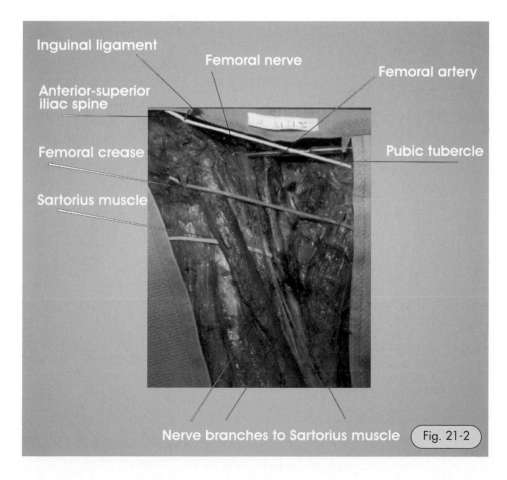

Inguinal ligament

Femoral nerve

Femoral artery

Anterior-superior iliac spine

Femoral crease

Pubic tubercle

Sartorius muscle

Nerve branches to Sartorius muscle

Fig. 21-2

At the femoral crease, the nerve is covered by the fascia iliaca and separated from the femoral artery and vein by a portion of the psoas muscle and the ligamentum iliopectineus **(Fig. 21-3)**. This physical separation of the femoral nerve from the vascular fascia explains the lack of spread of a "blind paravascular" injection of local anesthetics toward the femoral nerve.

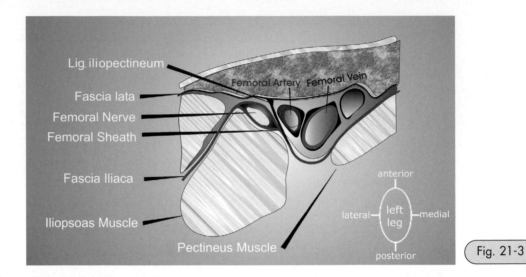

Fig. 21-3

TIP

▶ It is useful to think of the mnemonic "VAN" (vein, artery, nerve) going from medial to lateral, when recalling the relationship of the femoral nerve to the vessels in the femoral triangle.

The motor branches to the sartorius muscle depart from the anteromedial aspect of the femoral nerve toward the sartorius muscle. Because the anesthesiologist can never be sure whether stimulation of the sartorius muscle is obtained inside or outside the sheath of the femoral, this should always be confirmed by obtaining quadriceps stimulation before injecting local anesthetic.

Fig. 21-4

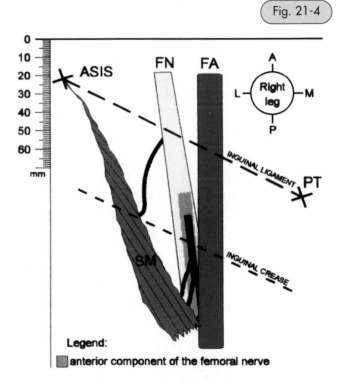

The relationship among the femoral artery, femoral nerve, and sartorius muscle. (ASIS) Anterior-superior iliac spine, (FN) femoral nerve, (FA) femoral artery, (SM) sartorius muscle, (PT) pubic tubercle.

The femoral nerve supplies the muscular branches of the iliacus and pectineus and the muscles of the anterior thigh except for the tensor fascia femoris. The nerve also provides cutaneous branches to the front and inner sides of the thigh and to the leg and foot (saphenous nerve), as well as to the articular branches of the hip and knee joints **(Table 21.1)**.

TABLE 21.1 Femoral Nerve Branches	
Anterior division	• Middle cutaneous • Medial cutaneous • Muscular (sartorius)
Posterior division	• Saphenous nerve (most medial) • Muscular (individual heads of the quadriceps muscle) • Articular branches (hip and knee)

Distribution of Anesthesia

A femoral block results in anesthesia of the entire anterior thigh and most of the femur and knee joint **(Fig. 21-5)**. The block also confers anesthesia of the skin on the medial aspect of the leg below the knee joint (saphenous nerve—a superficial terminal extension of the femoral nerve).

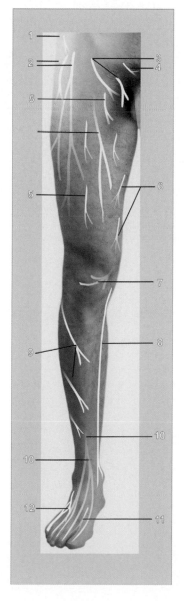

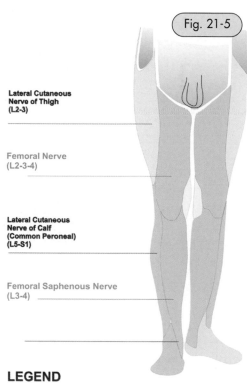

Fig. 21-5

Lateral Cutaneous
Nerve of Thigh
(L2-3)

Femoral Nerve
(L2-3-4)

Lateral Cutaneous
Nerve of Calf
(Common Peroneal)
(L5-S1)

Femoral Saphenous Nerve
(L3-4)

LEGEND

1. Subcostal nerve (lateral cutaneous branch)
2. Lateral femoral cutaneous nerve
3. Femoral branch of the genitofemoral nerve
4. Genital branch of the genitofemoral nerve
5. Anterior femoral cutaneous nerve (from femoral nerve)
6. Cutaneous branches of the obturator nerve
7. Infrapatellar branch of the saphenous nerve
8. Saphenous nerve (terminal cutaneous branch of the femoral nerve)
9. Lateral sural cutaneous nerves (from common peroneal nerve)
10. Superficial peroneal nerve
11. Deep peroneal nerve
12. Lateral dorsal cutaneous nerve (branch of sural nerve)

SINGLE-INJECTION FEMORAL NERVE BLOCK

Patient Positioning

The patient is in the supine position with both legs extended (Fig. 21-6). In obese patients, a pillow placed underneath the hips may facilitate palpation of the femoral artery and the block performance.

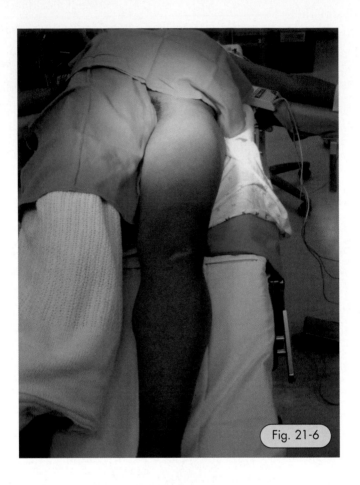

Fig. 21-6

Equipment

A standard regional anesthesia tray is prepared with the following equipment:

- Sterile towels and gauze packs

- 20-mL syringes containing local anesthetic

- Sterile gloves, marking pen, and surface electrode

- $1^{1}/_{2}$-in, 25-gauge needle for skin infiltration

- 5-cm, short-bevel, insulated stimulating needle

- Surface electrode

- Peripheral nerve stimulator

Surface Landmarks

The only significant surface landmark for this technique is **(Fig. 21-7)**:

1. Femoral crease

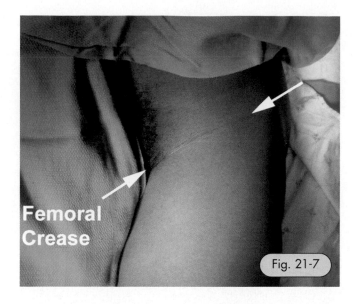

Femoral Crease

Fig. 21-7

Anatomic Landmarks

TIPS

► Note that this technique differs from common descriptions of a femoral nerve block in which the needle is inserted at the level of the inguinal ligament.

► Instead, with this technique the needle is inserted at the level of the femoral crease, a naturally occurring, oblique skin fold positioned a few centimeters below the inguinal ligament.

► The femoral crease can be accentuated in obese patients by having an assistant retract the lower abdomen laterally.

► Retraction of the abdomen should be maintained throughout the procedure to facilitate palpation of the femoral artery **(Fig. 21-8)** and performance of the block.

Anatomic landmarks for the femoral nerve block are easily recognizable in all patients and include **(Fig. 21-9)**:

1. Femoral crease

2. Femoral artery pulse.

The needle insertion site is labeled immediately lateral to the pulse of the femoral artery. All landmarks should be outlined with a marking pen.

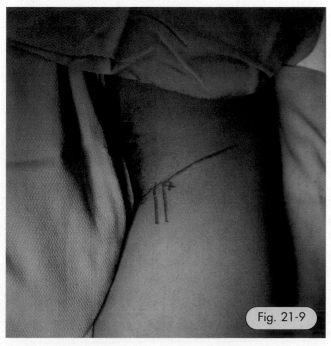

Fig. 21-9

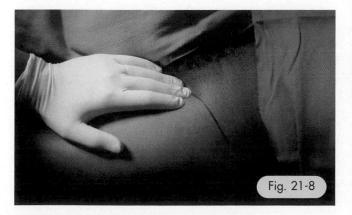

Fig. 21-8

Local Anesthetic Infiltration and Needle Insertion

After thorough preparation of the area with an antiseptic solution, local anesthetic is infiltrated subcutaneously at the estimated site of needle insertion **(Fig. 21-10)**. The injection for the skin anesthesia should be shallow and in a line extending laterally to allow a more lateral needle reinsertion when necessary. The anesthesiologist should stand on the side of the patient with the palpating hand on the femoral artery. The needle is introduced immediately at the lateral border of the artery and advanced in the sagittal, slightly cephalad plane **(Fig. 21-11)**.

> **TIP**
>
> ▶ The nerve stimulator is initially set to deliver 1.0 mA (2 Hz, 100–300 μs). With the proper needle position, advancement of the needle should not result in any local twitches; the first response is usually that of the femoral nerve.

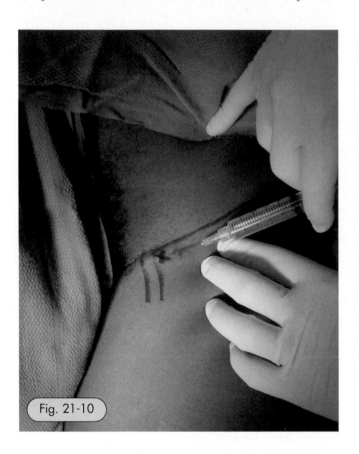

Fig. 21-10

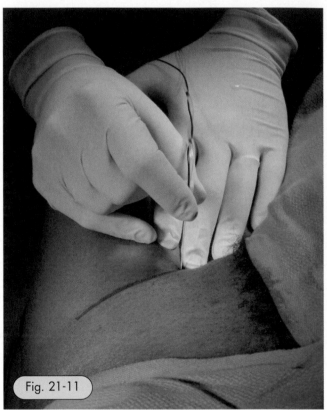

Fig. 21-11

> **GOAL**
>
> *The femoral nerve innervates several muscle groups (Fig 21-12). A visible or palpable twitch of the quadriceps muscle (a patella twitch) at 0.2 to 0.5 mA current is the most reliable response.*

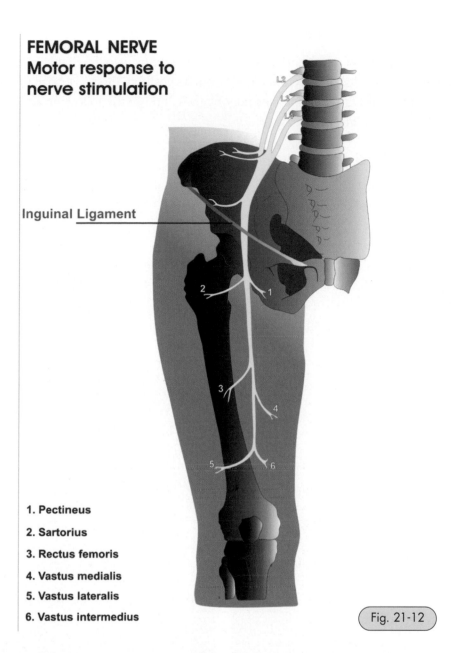

FEMORAL NERVE
Motor response to nerve stimulation

Inguinal Ligament

1. Pectineus
2. Sartorius
3. Rectus femoris
4. Vastus medialis
5. Vastus lateralis
6. Vastus intermedius

Fig. 21-12

TIPS

▶ The most common response to nerve stimulation with this technique is twitching of the sartorius muscle **(Fig. 21-12)**. This results in a bandlike contraction across the thigh without movement of the patella.

▶ It should be kept in mind that a sartorius muscle twitch is not reliable because the branches to the sartorius muscle may be outside the femoral sheath.

▶ When a sartorius muscle twitch occurs, the needle is simply redirected laterally and advanced several millimeters deeper.

Failure to Localize the Femoral Nerve

When stimulation of the quadriceps muscle is not obtained on the first needle pass, the palpating hand should not be moved from its position. First, visualize the needle plane in which stimulation was not obtained and use the following algorithm (**Fig. 21-13A** and **21-13B**):

• Ensure that the nerve stimulator is properly connected and functional.

• Withdraw the needle to skin level, redirect it 10° to 15° laterally, and repeat needle advancement.

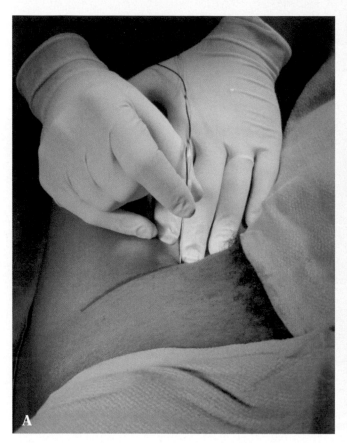
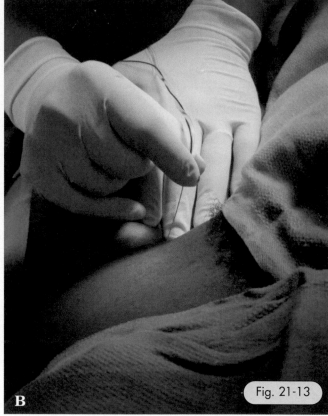

Fig. 21-13

When the above procedure fails to produce a twitch, the needle is withdrawn from the skin and reinserted 1 cm laterally, and the above steps are repeated with a progressively more lateral needle insertion **(Fig. 21-14A** and **21-14B)**. After initial stimulation of the femoral nerve is obtained, the stimulating current is gradually decreased until twitches are still seen or felt at 0.2 to 0.4 mA current. This typically occurs at a depth of 2 to 3 cm. After obtaining negative results from an aspiration test for blood, 20 to 25 mL of local anesthetic is slowly injected.

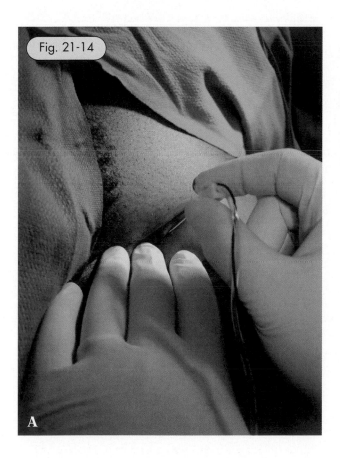

Fig. 21-14

A

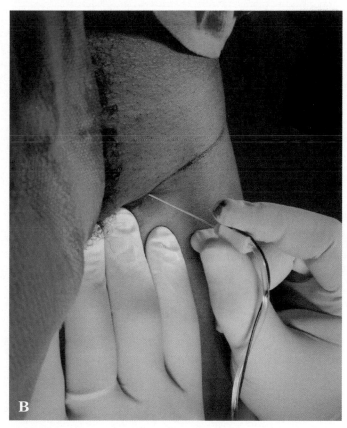

B

Interpreting the Responses to Nerve Stimulation

Some common responses to nerve stimulation and the course of action required to obtain the proper response are shown in **Table 21.2.**

TABLE 21.2

Some Common Responses to Nerve Stimulation and the Course of Action Required to Obtain the Proper Response

RESPONSE OBTAINED	INTERPRETATION	PROBLEM	ACTION
No response	Needle is inserted either too medially or too laterally	Femoral artery not properly localized or the palpating hand was moved during the procedure	Follow the systematic lateral angulation and reinsertion of the needle as described in the technique
Bone contact	Needle contacts hip or superior ramus of the pubic bone	Needle is inserted too deep	Withdraw needle to skin level and repeat the procedure
Local twitch	Direct stimulation of the iliopsoas or pectineus muscle	Needle is inserted too deep or too superiorly	Withdraw needle to skin level and repeat the procedure
Twitch of the sartorius muscle	Stimulation of the nerve branches to the sartorius muscle	Needle tip is slightly anterior and medial to main trunk of the femoral nerve	Redirect needle laterally and advance it deeper 1–3 mm
Vascular puncture	Blood in the invariably indicates placement into the femoral artery or vein	Needle is inserted too medially	Withdraw needle and reinsert it laterally 1 cm
Patella twitch	Stimulation of the main trunk of the femoral nerve	None	Accept and inject local anesthetic

Choice of Local Anesthetic

A femoral block can be accomplished with as little as 10 mL of local anesthetic. However, we use larger volumes (e.g., 20 to 25 mL) because it often disperses laterally underneath the fascia iliaca and also results in a block of the lateral femoral cutaneous nerve of the thigh. A block of this nerve in return confers anesthesia on the lateral aspect of the thigh, which nicely complements the femoral nerve block.

The choice of the type and concentration of local anesthetic should be based on whether the block is planned for surgical anesthesia or pain management. A long-acting local anesthetic should be avoided in ambulatory patients undergoing relatively minor procedures as ambulation is affected by prolonged motor blockade of the quadriceps muscle.

The onset times and the duration of anesthesia for different types and concentrations of local anesthetics and with the addition of a vasoconstrictor are listed in **Table 21.3.**

TABLE 21.3
Choice of Local Anesthetic For Femoral Nerve Block

ANESTHETIC	ONSET (min)	DURATION OF ANESTHESIA (h)	DURATION OF ANALGESIA (h)
3% 2-chloroprocaine (+ HCO_3)	10–15	1	2
3% 2-chloroprocaine (HCO_3 + epinephrine)	10–15	1.5–2	2–3
1.5% Mepivacaine (+ HCO_3)	15–20	2–3	3–5
1.5% Mepivacaine (HCO_3 + epinephrine)	15–20	2–5	3–8
2% Lidocaine ($HCO3_3$ + epinephrine)	10–20	2–5	3-8
0.5% Ropivacaine	15–30	4–8	5–12
0.75% Ropivacaine	10–15	5–10	6–24
0.5 Bupivacaine (or levobupivacaine)	15–30	5–15	6–30

Block Dynamics and Perioperative Management

This technique is associated with minimal patient discomfort because the needle passes only through the skin and adipose of the femoral inguinal region. However, many patients feel uncomfortable being exposed during palpation of the femoral artery, and appropriate sedation is necessary for the patient's comfort and acceptance. The administration of midazolam 1 to 2 mg after the patient is positioned and alfentanil 250 to 500 µg just before infiltration of the local anesthetic suffices for most patients. A typical onset time for this block is 10 to 15 minutes, depending on the type, concentration, and volume of anesthetic used. The first sign of onset of the blockade is a loss of sensation in the skin over the medial aspect of the leg below the knee (saphenous nerve). Weight bearing on the blocked side is impaired, which should be clearly explained to the patient to prevent the risk of falls.

CONTINUOUS FEMORAL NERVE BLOCK

The continuous femoral nerve block technique is quite similar to the single-injection procedure; however, insertion of the needle at a slightly more acute angle is necessary to facilitate threading of the catheter. The most common indications for use of this block are postoperative analgesia after knee arthroplasty, anterior cruciate ligament repair, and femoral fracture repair.

Equipment

A standard regional anesthesia tray is prepared with the following equipment:

- Sterile towels and gauze packs

- Two 20-mL syringes containing local anesthetic

- Sterile gloves, marking pen, and surface electrode

- $1^1/_2$-in, 25-gauge needle for skin infiltration

- 5-cm, insulated stimulating needle (Tuohy-style or regular tip)

- Catheter

- Peripheral nerve stimulator

Landmarks

The landmarks for a continuous femoral block include **(Fig. 21-15)**:

1. Femoral (inguinal crease)

2. Femoral artery

3. Needle insertion site is marked immediately lateral to the pulse of the femoral artery

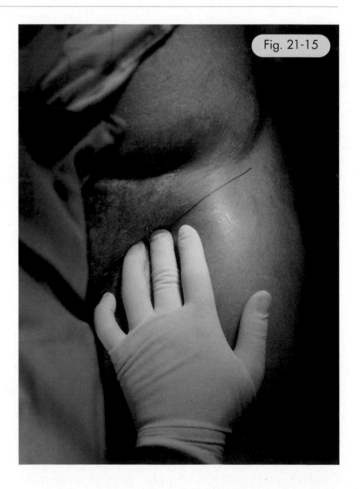

Fig. 21-15

Local Anesthetic Infiltration and Needle Insertion

With the patient in the supine position, infiltrate the skin with local anesthetic at the injection site using a 25-gauge needle. The palpating hand is used to keep the middle finger on the pulse of the femoral artery, while the entire hand slightly pulls the skin caudally to keep it from wrinkling on needle insertion **(Fig. 21-16)**. A 5-cm, stimulating needle connected to the nerve stimulator (1.0 mA, 2 Hz, 100–300 µs) is inserted and advanced at a 45° to 60° cephalad angle. Care should be taken to avoid medial insertion of the needle and consequent puncture of the femoral artery. After a quadriceps muscle twitch is obtained (patella twitch) at 0.5 mA current, the initial bolus of local anesthetic is injected (15 to 20 mL) and the catheter is inserted 5 to 10 cm beyond the tip of the needle **(Fig. 21-17A** and **21-17B)**. The catheter is then secured to the skin using a benzoin prep followed by application of a clear dressing.

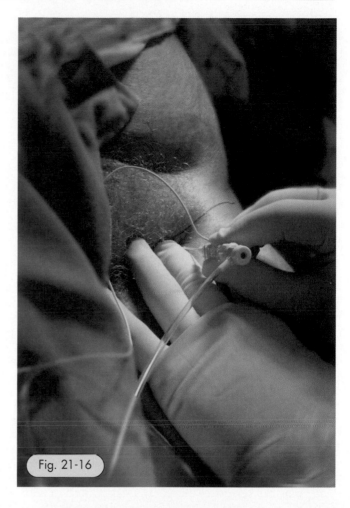

Fig. 21-16

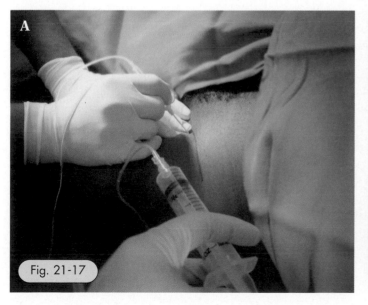

Fig. 21-17

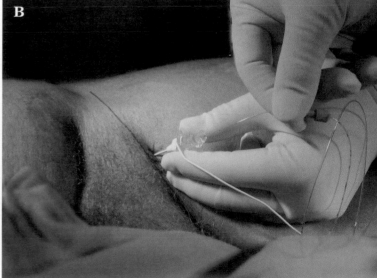

Continuous Infusion

Continuous infusion is always initiated following an initial bolus (15 to 20 mL) of dilute local anesthetic through the catheter. For this purpose, we routinely use 0.2% ropivacaine. Diluted bupivacaine or 0.25% levobupivacaine are also suitable, but may result in more pronounced motor blockade. The infusion is maintained at 8 mL/h or 5 mL/h when a patient-controlled anesthesia (PCA) dose is planned.

Complications and How to Avoid Them

Complications following a femoral block are uncommon. **Table 21.4** provides some general and specific instructions on possible complications and how to avoid them.

TABLE 21.4

Complications of Femoral Nerve Block and Preventive Techniques

Infection	• Use a strict aseptic technique. • At this location, catheters are difficult to keep sterile and should probably be removed after 48 h.
Hematoma	• Avoid advancement of the needle when the patient reports pain; this may indicate insertion of the needle through the iliopsoas or pectineus muscle. • When the femoral artery or vein is punctured, the procedure should be stopped and a firm, constant pressure applied over the femoral artery for 2–3 min before proceeding with the blockade. • In a patient with difficult anatomy or severe peripheral vascular disease, use a single-injection, smaller-gauge needle to localize the femoral nerve before proceeding with a larger-gauge needle for the continuous technique.
Vascular puncture	• The needle should never be redirected medially! • The needle is first inserted just laterally to the femoral artery, and consequent insertions and redirections should all be progressively more lateral.
Nerve injury	• Use nerve stimulation and slow needle advancement. • Distinct paresthesia is almost never elicited with a femoral nerve block and should not be sought. • Do not inject when the patient complains of pain or when high pressures are met on injection.
Other	• Instruct the patient on the inability to bear weight on the blocked extremity.

SUGGESTED READINGS

Single-injection Femoral Block

- Allen HW, Leu SS, Ware PD, NINR CS, Owens BD. Peripheral nerve blocks improve analgesia after total knee replacement surgery. *Anesth Analog* 1998; 87:93–97.

- Chadic A, Volk JD, Kurova MM, Korin R, Birdbath DJ. The practice of peripheral nerve blocks in the United States: a national survey. *Reg Anesth Pain Med* 1998; 23:241–246.

- Lang SA, Yip RW, Chang PC. The femoral 3-in-1 blocks revisited. *J CLIM Anethi* 1993; 5:292–296.

- Made TH, Ellis FR, Hassall PJ. Evaluation of "3 in 1" lumbar plexus block in patients having muscle biopsy. *Br J Anaest* 1989; 62:515–517.

- Machover P, NaSal C, Sitz Ohl C, Karla S. Magnetic resonance imaging of the distribution of local anesthetic during the three-in-one block. *Anesth Analog* 2000; 90:119–124.

- Milroy MF, Larkin KL, Bart MS, Hodgson PS, Owens BD. Femoral nerve block with 0.25% or 0.5% bupivacaine improves postoperative analgesia following outpatient arthroscopic anterior cruciate ligament repair. *Reg Anesth Pain Med* 2001; 26:24–29.

- Parkinson SK, Mueller JB, Little WL, Bailey SL. Extent of blockade with various approaches to the lumbar plexus. Anesth Analg 1989;68:243–248.

- Ritter JW. Femoral nerve "sheath" for inguinal paravascular lumbar plexus block is not found in human cadavers. *J Clin Anesth* 1995;470–473.

- Seeberger MD, Urwyler A. Paravascular lumbar plexus block: block extension after femoral nerve stimulation and injection of 20 vs. 40 ml mepivacaine 10 mg/ml. *Acta Anaesthesiol Scand* 1995;39:769–773.

- Singelyn FJ, Vanderelst PE, Gouverneur JM. Extended femoral nerve sheath block after total hip arthroplasty: continuous versus patient-controlled techniques. *Anesth Analg* 2001;92:455–459.

- Vloka JD, Hadžić A, Drobnik L, Ernest A, Reiss W, Thys DM. Anatomical landmarks for femoral nerve block: a comparison of four needle insertion sites. *Anesth Analg* 1999; 89:1467–1470.

- Vloka JD, Hadžić A, Mulcare R, Lesser JB, Kitain E, Thys DM. Femoral and genitofemoral nerve blocks versus spinal anesthesia for outpatients undergoing long saphenous vein stripping surgery. *Anesth Analg* 1997;84:749–752.

- Wang H, Boctor B, Verner J. The effect of single-injection femoral nerve block on rehabilitation and length of hospital stay after total knee replacement. *Reg Anesth Pain Med* 2002;27:139–144.

- Winnie AP, Ramamurthy S, Durrani Z. The inguinal paravascular technic of lumbar plexus anesthesia: the "3-in-1 block." *Anesth Analg* 1973;52:989–996.

Continuous Femoral Nerve Block

- Allen JG, Denny NM, Oakman N. Postoperative analgesia following total knee arthroplasty: a study comparing spinal anesthesia and combined sciatic femoral 3-in-1 block. *Reg Anesth Pain Med* 1998;23:142–146.

- Capdevila X, Barthelet Y, Biboulet P, Ryckwaert Y, Rubenovitch J, d'Athis F. Effects of perioperative analgesic technique on the surgical outcome and duration of rehabilitation after major knee surgery. *Anesthesiology* 1999;91:8–15.

- Capdevila X, Biboulet P, Morau D, Bernard N, Deschodt J, Lopez S, d'Athis F. Continuous three-in-one block for postoperative pain after lower limb orthopedic surgery: where do the catheters go? *Anesth Analg* 2002;94:1001–1006.

- Chelly JE, Casati A, Fanelli G. *Continuous Peripheral Nerve Block Techniques: An Illustrated Guide.* London, England: Mosby International; 2001.

- Cuvillon P, Ripart J, Lalourcey L, Veyrat E, L'Hermite J, Boisson C, Thouabtia E, Eledjam JJ. The continuous femoral nerve block catheter for postoperative analgesia: bacterial colonization, infectious rate and adverse effects. *Anesth Analg* 2001;93:1045–1049.

- Hirst GC, Lang SA, Dust WN, Cassidy JD, Yip RW. Femoral nerve block: single injection versus continuous infusion for total knee arthroplasty. *Reg Anesth* 1996; 21:292–297.

- Singelyn FJ, Gouverneur JM. Extended "three-in-one" block after total knee arthroplasty: continuous versus patient-controlled techniques. *Anesth Analg* 2000;91: 176–180.

- Singelyn FJ, Vanderelst PE, Gouverneur JM. Extended femoral nerve sheath block after total hip arthroplasty: continuous versus patient-controlled techniques. *Anesth Analg* 2001; 92:455–45

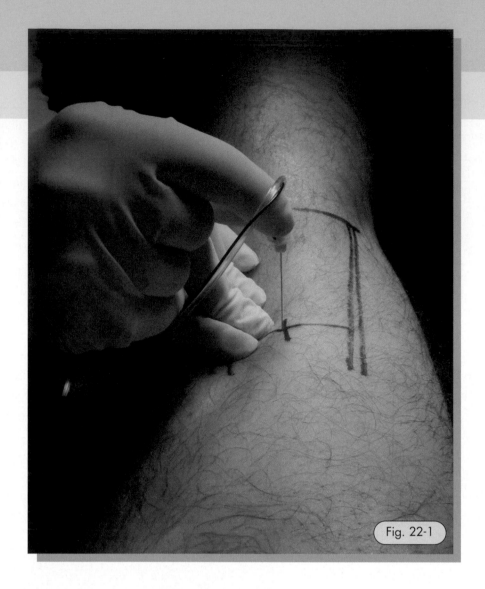

Fig. 22-1

BLOCK AT A GLANCE

- Indications: ankle and foot surgery

- Landmarks: popliteal fossa crease, tendons of the semitendinosus and semimembranosus, and tendon of biceps femoris muscle

- Needle: 5 cm

- Nerve stimulation: twitch of the foot or toes at 0.2 to 0.5 mA current

- Local anesthetic: 35 to 45 mL

- Complexity level: intermediate

22 POPLITEAL BLOCK:
INTERTENDINOUS APPROACH

GENERAL CONSIDERATIONS

The popliteal block is a block of the sciatic nerve at the level of the popliteal fossa. This block is one of the regional anesthesia techniques most often used in our practice. Some common indications include corrective foot surgery, foot debridement, and Achilles tendon repair. A sound knowledge of the principles of nerve stimulation and the anatomic characteristics of the sciatic nerve in the popliteal fossa are essential for its successful implementation.

Anatomy

The *sciatic nerve* is a nerve bundle consisting of two separate nerve trunks, the tibial and the common peroneal nerves **(Fig. 22-2)**. A common epineural sheath envelops these two nerves at their outset in pelvis. As the sciatic nerve descends toward the knee, the two components eventually diverge in the popliteal fossa, giving rise to the tibial and the common peroneal nerves. This division of the sciatic nerve usually occurs between 50 and 70 mm proximal to the popliteal fossa crease. From its divergence from the sciatic nerve, the *common peroneal nerve* continues its path downward and descends along the head and neck of the fibula. Its major branches in this region are branches to the knee joint and cutaneous branches that form the sural nerve. Its terminal branches are the superficial and deep peroneal nerves. The *tibial nerve* is the larger of the two divisions of the sciatic nerve. It continues its path vertically through the popliteal fossa, and its terminal branches are the medial and lateral plantar nerves. Its collateral branches give rise to the cutaneous sural nerves, muscular branches to the muscles of the calf, and articular branches to the ankle joint. It is important to note that in contrast to common assumption, the sciatic nerve in the popliteal fossa is lateral and superficial to the popliteal artery and vein and is *not*

enveloped by the same tissue sheath (neurovascular sheath). This anatomic characteristic is important in understanding why systemic toxicity and vascular punctures are infrequent following a popliteal block.

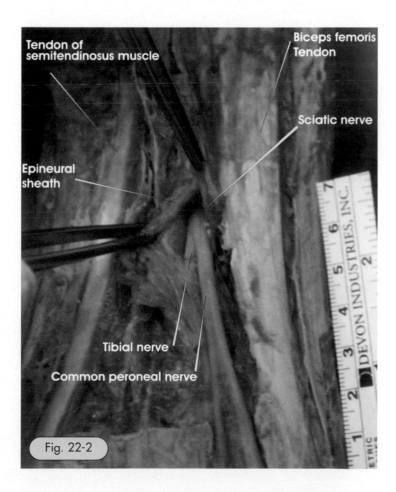

Tendon of semitendinosus muscle

Biceps femoris Tendon

Sciatic nerve

Epineural sheath

Tibial nerve

Common peroneal nerve

DEVON INDUSTRIES, INC.

Fig. 22-2

Distribution of Anesthesia

A popliteal block results in anesthesia of the entire distal two-thirds of the lower extremity, with the exception of the medial aspect of the leg (see the shaded area) **(Fig. 22-3)**. Cutaneous innervation of the medial leg below the knee is provided by the saphenous nerve, a superficial terminal extension of the femoral nerve. Depending on the level of sur-

gery, the addition of a saphenous nerve block may be required for surgery. Popliteal block alone is typically sufficient enough to achieve anesthesia for tourniquet pain because this pain is the result of pressure and ischemia of the deep muscle beds and not of the skin and subcutaneous tissues.

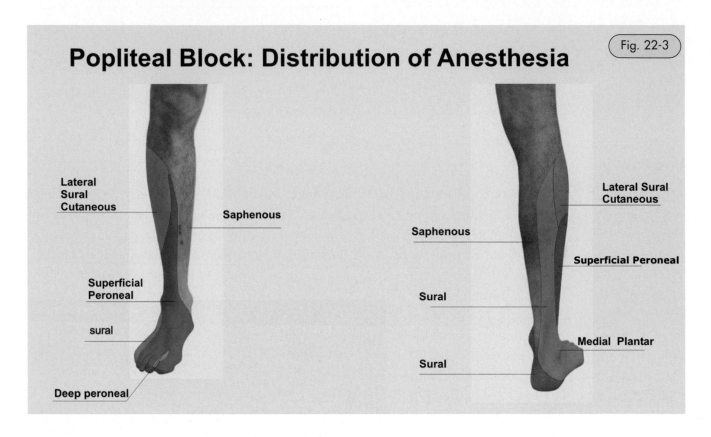

Popliteal Block: Distribution of Anesthesia

Fig. 22-3

Lateral Sural Cutaneous

Saphenous

Superficial Peroneal

sural

Deep peroneal

Saphenous

Sural

Sural

Lateral Sural Cutaneous

Superficial Peroneal

Medial Plantar

SINGLE-INJECTION POPLITEAL BLOCK (INTERTENDINOUS APPROACH)

Patient Positioning

The patient is in the prone position **(Fig. 22-4)**. The foot on the side to be blocked should be positioned so that even the slightest movements of the foot or toes can be easily observed. This is best achieved by allowing the foot to extend beyond the operating room bed.

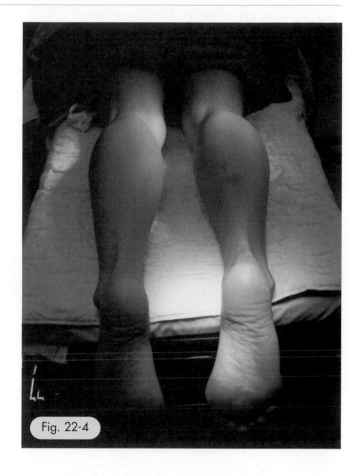

Fig. 22-4

Equipment

A standard regional anesthesia tray is prepared with the following equipment **(Fig. 22-5)**:

- Sterile towels and gauze packs

- 20-mL syringes containing local anesthetic

- Sterile gloves, marking pen, and surface electrode

- 1$^{1}/_{2}$-in, 25-gauge needle for skin infiltration

- 5-cm, short-bevel, insulated stimulating needle

- Peripheral nerve stimulator

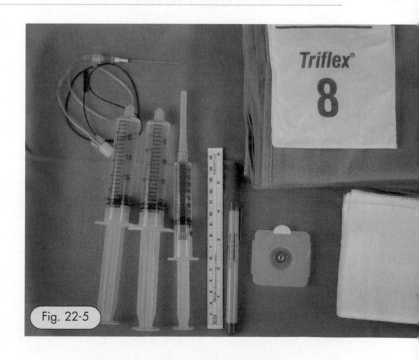

Fig. 22-5

Surface Landmarks

The following surface anatomy landmarks are used to determine the insertion point for the needle **(Fig. 22-6)**.

1. Popliteal fossa crease

2. Tendon of the biceps femoris muscle (laterally)

3. Tendons of the semitendinosus and semimembranosus muscles (medially)

These anatomical structures are best accentuated by asking the patient to elevate the foot while palpating **(Fig. 22-6)**.

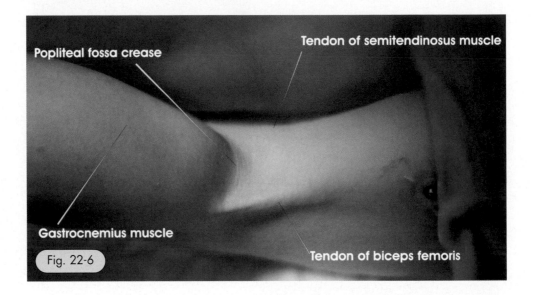

Fig. 22-6

Anatomic Landmarks

Landmarks for the intertendinous approach to a popliteal block are easily recognizable even in obese patients. All three landmarks should be outlined with a marking pen **(Fig. 22-7)**:

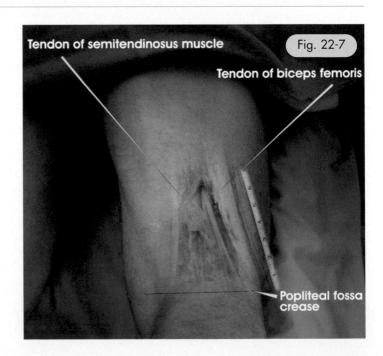

Fig. 22-7

1. Popliteal fossa crease

2. Tendon of the biceps femoris muscle (laterally)

3. Tendons of the semitendinosus and semimembranosus muscles (medially)

▶ Relying on tendons rather than on a subjective interpretation of the popliteal fossa triangle gives a more precise, consistent localization of the sciatic nerve.

▶ The tendons of the semitendinosus and semimembranosus (**Fig. 22-8A**) and biceps femoris (**Fig. 22-8B**) are palpated using a two-finger technique.

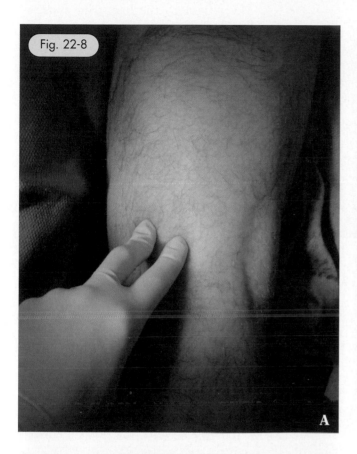

Fig. 22-8

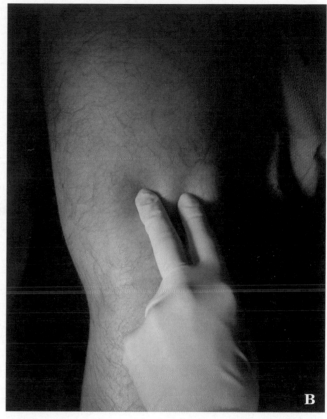

A

B

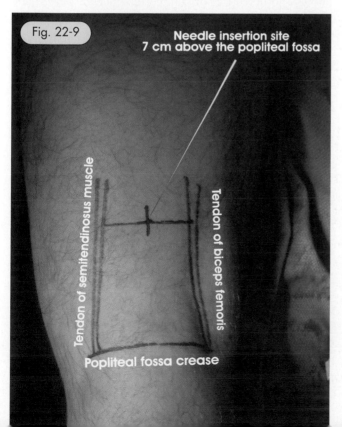

Fig. 22-9

Needle insertion site
7 cm above the popliteal fossa

Tendon of semitendinosus muscle

Tendon of biceps femoris

Popliteal fossa crease

The needle insertion point is marked at 7 cm above the popliteal fossa crease at the midpoint between the two tendons (**Fig. 22-9**).

▶ It should be noted that these landmarks differ from those in the popliteal fossa triangle approach in that they are based on easily palpable anatomic structures rather than on the imaginary lines of the triangle.

▶ Relying on the tendons of the biceps femoris and semitendinosus as landmarks makes this approach easy to use even in obese patients.

▶ In obese patients, it is easier to start tracing the tendons cephalad from their attachment at the knee.

Maneuvers to Accentuate the Landmarks

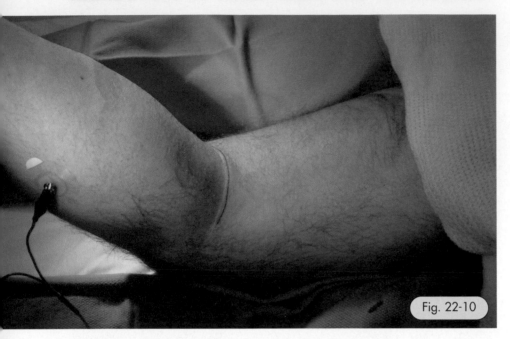

Fig. 22-10

When not visually apparent, these landmarks can be accentuated by having the patient flex the leg at the knee joint **(Fig. 22-10)**. This maneuver tightens the hamstring muscles and allows easy, accurate palpation of the tendons.

Local Anesthetic Infiltration and Needle Insertion

After thorough cleaning of the injection site with an antiseptic solution, local anesthetic is infiltrated subcutaneously. The anesthesiologist stands on the side of the patient with the palpating hand on the biceps femoris muscle. The needle is introduced at the midpoint between the tendons **(Fig. 22-11)**. This position allows the anesthesiologist to both observe the responses to nerve stimulation and monitor the patient. The nerve stimulator should be initially set to deliver a current of 1.5 mA (2 Hz, 100 μs) because this higher current allows the detection of inadvertent needle placement into the hamstring muscles (local twitches). When the needle is inserted in the correct plane, its advancement should not result in any local muscle twitches; the first response to nerve stimulation is typically that of the sciatic nerve (a foot twitch).

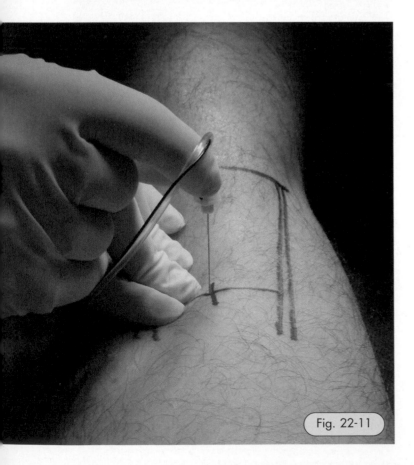

Fig. 22-11

The correct hand position and needle orientation during block placement.

▶ Keeping the fingers of the palpating hand on the biceps muscle is important for the early detection of twitches of the biceps or semitendinosus muscle beneath the fingers **(Fig. 22-11)**.

▶ These local twitches are the result of direct muscle stimulation when the needle is placed too laterally or medially, respectively **(Fig. 22-12)**.

▶ When local stimulation of the biceps muscle is felt under the fingers, the needle should be redirected medially **(Fig. 22-12)**.

▶ Local twitches of the semitendinosus muscle indicate that the needle has been inserted too medially. The needle should be withdrawn to skin level and reinserted laterally **(Fig. 22-12)**.

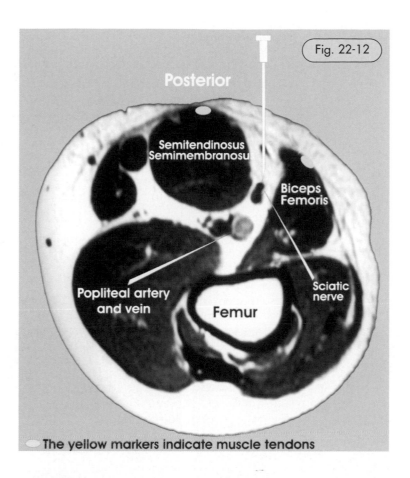

Fig. 22-12

Posterior

Semitendinosus
Semimembranosu

Biceps
Femoris

Popliteal artery
and vein

Femur

Sciatic
nerve

The yellow markers indicate muscle tendons

After initial stimulation of the sciatic nerve is obtained, the stimulating current is gradually decreased until twitches are still seen or felt at 0.2 to 0.5 mA. This typically occurs at a depth of 3 to 5 cm. After obtaining negative results from an aspiration test for blood, 35 to 45 mL of local anesthetic is slowly injected.

▶ Stimulation at a current intensity of less than 0.5 mA may not be possible in some patients. This is occasionally (but not frequently) the case in patients with long-standing diabetes mellitus, peripheral neuropathy, sepsis, or severe peripheral vascular disease. In these cases, stimulating currents up to 1.0 mA should be accepted as long as the motor response is specific and clearly seen or felt.

▶ Occasionally, a very small (e.g., 1-mm) movement of the needle results in a change in the motor response from that of the popliteal nerve (plantar flexion of the foot) to that of the common peroneal nerve (dorsiflexion of the foot). This indicates an intimate needle–nerve relationship at a level before the divergence of the sciatic nerve and should be accepted as the most reliable sign of localization of the common trunk of the sciatic nerve.

Troubleshooting:

When insertion of the needle does not result in stimulation of the sciatic nerve (foot twitches), implement the following maneuvers:

1. Keep the palpating hand in the same position.

2. Withdraw the needle to skin level, redirect it 15° laterally, and reinsert it **(Fig.22-13A)**.

3. When step 2 fails to result in sciatic nerve stimulation, withdraw the needle to skin level, reinsert it 1 cm laterally, and repeat the procedure first with perpendicular needle insertion.

4. When the step 3 fails, reinsert the needle 15° laterally.

These maneuvers should invariably result in localization of the sciatic nerve.

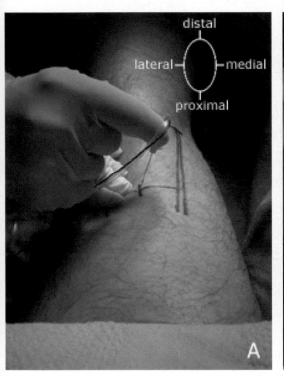
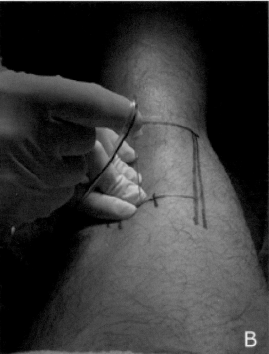
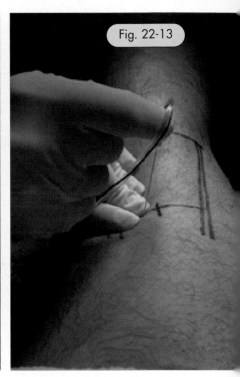

Fig. 22-13

A

B

GOAL

Visible or palpable twitches of the foot or toes at 0.2 to 0.5 mA current. There are two common types of twitches (Fig. 22-14):

• *Common peroneal nerve stimulation results in dorsiflexion and eversion.*

• *Stimulation of the tibial nerve results in plantar flexion and inversion.*

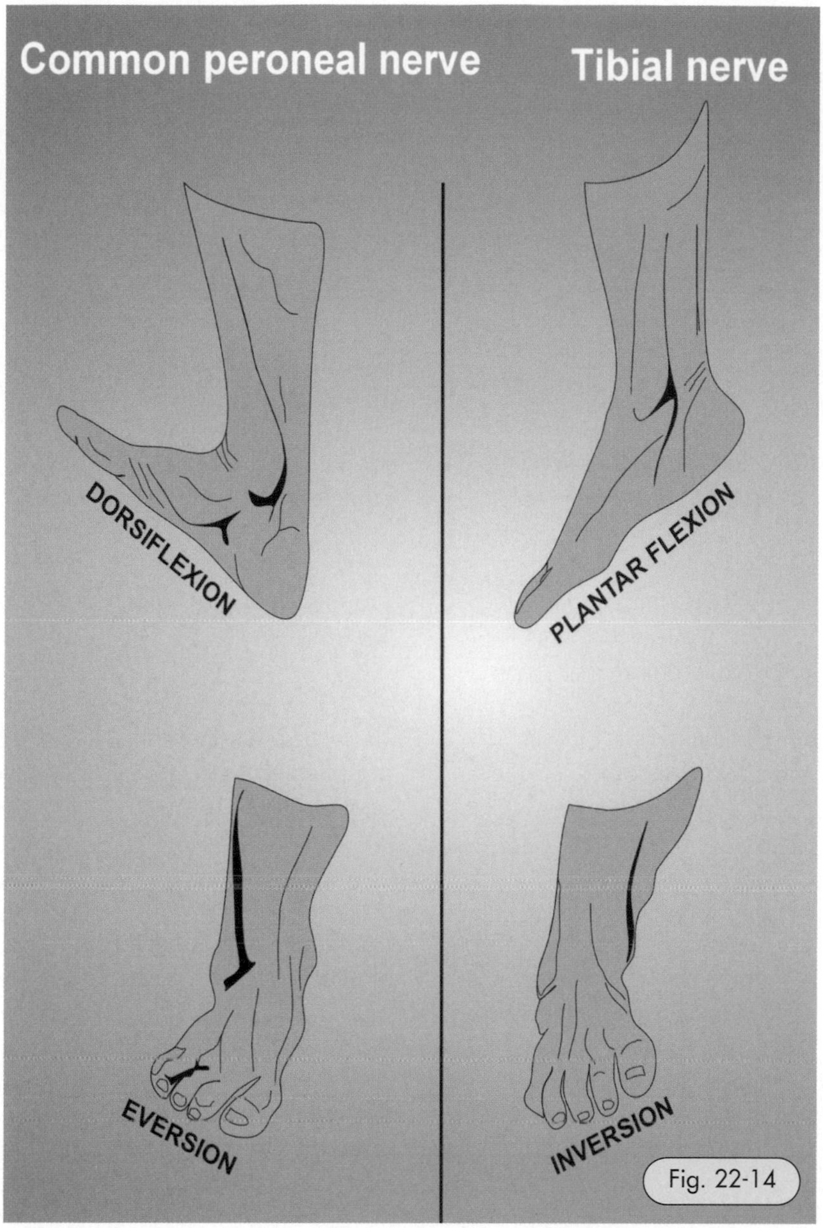

Common peroneal nerve   Tibial nerve

DORSIFLEXION   PLANTAR FLEXION

EVERSION   INVERSION

Fig. 22-14

► It may be difficult to obtain stimulation with currents less than 0.7 mA. In these cases, stimulation of the tibial nerve (plantar flexion) proves to be more reliable.

► Some authors recommend a double-injection technique to increase the success rate of blockade of both divisions of the sciatic nerve (tibial and common peroneal). Briefly, this involves stimulating and injecting both trunks of the nerve. This technique may be beneficial

when the needle is inserted at the level of the patella, but is not necessary with the approach described here.

► After obtaining a response of either trunk of the sciatic nerve, a large volume of injected local anesthetic will spread within the sheath to block the entire nerve.

► Isolated twitches of the calf muscles should not be accepted because they may result from stimulation of the sciatic nerve branches to calf muscles outside the sciatic nerve sheath.

Interpreting the Responses to Nerve Stimulation

Some common responses to nerve stimulation and the course of action to take to obtain the proper response are listed in **Table 22.1.**

TABLE 22.1
Some Common Responses to Nerve Stimulation and the Course of Action to Take to Obtain the Proper Response

RESPONSE OBTAINED	INTERPRETATION	PROBLEM	ACTION
Local twitch of the biceps femoris muscle	Direct stimulation of the biceps femoris muscle	Too lateral a placement of needle	Withdraw the needle and redirect it slightly medially (5º–10º)
Local twitch of the semitendinosus or semimembranosus muscle	Direct stimulation of the semitendinosus or semimembranosus muscle	Too medial a placement of needle	Withdraw the needle and redirect it slightly laterally (5º–10º)
Twitch of the calf muscles without foot or toe movement	Stimulation of the muscular branches of the sciatic nerve	These small branches are often outside the sciatic sheath	Disregard and continue advancing the needle until foot or toe twitches are obtained
Vascular puncture	Blood in the syringe most commonly indicates placement into the popliteal artery or vein	Too medial a placement of needle	Withdraw the needle and redirect it laterally
Bone contact	Needle has encountered the femur	Too deep a needle insertion; the nerve was missed or twitches not noticed	Withdraw the needle slowly and look for a foot twitch; if twitches are not seen follow the previously described trouble-shooting procedure

Choice of Local Anesthetic

A popliteal block requires a larger volume of local anesthetic (35 to 45 mL) to achieve anesthesia of both divisions of the sciatic nerve. The choice of the type, volume, and concentration of local anesthetic should be based on the patient's weight and general condition and whether the block is planned for surgical anesthesia or pain management.

The type and concentration of local anesthetic and the choice of additives influence the onset and, particularly, the duration of the blockade **(Table 22.3).**

TABLE 22.2
Choice of Local Anesthetic for Popliteal Block

ANESTHETIC	ONSET (min)	DURATION OF ANESTHESIA (h)	DURATION OF ANALGESIA (h)
3% 2-Chloroprocaine (+ HCO$_3$)	10–15	1–1.5	2
3% 2-Chloroprocaine (HCO$_3$ + epinephrine)	10–15	1.5–2	2–3
1.5% Mepivacaine (+ HCO$_3$)	15–20	2–3	3–5
1.5% Mepivacaine (HCO$_3$ + epinephrine)	15–20	2–5	3–8
2% Lidocaine (HCO$_3$ + epinephrine)	10–20	2-5	3–8
0.5% Ropivacaine	15–30	4-8	5–12
0.75% Ropivacaine	10–15	5–10	8–24
0.5 Bupivacaine (or levobupivacaine)	15–30	5–15	8–30

Block Dynamics and Perioperative Management

This technique is associated with minimal patient discomfort because the needle passes only through the adipose tissue of the popliteal fossa. Although adequate sedation and analgesia are always important to ensure a still, tranquil patient, midazolam 1 to 2 mg after the patient is positioned and alfentanil 250 to 500 µg just before block placement suffice for most patients. A typical onset time for this block is 10 to 25 minutes, depending on the type, concentration, and volume of local anesthetic used. The first signs of the onset of blockade are usually reports by the patient of inability to move their toes or that the foot "feels different". With this block, sensory anesthesia of the skin is often the last to develop. Inadequate skin anesthesia despite the apparently timely onset of the blockade is common and it may take up to 30 minutes to develop. Thus, local infiltration by the surgeon at the site of the incision is often all that is needed to allow the surgery to proceed.

CONTINUOUS POPLITEAL BLOCK (INTERTENDINOUS APPROACH)

A continuous popliteal block is an advanced regional anesthesia technique, and solid experience with the single-injection technique is recommended to ensure its efficacy. The technique is similar to a single-injection procedure, however, slight angulation of the needle cephalad is necessary to facilitate threading the catheter. Securing and maintaining the catheter are easy and convenient. This technique can be used for surgery and postoperative pain management in patients undergoing a wide variety of lower leg, foot, and ankle surgeries.

Patient Positioning

The patient is positioned in the prone position with the feet extending beyond the table to facilitate monitoring of foot or toe responses to nerve stimulation **(Fig. 22-15)**.

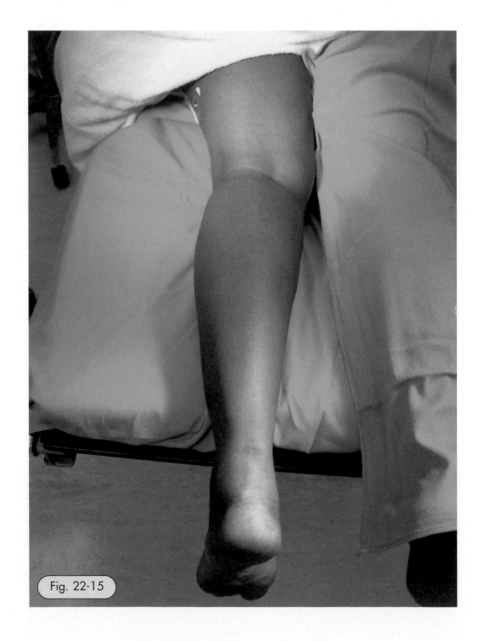

Fig. 22-15

Equipment

A standard regional anesthesia tray is prepared with the following equipment **(see Fig. 22-5)**:

- Sterile towels and gauze packs

- 20-mL syringes containing local anesthetic

- Sterile gloves, marking pen, and surface electrode

- $1^{1}/_{2}$-in, 25-gauge needle for skin infiltration

- 5-cm, insulated stimulating needle

- Catheter

- Peripheral nerve stimulator

Landmarks

The landmarks for a continuous popliteal block are essentially the same as those for the single-injection technique **(Fig. 22-16)**. These include:

1. Popliteal fossa crease

2. Tendon of the biceps femoris muscle (laterally)

3. Tendons of the semitendinosus and semimembranosus muscles (medially)

The needle insertion site is marked 7 cm proximal to the popliteal fossa crease and between the tendons of the biceps femoris and semitendinosus muscles **(Fig. 22-17)**

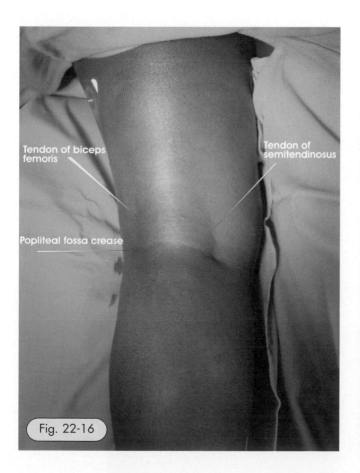

Tendon of biceps femoris

Tendon of semitendinosus

Popliteal fossa crease

Fig. 22-16

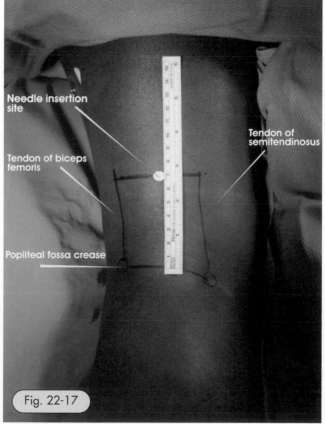

Needle insertion site

Tendon of biceps femoris

Tendon of semitendinosus

Popliteal fossa crease

Fig. 22-17

Local Anesthetic Infiltration and Needle Insertion

The continuous popliteal block technique is similar to the single-injection technique. With the patient in the prone position, infiltrate the skin with local anesthetic using a 25-gauge needle at an injection site 7 cm above the popliteal fossa crease and between the tendons of biceps femoris and semitendinosus muscles **(Fig. 22-18)**. A 5-cm needle connected to the nerve stimulator (1.5 mA current) is inserted at the midpoint between the tendons of the biceps femoris and semitendinosus muscles. Advance the block needle slowly in a slightly cranial direction while observing the patient for plantar or dorsiflexion of the foot or toes. After appropriate twitches are noted, continue manipulating the needle until the desired response is seen or felt using a current of 0.5 to 0.2 mA. After obtaining negative results from an aspiration test for blood, inject 35 to 45 mL of a local anesthetic of choice.

The catheter should be advanced about 5 cm beyond the needle tip **(Fig. 22-19)**. The needle is then withdrawn back to the skin level while the catheter is simultaneously advanced to prevent its inadvertent removal.

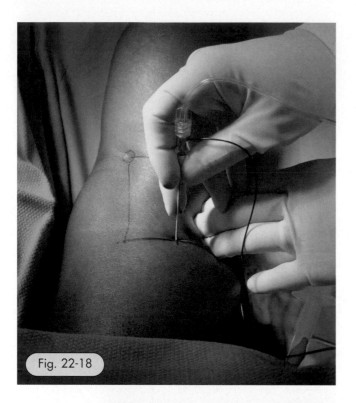

Fig. 22-18

TIP

▶ When insertion of the catheter proves difficult, lowering the angle of the needle or rotating the needle should be attempted.

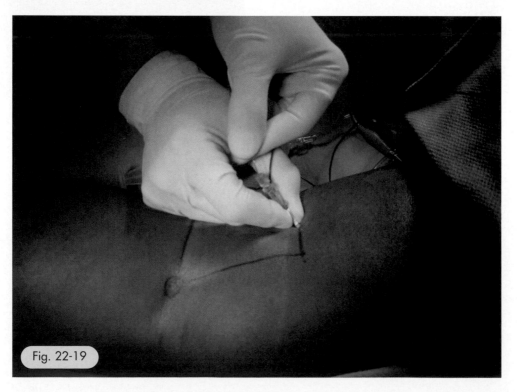

Fig. 22-19

Before it is activated, the catheter is checked for inadvertent intravascular placement by obtaining negative results from an aspiration test for blood and injecting an epinephrine-containing local anesthetic. Several techniques to secure the catheter to the skin have been proposed. A benzoin skin preparation followed by application of a clear dressing is one of simplest and most efficacious methods **(Fig. 22-20)**. The infusion port should be clearly marked "continuous popliteal block."

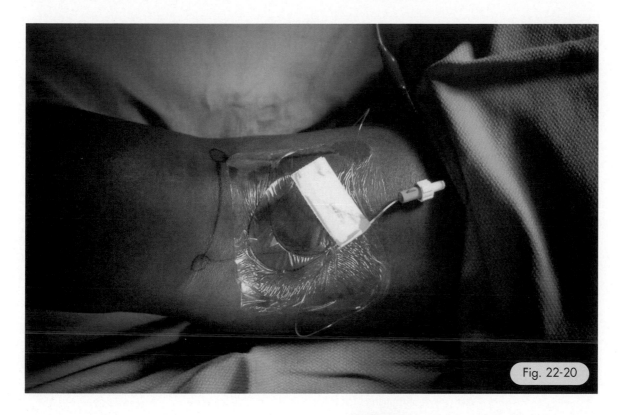

Fig. 22-20

Continuous Infusion

Continuous infusion is initiated after introduction of an initial bolus of local anesthetic through the catheter. For this purpose, we routinely use 0.2% ropivacaine 15 to 20 mL. Diluted bupivacaine or levobupivacaine are also suitable, but may result in additional motor blockade. The infusion is maintained at 10 ml/h or 5 mL/h when a patient-controlled analgesia (PCA) dose (5 mL/h) is planned.

TIPS

▶ Breakthrough pain in patients undergoing continuous infusion is always managed by administering a bolus of local anesthetic. Just increasing the rate of infusion is never adequate. With patients on the ward, a higher concentration of a shorter-acting local anesthetic (e.g., 1% mepivacaine or lidocaine) is useful to both manage the pain and test the position of the catheter.

▶ When a bolus injection through the catheter fails to result in a blockade after 30 minutes, the catheter should be considered dislodged and should be removed.

▶ Patients undergoing continuous nerve block infusion should also be prescribed an alternative pain management protocol because incomplete analgesia and catheter dislodgment can occur. For inpatients, this is probably best done using backup IV PCA.

Complications and How to Avoid Them

Complications following a popliteal block are rare. Some general and specific instructions on possible complications and how to avoid them are given in **Table 22.3.**

TABLE 22.3
Complications of Femoral Nerve Block and Preventive Techniques

Infection	• Use a strict aseptic technique.
Local anesthetic toxicity	• Systemic toxicity after a popliteal block is uncommon. • Absorption of the local anesthetic from the popliteal fossa is slow because of the low vascularity of the adipose tissue in the fossa.
Hematoma	• Stop insertion of the needle when the patient complains of pain. This typically indicates that the needle has been inserted through the biceps or semitendinosus muscle. Increasing the current output of the nerve stimulator helps distinguish between the two.
Vascular puncture	• Avoid medial redirection of the needle because the vascular sheath is positioned medially and deeper as compared to the sciatic nerve.
Nerve injury	• Injury is exceedingly rare. • Use nerve stimulation and slow needle advancement. • Do not inject when the patient complains of pain or high pressures are met on injection; do not inject when stimulation is obtained at <0.2 mA current (100 μs). • Avoid application of a tourniquet over the injection site to decrease the risk of prolonged ischemia of the nerve.
Other	• Instruct the patient on care of the insensate extremity.

SUGGESTED READINGS

Popliteal Block, Intertendinous Approach, Single-injection Technique

- Benzon HT, Kim C, Benzon HP, et al. Correlation between evoked motor response of the sciatic nerve and sensory blockade. *Anesthesiology* 1997;87:548–552.
- Gouverneur JM. Sciatic nerve block in the popliteal fossa with atraumatic needles and nerve stimulation. *Acta Anaesthesiol Belg* 1985;36:391–399.
- Hadžić A, Vloka JD. A comparison of the posterior versus lateral approaches to the block of the sciatic nerve in the popliteal fossa. *Anesthesiology* 1998;88:1480–1486.
- Hadžić A, Vloka JD, Singson R, Santos AC, Thys DM. A comparison of intertendinous and classical approaches to popliteal nerve block using magnetic resonance imaging simulation. Anesth Analg 2002;94:1321–1324.
- Kilpatrick AW, Coventry DM, Todd JG. A comparison of two approaches to sciatic nerve block. *Anaesthesia* 1992;47:155–157.
- Rorie DK, Byer DE, Nelson DO, et al. Assessment of block of the sciatic nerve in the popliteal fossa. Anesth Analg 1980;59:371–376.
- Sunderland S. The sciatic nerve and its tibial and common peroneal divisions: anatomical features. In: Sunderland S. *Nerves and Nerve Injuries*. Edinburgh, Scotland: E&S Livingstone, 1968;1012–1095.
- Vloka JD, Hadžić A, April EW, Geatz H, Thys DM. Division of the sciatic nerve in the popliteal fossa and its possible implications in the popliteal nerve blockade. *Anesth Analg* 2001;92:215–217.
- Vloka JD, Hadžić A, Koorn R, Thys D. Supine approach to the sciatic nerve in the popliteal fossa. *Can J Anaesth* 1996;43:964–967.
- Vloka JD, Hadžić A, Lesser JB, Kitain E, Geatz H, April EW, Thys DM. A common epineural sheath for the nerves in the popliteal fossa and its possible implications for sciatic nerve block. *Anesth Analg* 1997;84: 387–390.
- Vloka JD, Hadžić A, Mulcare R, Lesser JB, Koorn R, Thys DM. Combined blocks of the sciatic nerve at the popliteal fossa and posterior cutaneous nerve of the thigh for short saphenous vein stripping in outpatients: an alternative to spinal anesthesia. *J Clin Anesth* 1997;9:618–622.

Popliteal Block, Continuous Technique

- di Benedetto P, Casati A, Bertini L, Fanelli G, Chelly JE. Postoperative analgesia with continuous sciatic nerve block after foot surgery: a prospective, randomized comparison between the popliteal and subgluteal approaches. *Anesth Analg* 2002;94:996–1000.
- Ilfeld BM, Morey TE, Wang RD, Enneking FK. Continuous popliteal sciatic nerve block for postoperative pain control at home: a randomized, double-blinded, placebo-controlled study. *Anesthesiology* 2002; 97:959–965.
- Singelyn FJ, Aye F, Gouverneur JM. Continuous popliteal sciatic nerve block: an original technique to provide postoperative analgesia after foot surgery. *Anesth Analg* 1997;84:383–386.

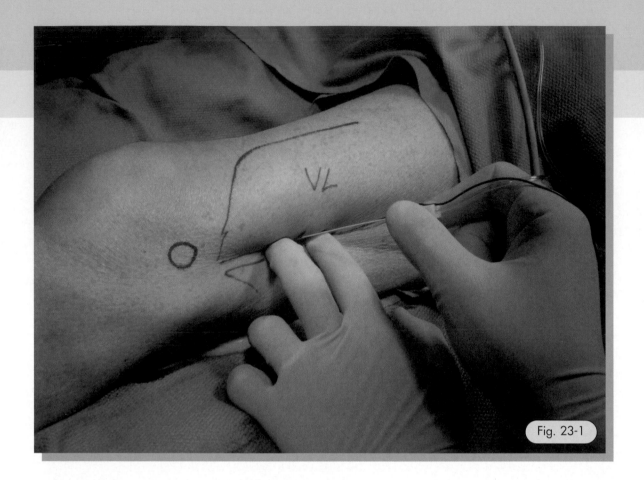

Fig. 23-1

BLOCK AT A GLANCE

- Indications: ankle and foot surgery

- Landmarks: popliteal fossa crease, vastus lateralis and biceps femoris muscles

- Needle: 10 cm

- Nerve stimulation: twitch of the foot or toes at 0.2 to 0.5 mA current

- Local anesthetic: 35 to 45 mL

- Complexity level: intermediate

23 POPLITEAL BLOCK:
LATERAL APPROACH

GENERAL CONSIDERATIONS

The lateral approach to a popliteal blockade is a block of the sciatic nerve at the level of the popliteal fossa. This is an intermediate nerve block technique, and sound knowledge of the principles of nerve stimulation and the anatomic characteristics of the sciatic nerve are needed for its successful implementation. This block is well-suited for surgery on the calf, Achilles tendon, ankle, and foot. It also provides adequate analgesia for a calf tourniquet without the need for supplementary blocks of the saphenous nerve.

Regional Anesthesia Anatomy

The *sciatic nerve* consists of two separate nerve trunks, the tibial and common peroneal nerves **(Fig. 23-2)**. A common epineural sheath envelops these two nerves at their outset in the pelvis. As the sciatic nerve descends toward the knee, the two components eventually diverge in the popliteal fossa, giving rise to the tibial and common peroneal nerves. This division of the sciatic nerve usually occurs 70 mm proximal to the popliteal fossa crease **(Fig. 23-3)**.

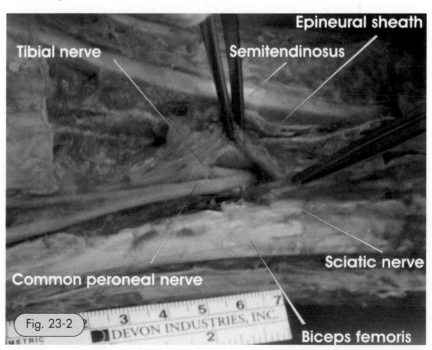

Fig. 23-2

Tibial nerve · Epineural sheath · Semitendinosus · Sciatic nerve · Common peroneal nerve · Biceps femoris

A magnetic resonance (MR) image of the popliteal fossa at the level of the blockade (8 cm above the popliteal fossa crease). Note the position of the sciatic nerve between the biceps femoris and semitendinosus muscles. During block placement, stimulation of the common peroneal nerve is usually obtained first (65%) because this nerve is positioned laterally and more superficially than the tibial nerve.

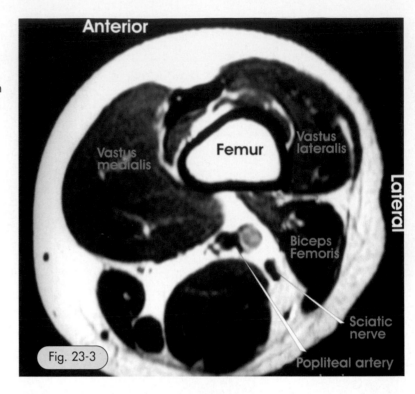

Fig. 23-3

Distribution of Anesthesia

A popliteal block results in anesthesia of the entire distal two-thirds of the lower extremity with the exception of the medial aspect of the leg (see the shaded are on **Fig. 23-4**). Cutaneous innervation of the medial leg below the knee is provided by the saphenous nerve, a cutaneous extension of the femoral nerve. Depending on the level of surgery, the addition of a saphenous nerve block may be required for complete surgical anesthesia.

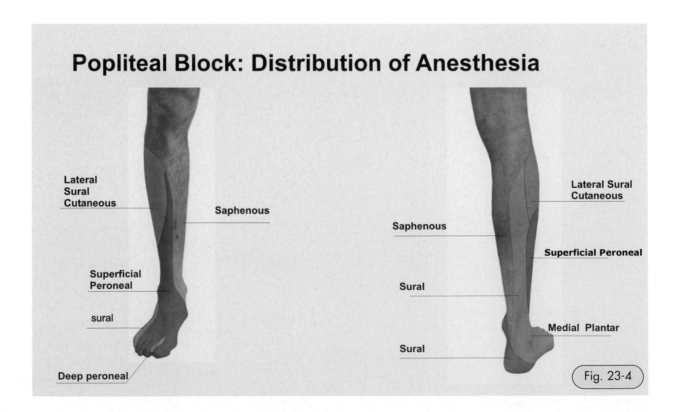

Popliteal Block: Distribution of Anesthesia

Lateral Sural Cutaneous

Saphenous

Superficial Peroneal

sural

Deep peroneal

Lateral Sural Cutaneous

Saphenous

Superficial Peroneal

Sural

Medial Plantar

Sural

Fig. 23-4

SINGLE-INJECTION POPLITEAL BLOCK (LATERAL APPROACH)

Patient Positioning

The patient is in the lateral position. The foot on the side to be blocked should be positioned so that even the slightest movement of the foot or toes can be easily observed **(Fig. 23-5)**. In some patients this is best achieved by placing the foot on a footrest, making certain that the Achilles tendon protrudes beyond the footrest. This positioning allows easy visualization of any foot movement during nerve stimulation. The foot should form a 90° angle to the horizontal plane of the table.

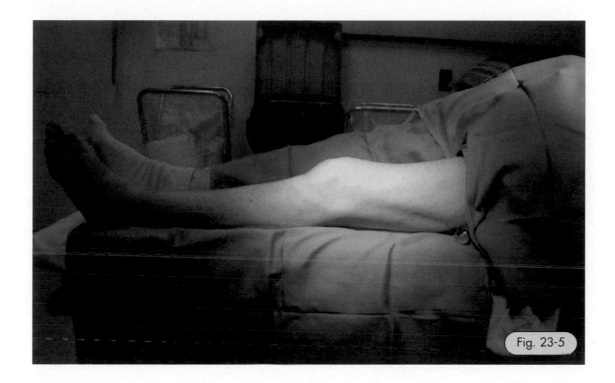

Fig. 23-5

Equipment

A standard regional anesthesia tray is prepared with the following equipment:

- Sterile towels and gauze packs

- Three 20-mL syringes containing local anesthetic

- Sterile gloves, marking pen, and surface electrode

- $1^{1}/_{2}$-in, 25-gauge needle for skin infiltration

- 10-cm, short-bevel, insulated stimulating needle

- Peripheral nerve stimulator

Surface Landmarks

The following surface landmarks are used to determine the insertion point for the needle **(Fig. 23-6)**:

1. Vastus lateralis muscle

2. Biceps femoris muscle

3. Patella

4. Popliteal fossa crease

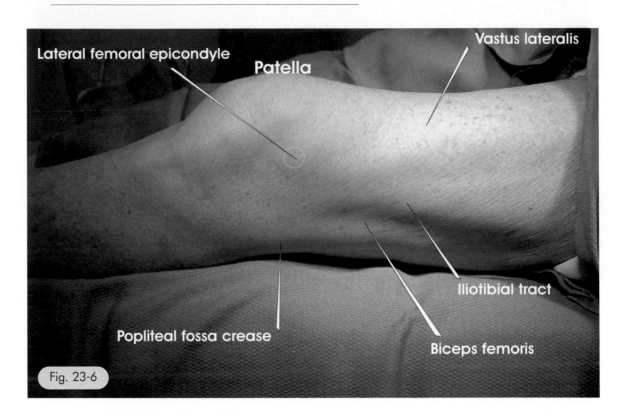

Fig. 23-6

Anatomic Landmarks

Landmarks for the lateral approach to a popliteal block include **(Fig. 23-7)**:

1. Popliteal fossa crease

2. Vastus lateralis muscle

3. Biceps femoris muscle

The needle insertion site is marked in the groove between the vastus lateralis and biceps femoris muscles 8 cm above the popliteal fossa crease. Note that the lateral femoral epicondyle is another landmark that can be used in this technique **(Fig. 23-6)**.

It is easily palpated on the lateral aspect of the knee 1 cm cephalad to the popliteal fossa crease, thus the needle insertion site is marked 7 cm cephalad when using this landmark.

TIP

▶ In some patients, the biceps femoris muscle may be atrophic and the iliotibial aponeurosis tract may be more prominent **(Fig 23-6)**. In such cases, the needle insertion site is labeled in the groove between the vastus lateralis and the iliotibial tract.

▶ Patients in whom these landmarks are not immediately apparent can be asked to lift their foot off the table to make them more prominent **(Fig. 23-7)**.

▶ This maneuver requires that both the quadriceps (vastus lateralis) muscle (leg extension) and biceps femoris muscle (leg flexion) be tensed and opposing, which nicely accentuates the groove between the two muscles **(Fig. 23-7)**.

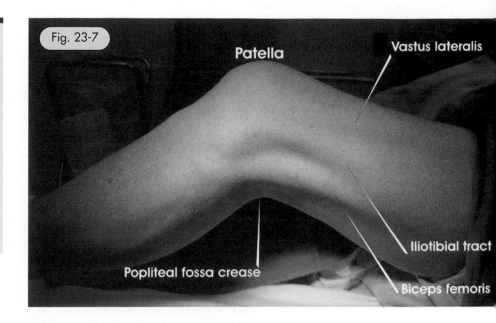

Fig. 23-7

Patella

Vastus lateralis

Iliotibial tract

Biceps femoris

Popliteal fossa crease

Maneuvers to Accentuate Anatomic Landmarks

When not immediately, visually apparent, the groove between the vastus lateralis and biceps femoris is examined by firmly pressing the fingers of the palpating hand against the adipose tissue in the groove approximately 7 cm above the popliteal fossa crease **(Fig. 23-8)**.

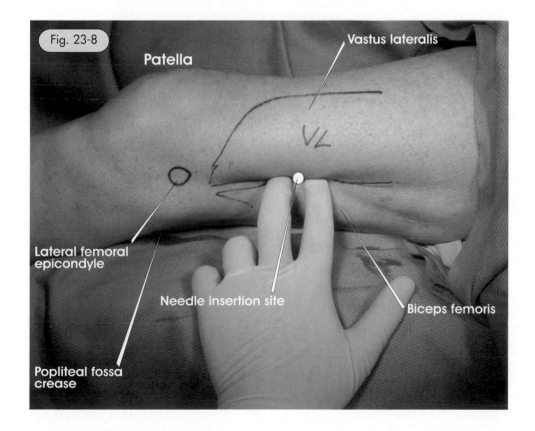

Fig. 23-8

Patella

Vastus lateralis

Lateral femoral epicondyle

Needle insertion site

Biceps femoris

Popliteal fossa crease

Local Anesthetic Infiltration and Needle Insertion

The operator should be seated facing the side to be blocked. The height of the patient's bed is adjusted to allow for a more ergonomic position and greater precision during block placement. This position also allows the operator to simultaneously monitor both the patient and the responses to nerve stimulation.

The site of estimated needle insertion is prepared with an antiseptic solution and infiltrated with local anesthetic using a 1$^1/_2$-in, 25-gauge needle **(Fig. 23-9)**. It is useful to infiltrate the skin along a line rather than raise a single skin wheal. This allows needle reinsertion at a different site when necessary without the need to anesthetize the skin again.

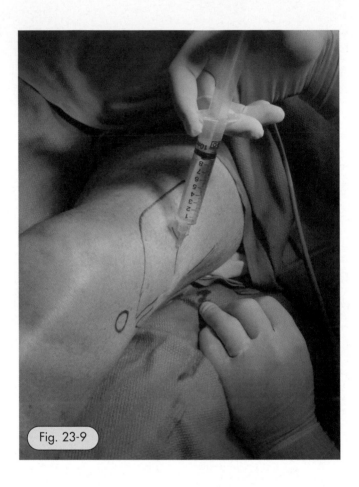

Fig. 23-9

A 10-cm, 22-gauge needle is connected to a nerve stimulator, inserted in a horizontal plane and perpendicular to the long axis of the leg between the vastus lateralis and biceps femoris muscles, and advanced to contact the femur **(Fig. 23-10)**. Contact with the femur is important because it provides information on the depth of the nerve (typically 1 to 2 cm beyond the skin-femur distance) as well as on the angle the needle must be redirected posteriorly in order to stimulate the nerve. The current intensity is initially set at 1.5 mA. With the fingers of the palpating hand firmly pressed and immobile in the groove, the needle is then withdrawn to skin level,

redirected 30° posteriorly to the angle at which the femur was contacted, and advanced toward the nerve **(Fig. 23-11)**.

GOAL

The ultimate goal of nerve stimulation is to obtain visible or palpable twitches of the foot or toes at a current of 0.2 to 0.5 mA.

TIPS

► Note that after redirection the needle passes through the biceps femoris muscle. Consequently, local twitches of this muscle are often obtained during needle advancement **(Fig. 23-12)**. Cessation of these twitches should prompt slower needle advancement, as this signifies that the needle has entered the popliteal fossa and it should be in close proximity to the sciatic nerve.

► When stimulation of the sciatic nerve is not obtained within 2 cm after cessation of the biceps femoris twitches, the needle is probably not in plane with the nerves and should not be advanced further because of the risk of puncturing the popliteal vessels **(Fig. 23-12)**.

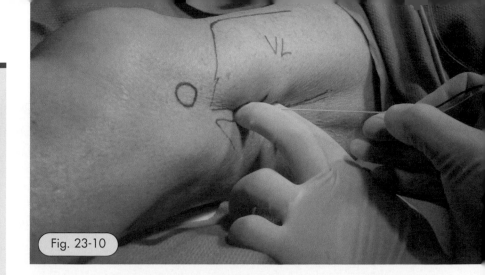

Fig. 23-10

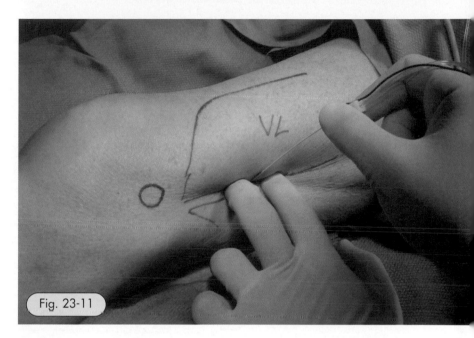

Fig. 23-11

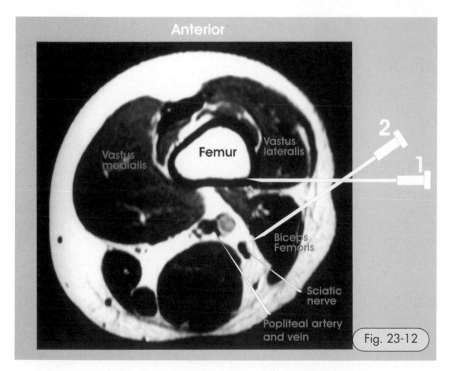

Fig. 23-12

The MR image demonstrates (1) the initial plane of needle insertion between the vastus lateralis and biceps femoris muscles required to reach the sciatic nerve in the popliteal fossa and (2) the angle of approximately 30° at which the needle is redirected to reach the sciatic nerve **(Fig. 22-2)**.

Troubleshooting

When the sciatic nerve is not localized on the first needle pass, the needle is withdrawn to skin level and the following algorithm is used:

1. Ensure that the nerve stimulator is functional, properly connected to the patient and to the needle, and set to deliver current of desired intensity.

2. Ensure that the leg is not externally rotated at the hip joint and that the foot forms a 90° angle to the horizontal plane of the table. Any deviation from this angle changes the relationship of the sciatic nerve to the femur and the biceps femoris muscle.

3. Mentally visualize the plane of the initial needle insertion and redirect the needle in a slightly posterior direction (5° to 10° posterior angulation).

4. If step 3 fails, withdraw the needle and reinsert it with an additional 5° to 10° posterior redirection.

5. Failure to obtain a foot response to nerve stimulation should prompt reassessment of the landmarks and leg position. In addition, the stimulating current should be increased to 2 mA.

TIPS

▶ Stimulation of the sciatic nerve can result in a tibial (plantar flexion) or common peroneal (dorsiflexion) response (**Fig. 23-13**). Either of these is acceptable when a low-intensity current stimulation is obtained and a large volume of local anesthetic is used. A large volume of injected local anesthetic spreads within the sheath to block both divisions of the nerve.

▶ Some authors recommend a double-injection technique to increase the success rate of blockade of both divisions of the nerve. This involve stimulating and separately injecting both divisions of the sciatic nerve (tibial and common peroneal). This, however, is not necessary with the technique described in this book.

▶ Isolated twitches of the calf muscles should not be accepted because they may be the result of stimulation of the sciatic nerve branches to the calf muscles that may be outside the sciatic nerve sheath.

▶ In some patients with long-standing diabetes mellitus, renal failure, or peripheral neuropathy, it may not be possible to obtain stimulation with low current intensity. In this case, stimulating currents of up to 1.0 mA should be accepted as long as the motor response is specific and clearly seen or felt.

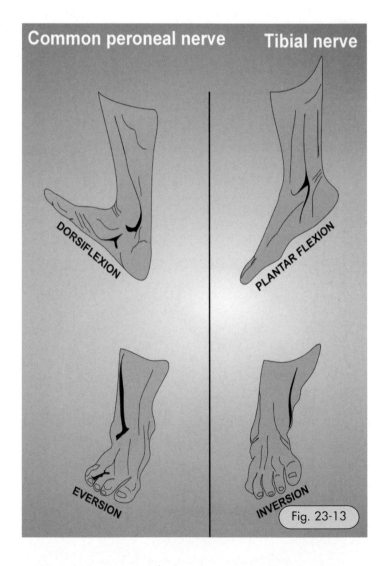

Common peroneal nerve · Tibial nerve

DORSIFLEXION

PLANTAR FLEXION

EVERSION

INVERSION

Fig. 23-13

After initial stimulation of the sciatic nerve is obtained, the stimulating current is gradually decreased until twitches are still seen or felt at 0.2 to 0.5 mA. This typically occurs at a depth of 5 to 7 cm. At this point, the needle should be stabilized and, after obtaining negative results from an aspiration test for blood, 35 to 45 mL of local anesthetic is slowly injected **(Fig. 23-14)**. The hands should be kept as immobile as possible to prevent injection outside the sheath of the sciatic nerve.

Interpreting the Responses to Nerve Stimulation

Some common responses occurring during block placement using a nerve stimulator and the proper course of action needed to obtain twitches of the foot are listed in **Table 23.1**.

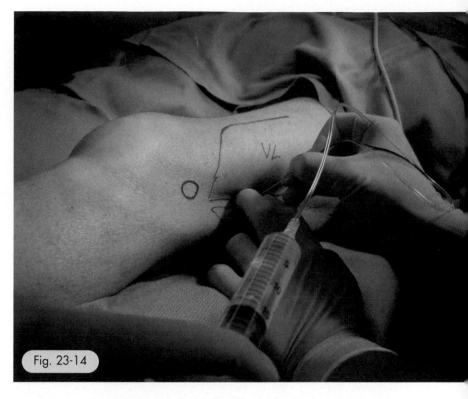

Fig. 23-14

TABLE 23.1
Some Common Responses Occurring During Block Placement Using A Nerve Stimulator and the Proper Course of Action Needed to Obtain Twitches of the Foot

RESPONSE OBTAINED	INTERPRETATION	PROBLEM	ACTION
Local twitch of the biceps femoris muscle	Direct stimulation of the biceps femoris muscle	Too shallow a placement of the needle	Advance the needle deeper
Local twitch of the vastus lateralis muscle	Direct stimulation of the vastus lateralis muscle	Too anterior a placement of the needle	Withdraw the needle and reinsert it posteriorly
Twitch of the calf muscles without foot or toe movement	Stimulation of the motor branches of the sciatic nerve	These small branches are often outside the sciatic sheath.	Disregard and continue advancing the needle until foot or toe twitches are obtained
Vascular puncture	Blood in the syringe most commonly indicates placement into the popliteal artery or vein	Too deep and too anterior a placement of the needle	Withdraw the needle and redirect it laterally
Twitches of the foot or toes	Stimulation of the sciatic nerve	None	Accept and inject local anesthetic

Choice of Local Anesthetic

A popliteal block requires a larger volume of local anesthetic in order to achieve anesthesia of both divisions of the nerve (tibial and common peroneal nerves). The choice of the type and concentration of local anesthetic should be based on whether the block is planned for surgical anesthesia or pain management. As can be seen in **Table 23.2**, the type and concentration of local anesthetic, as well as the choice of additives used, influence the onset and, particularly, the duration of the blockade.

TABLE 23.2
Choice of Local Anesthetic For Popliteal Block

ANESTHETIC	ONSET (min)	DURATION OF ANESTHESIA (h)	DURATION OF ANALGESIA (h)
3% 2-Chloroprocaine (+ HCO$_3$)	10–15	1–1.5	2
3% 2-Chloroprocaine (HCO$_3$ + epinephrine)	10–15	1.5–2	2–3
1.5% Mepivacaine (+ HCO$_3$)	15–20	2–3	3–5
1.5% Mepivacaine (HCO$_3$ + epinephrine)	15–20	2–5	3–8
2% Lidocaine (HCO$_3$ + epinephrine)	10–20	2–5	3–8
0.5% Ropivacaine	15–30	4–8	8–12
0.75% Ropivacaine	10–15	5–10	8–24
0.5% Bupivacaine (or levobupivacaine)	15–30	5–15	8–30

Block Dynamics and Perioperative Management

This technique is associated with moderate patient discomfort because the needle transverses the biceps femoris muscle, and adequate sedation and analgesia are necessary. Administration of midazolam (2 to 4 mg intravenously) and a short-acting narcotic (alfentanil 250 to 750 µg) ensures patient comfort and prevents patient movement during needle advancement. Failure to administer appropriate premedication makes it difficult to interpret the response to nerve stimulation because of patient movement during needle advancement. A typical onset time for this block is 10 to 25 minutes, depending on the type, concentration, and volume of local anesthetic used. The first signs of onset of the blockade are usually a report by the patient that the foot "feels different" or that they are unable to wiggle their toes. With this block, sensory anesthesia of the skin is often the last to develop. Inadequate skin anesthesia despite an apparently timely onset of the blockade is common, and it may take up to 30 minutes to develop. Thus, local infiltration by the surgeon at the site of the incision is often all that is needed to allow the surgery to proceed.

CONTINUOUS POPLITEAL BLOCK (LATERAL APPROACH)

Continuous popliteal blockade is an advanced regional anesthesia technique, and expertise with the single-injection technique is necessary to ensure its efficacy and patient comfort and safety. The technique is similar to the single-injection procedure; however, slight angulation of the needle cephalad is necessary to facilitate threading the catheter. Securing and maintaining the catheter are easy and convenient with this technique. A lateral popliteal block is suitable for surgery and postoperative pain management in patients undergoing a wide variety of lower leg, foot, and ankle surgeries.

Equipment

A standard regional anesthesia tray is prepared similar to that of the single injection technique. A 17 – 18 guage needle and catheter are added

Landmarks

The landmarks for a continuous popliteal block with the lateral approach are essentially the same as for the single-injection technique and include **(Fig. 23-15)**:

1. Popliteal fossa crease

2. Vastus lateralis

3. Biceps femoris

The needle insertion site is marked at 8 cm proximal to the popliteal fossa crease in the groove between the vastus lateralis and biceps femoris.

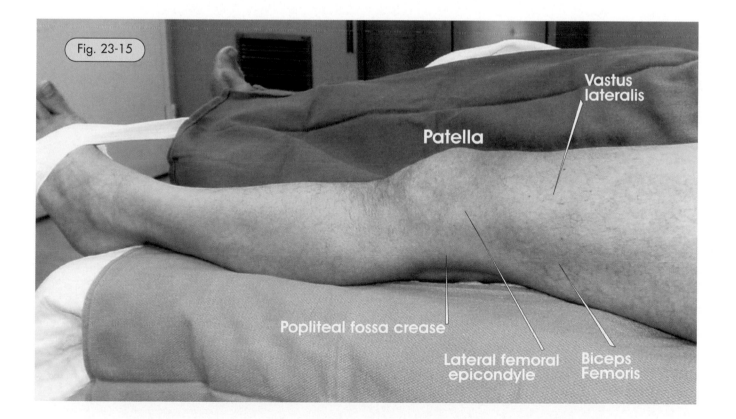

Fig. 23-15

Vastus lateralis

Patella

Popliteal fossa crease

Lateral femoral epicondyle

Biceps Femoris

Local Anesthetic Infiltration and Needle Insertion

The continuous popliteal block technique is similar to the single-injection technique. The patient is in the prone position. Using a 25-guage needle, infiltrate the skin with local anesthetic at the injection site 8 cm proximal to the lateral femoral epicondyle in the groove between the biceps femoris and vastus lateralis muscles. A 10-cm needle with a Tuohy-style tip for a continuous nerve block is connected to the nerve stimulator (1.5 mA) and inserted to contact the femur **(Fig. 23-16)**. Once the femur is contacted, the needle is withdrawn to skin level and redirected in a slightly posterior direction 30° **(Fig. 23-17)**. It is then advanced slowly while observing the patient for plantar flexion or dorsiflexion of the foot or toes. After obtaining the appropriate twitches, continue manipulating the needle until the desired response is still seen or felt using a current of 0.5 mA. After obtaining negative results from an aspiration test for blood, 35 to 45 mL of the local anesthetic of choice is injected.

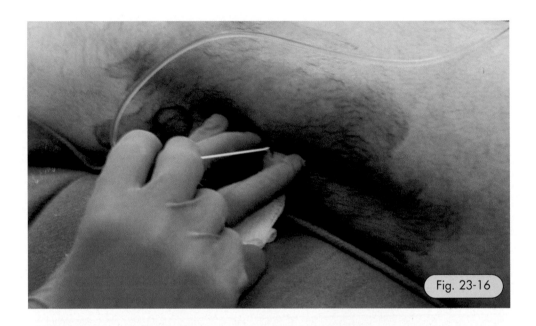

Fig. 23-16

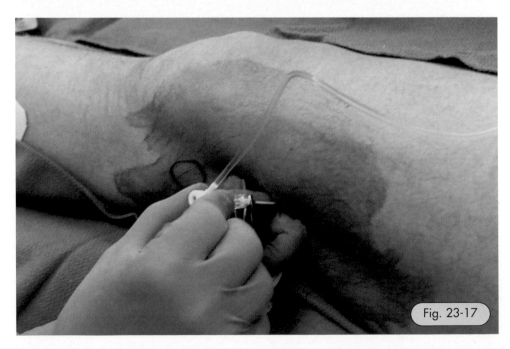

Fig. 23-17

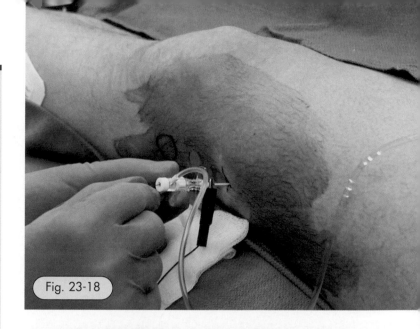

Fig. 23-18

Catheter Insertion

The catheter should be advanced about 5 to 7 cm beyond the tip of the needle **(Fig. 23-18)**. The needle is then withdrawn back to skin level, while the catheter is simultaneously advanced to prevent it from being accidently dislodged **(Fig. 23-19)**. The needle is then withdrawn while continuously advancing the catheter to prevent accidental withdrawal of the catheter. The catheter is left 5 to 10 cm beyond the tip of the needle. The insertion site is dressed, and the catheter secured to the skin **(Fig. 23-20)**. Before activating, the catheter is checked for inadvertent intravascular placement by obtaining negative results from an aspiration test for blood and injection of an epinephrine-containing local anesthetic.

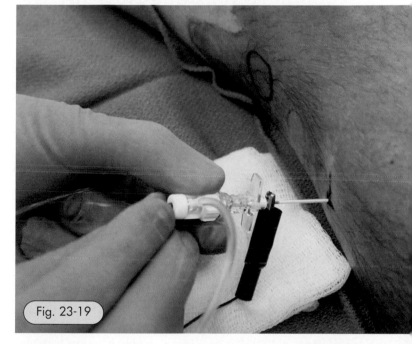

Fig. 23-19

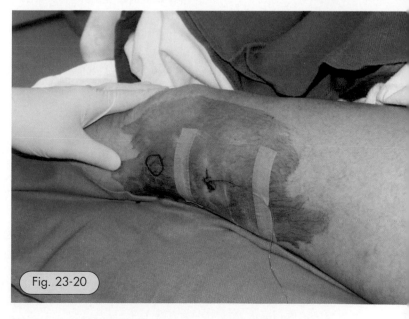

Fig. 23-20

Management of a Continuous-Infusion Catheter

Continuous infusion is initiated after an initial bolus of dilute local anesthetic is administered through the catheter. For initiation of the block, the bolus is first administered through the needle using a higher concentration of local anesthetic. For the initial bolus, 20 mL of 0.5% ropivacaine or 0.5% bupivacaine (levobupivacaine) is the most appropriate. This is followed by continuous infusion of a dilute concentration of local anesthetic (e.g., 0.2% ropivacaine). The infusion is maintained at 10 mL/hr or 5 mL/h when a patient-controlled analgesia (PCA) dose (5 mL/h) is planned.

Complications and How to Avoid Them

Complications following a popliteal block are rare. **Table 23.3** provides specific instructions on some complications and how to avoid them.

TABLE 23.3

Complications of Popliteal Block Through the Lateral Approach and Preventive Techniques

Infection	• Use a strict aseptic technique.
Hematoma	• Avoid multiple needle passes with a continuous block needle; the larger needle diameter and/or Tuohy design may result in a hematoma of the biceps femoris or vastus lateralis muscle.
	• When the nerve is not localized on first the two or three needle passes, use a smaller-gauge, single-injection needle first and then reinsert the continuous block needle using the same angle; this logic is similar to localization of the internal jugular vein with a "localization needle" before inserting a large needle for canalization.
Vascular puncture	• Avoid too deep an insertion of the needle because the vascular sheath is positioned medially and deeper to the sciatic nerve.
	• When the nerve is not localized within 2 cm after local twitches of the biceps femoris muscle cease, the needle should be withdrawn and reinserted at a different angle rather than advanced deeper.
Nerve injury	• Rare
	• Use nerve stimulation and slow needle advancement
	• Do not inject when the patient complains of pain or high pressures are met on injection
	• Do not inject when stimulation is obtained at <0.2 mA current (100 μs).
	• Avoid application of a tourniquet over the injection site to decrease the risk of prolonged ischemia of the nerve.
Pressure necrosis of the heel	• Instruct the patient on care of the insensate extremity.
	• Use heel padding and frequent repositioning.

SUGGESTED READINGS

Popliteal Block, Lateral Approach, Single-injection Technique

- Benzon HT, Kim C, Benzon HP, et al. Correlation between evoked motor response of the sciatic nerve and sensory blockade. *Anesthesiology* 1997; 87:548–552.
- Hadžić A, Vloka JD. A comparison of the posterior versus lateral approaches to the block of the sciatic nerve in the popliteal fossa. *Anesthesiology* 1998;88:1480–1486.
- Hadžić A, Vloka JD, Singson R, Santos AC, Thys DM. A comparison of intertendinous and classical approaches to popliteal nerve block using magnetic resonance imaging simulation. *Anesth Analg* 2002; 94:1321–1324.
- McLeod DH, Wong DH, Claridge RJ, Merrick PM. Lateral popliteal sciatic nerve block compared with subcutaneous infiltration for analgesia following foot surgery. *Can J Anaesth* 1994;41:673–676.
- McLeod DH, Wong DH, Vaghadia H, Claridge RJ, Merrick PM. Lateral popliteal sciatic nerve block compared with ankle block for analgesia following foot surgery. *Can J Anaesth* 1995;42:765–769.
- Sunderland S. The sciatic nerve and its tibial and common peroneal divisions: anatomical features. In: Sutherland, *Nerves and Nerve Injuries*. Edinburgh, Scotland: E&S Livingstone, 1968;1012–1095.
- Vloka JD, Hadžić A, April EW, Geatz H, Thys, DM. Division of the sciatic nerve in the popliteal fossa and its possible implications in the popliteal nerve blockade. *Anesth Analg* 2001;92:215–217.
- Vloka JD, Hadžić A, Kitain E, Lesser JB, Kuroda M, April EW, Thys DM. Anatomic considerations for sciatic nerve block in the popliteal fossa through the lateral approach. *Reg Anesth* 1996;21:414–418.
- Vloka JD, Hadžić A, Lesser JB, Kitain E, Geatz H, April EW, Thys DM. A common epineural sheath for the nerves in the popliteal fossa and its possible implications for sciatic nerve block. *Anesth Analg* 1997;84:387–390.
- Zetlaoui PJ, Bouaziz H. Lateral approach to the sciatic nerve in the popliteal fossa. *Anesth Analg* 1998;87:79–82.

Popliteal Block, Lateral Approach, Continuous Technique

- Chelly JE, Casati A, Fanelli G. Continuous *Peripheral Nerve Block Technique: An Illustrated Guide*. London, England: Mosby International; 2001.
- di Benedetto P, Casati A, Bertini L, Fanelli G, Chelly JE. Postoperative analgesia with continuous sciatic nerve block after foot surgery: a prospective, randomized comparison between the popliteal and subgluteal approaches. *Anesth Analg* 2002;94:996–1000.
- Ilfeld BM, Morey TE, Wang RD, Enneking FK. Continuous popliteal sciatic nerve block for postoperative pain control at home: a randomized, double-blinded, placebo-controlled study. *Anesthesiology* 2002; 97.959–965.
- Singelyn FJ, Aye F, Gouverneur JM. Continuous popliteal sciatic nerve block: an original technique to provide postoperative analgesia after foot surgery. *Anesth Analg* 1997; 84:383–38.

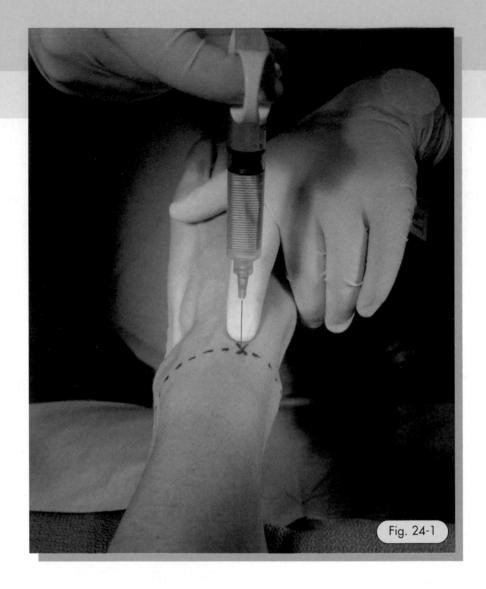

Fig. 24-1

BLOCK AT A GLANCE

- Indications: surgery of the foot and toes

- Two deep nerves: posterior tibial, deep peroneal

- Three superficial nerves: superficial peroneal, sural, saphenous

- Needle: $1\frac{1}{2}$ inch

- Local anesthetic: 6 mL per nerve

- Epinephrine-containing local anesthetic should not be used

- Complexity level: basic

GENERAL CONSIDERATIONS

An ankle block is essentially a block of four branches of the sciatic nerve (deep and superficial peroneal, tibial, and sural) and one cutaneous branch of the femoral nerve (saphenous). An ankle block is a basic peripheral nerve block technique. It is simple to perform, essentially devoid of systemic complications, and highly effective for a wide variety of procedures on the foot and toes. For this reason, this technique should be in the armamentarium of every anesthesiologist. At our institution, an ankle block is most commonly used in podiatric surgery and foot and toe debridement or amputation.

Regional Anesthesia Anatomy

An ankle block is essentially a block of the terminal branches of the sciatic nerve except for the saphenous nerve (the sensory branch of the femoral nerve). It is useful to think of the ankle block as a block of two deep nerves (posterior tibial and deep peroneal) and three superficial nerves (saphenous, sural, and superficial peroneal **Fig. 24-2**). This concept is crucial for success of the block because the two deep nerves are anesthetized by injecting local anesthetic under the superficial fascia, whereas the three superficial nerves are anesthetized by a simple subcutaneous injection of local anesthetic.

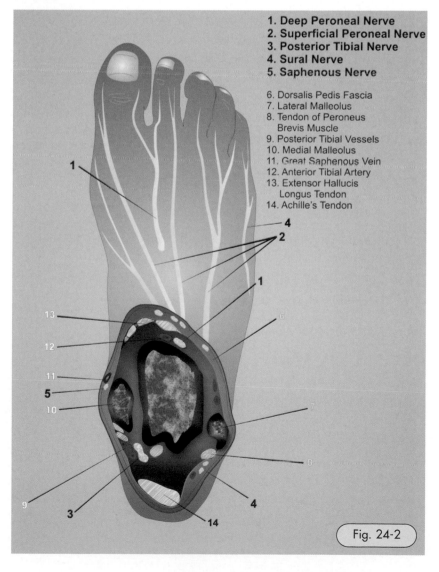

1. Deep Peroneal Nerve
2. Superficial Peroneal Nerve
3. Posterior Tibial Nerve
4. Sural Nerve
5. Saphenous Nerve

6. Dorsalis Pedis Fascia
7. Lateral Malleolus
8. Tendon of Peroneus Brevis Muscle
9. Posterior Tibial Vessels
10. Medial Malleolus
11. Great Saphenous Vein
12. Anterior Tibial Artery
13. Extensor Hallucis Longus Tendon
14. Achille's Tendon

Fig. 24-2

Common Peroneal Nerve

The common peroneal (lateral popliteal) nerve separates from the tibial nerve (L4 and L5, S1 and S2) and descends along the tendon of the biceps femoris muscle and around the neck of the fibula. Just below the head of the fibula, the common peroneal nerve divides into its terminal branches: the deep peroneal and superficial peroneal nerves **(Figs. 24-2 and 24-3)**. The peroneus longus muscle covers both nerves.

Deep Peroneal Nerve

The deep peroneal nerve runs downward below the layers of the peroneus longus, extensor digitorum longus, and extensor hallucis longus muscles to the front of the leg **(Fig. 24.2)**. At the ankle level, the nerve lies anterior to the tibia and the interosseous membrane and close to the anterior tibial artery. It is usually "sandwiched" between the tendons of the anterior tibial and extensor digitorum longus muscles. At this point, it divides into two terminal branches for the foot: the medial and the lateral. The medial branch passes over the dorsum of the foot, along the medial side of the dorsalis pedis artery, to the first interosseous space, where it divides into two dorsal digital branches for the nerve supply to the first web space between the big toe and the second toe. The lateral branch of the deep peroneal nerve is directed anterolaterally, penetrates and innervates the extensor digitorum brevis muscle, and terminates as the second, third, and fourth dorsal interosseous nerves. These branches provide the nerve supply to the tarsometatarsal, metatarsophalangeal, and interphalangeal joints of the lesser toes.

Superficial Peroneal Nerve

The superficial peroneal nerve (also called the musculocutaneous nerve of the leg) is a branch of the common peroneal nerve **(Fig. 24-3)**. The superficial peroneal nerve provides muscular branches to the peroneus longus and brevis muscles. After piercing the deep fascia covering the muscles, the nerve eventually emerges from the anterolateral compartment of the lower part of the leg and surfaces from beneath the fascia 5 to 10 cm above the lateral malleolus. At this point, it divides into terminal cutaneous branches: the medial and the lateral dorsal cutaneous nerves. These branches carry sensory innervation to the dorsum of the foot and communicate with the saphenous nerve medially, with the deep peroneal nerve in the first web space and

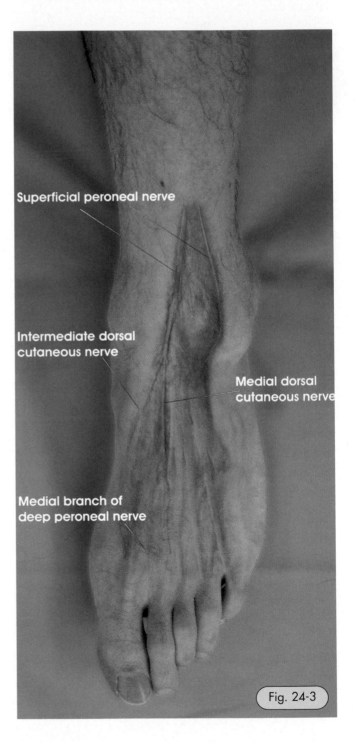

Fig. 24-3

the sural nerve on the lateral aspect of the foot.

Tibial Nerve

The tibial nerve (medial popliteal or posterior tibial nerve) separates from the common popliteal nerve at various distances from the popliteal fossa crease and joins the tibial artery behind the knee joint. The nerve runs distally in the thick neurovascular fascia and emerges at the inferior third of the leg from beneath the soleus and gastrocnemius muscles on the medial border of the Achilles tendon **(Fig. 24-4)**. At the level of the medial malleolus, the tibial nerve is covered by the superficial and deep fasciae of the leg. It is positioned laterally and posteriorly to the posterior tibial artery and midway between the posterior aspect of the medial malleolus and the posterior aspect of the Achilles tendon. Just beneath the malleolus, the nerve divides into lateral and medial plantar nerves. The posterior tibial nerve provides cutaneous, articular, and vascular branches to the ankle joint, medial malleolus, inner aspect of the heel, and Achilles tendon. It

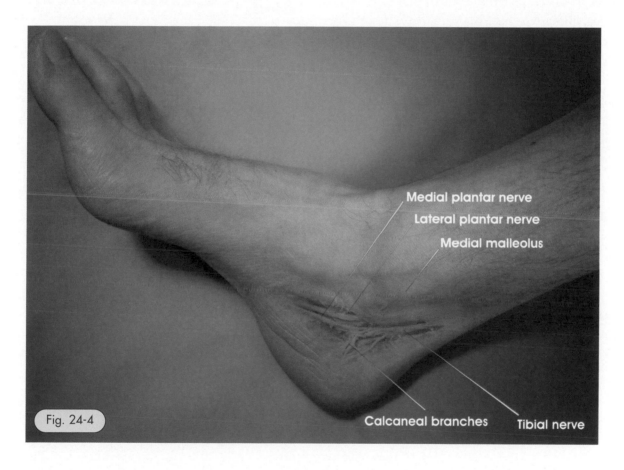

Medial plantar nerve
Lateral plantar nerve
Medial malleolus

Calcaneal branches   Tibial nerve

Fig. 24-4

also branches to the skin, subcutaneous tissue, muscles, and bones of the sole.

Sural Nerve

The sural nerve is a sensory nerve formed by a union of the medial sural nerve (a branch of the tibial nerve) and the lateral sural nerve (a branch of the common peroneal nerve). The sural nerve courses between the heads of the gastrocnemius muscle, and after piercing the fascia covering the muscles, emerges on the lateral aspect of the Achilles tendon 10 to 15 cm above the lateral malleolus **(Fig. 24-5)**. After providing lateral calcaneal branches to the heel, the sural nerve descends 1 to 1.5 cm behind the lateral malleolus anterolaterally to the short saphenous vein and on the surface of the fascia covering the muscles and tendons. At this level, it supplies the lateral malleolus, Achilles tendon, and ankle joint. The sural nerve continues on the lateral

aspect of the foot, innervating the skin, subcutaneous tissue, fourth interosseous space, and fifth toe.

Saphenous Nerve

The saphenous nerve is a terminal cutaneous branch (or branches) of the femoral nerve. Its course is in the

TIP

▶ All superficial (cutaneous) nerves of the foot should be thought of as a neuronal network rather than as single strings of nerves with a well-defined, consistent anatomic position **(Fig. 24-5)**.

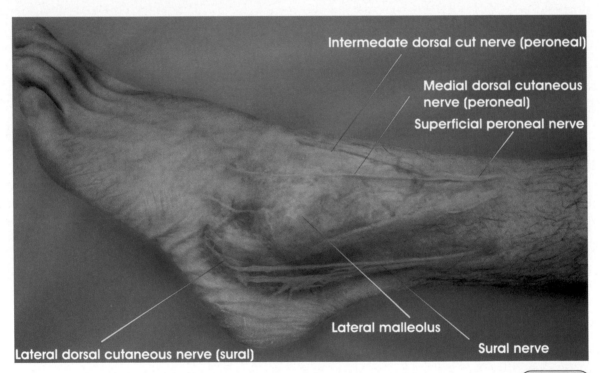

Intermedate dorsal cut nerve (peroneal)

Medial dorsal cutaneous nerve (peroneal)

Superficial peroneal nerve

Lateral malleolus

Sural nerve

Lateral dorsal cutaneous nerve (sural)

Fig. 24-5

subcutaneous tissue of the skin on the medial aspect of the ankle and foot **(Fig. 24-2)**.

Distribution of Anesthesia

An ankle block results in anesthesia of the foot. However, it should be noted that an ankle block does not result in anesthesia of the ankle itself. The proximal extension of the blockade is to the level at which the block is performed. The more proximal branches of the tibial and peroneal nerves innervate the deep structures of the ankle joint (see "Anatomy"). Cutaneous innervation of the foot is provided by three superficial nerves (saphenous, sural, superficial peroneal). The two deep nerves (tibial, deep peroneal) provide innervation to the deep structures, bones, and cutaneous coverage of the

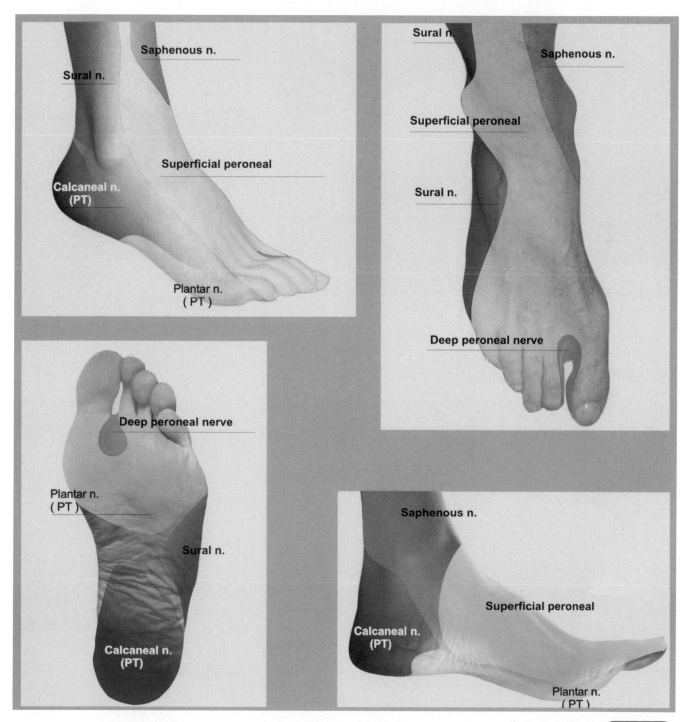

Fig. 24-6

sole and web between the first and second toes **(Fig. 24-6)**.

Patient Positioning

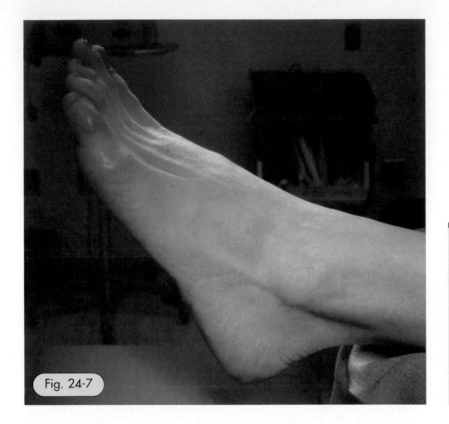

Fig. 24-7

The patient is in the supine position with the foot on a footrest **(Fig. 24-7)**.

Equipment

A standard regional anesthesia tray is prepared with the following equipment:

- Sterile towels and gauze packs

- Three 10-mL syringes containing local anesthetic

- Sterile gloves, marking pen

- $1\frac{1}{2}$-in, 25-gauge needle

Anatomic and Surface Landmarks

The deep peroneal nerve is located immediately lateral to the tendon of the extensor hallucis longus muscle (between the extensor hallucis longus and the extensor digitorum longus, **Fig. 24-8**). The pulse of the anterior tibial artery (dorsalis pedis) can be felt at this location; the nerve is immediately lateral to the artery.

TIP

▶ This landmark is easily palpated and can be accentuated by asking the patient to dorsiflex the foot or toe (**Fig. 24-8**).

The posterior tibial nerve is located just behind and distal to the medial malleolus. The pulse of the posterior tibial artery can be felt at this location; the nerve is just posterior to the artery.

The superficial peroneal, sural, and saphenous nerves are located in the subcutaneous tissue along a circular line stretching from the lateral aspect of the Achilles tendon across the lateral malleolus, anterior aspect of the foot, and medial malleolus to the medial aspect of the Achilles tendon (**Fig. 24-2**).

TIP

▶ The superficial nerves branch out and anastomose extensively; they do not have a single, consistently positioned nerve trunk that can be anesthetized by a single, precise injection as often taught.

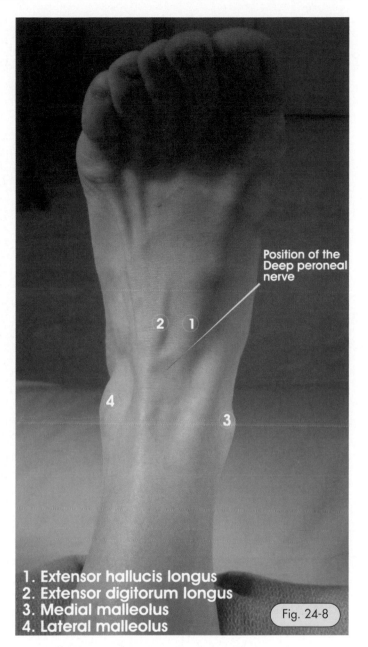

Position of the Deep peroneal nerve

1. Extensor hallucis longus
2. Extensor digitorum longus
3. Medial malleolus
4. Lateral malleolus

Fig. 24-8

Anatomic landmarks for the ankle block.

To accomplish proper blockade of all five nerves, it is important that the anesthesiologist walk from one side of the foot to the other during the block procedure instead of bending and leaning over to reach the opposite side. Before beginning the procedure, the entire foot should be cleaned with a disinfectant.It makes sense to begin this procedure with blocks of the two deep nerves because subcutaneous injections for the superficial blocks inevitably deform the anatomy. A controlled or regular syringe can be used.

Deep Peroneal Block

The finger of the palpating hand is positioned in the groove just lateral to the extensor hallucis longus (Fig. 24-9). The needle is inserted under the skin and advanced until stopped by the bone. At this point, the needle is withdrawn back 1 to 2 mm and 2 to 3 mL of local anesthetic is injected.

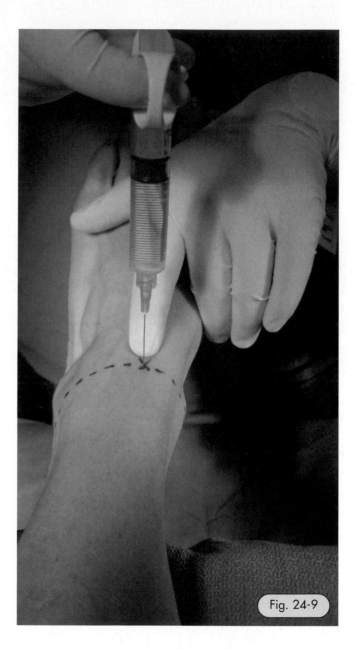

Fig. 24-9

TIPS

▶ A deep peroneal block is essentially a "blind" injection of local anesthetic. Instead of relying on a single injection, a "fan" technique is recommended to increase the success rate after the injection. After the initial injection the needle is withdrawn back to skin level, redirected 30° laterally **(Fig. 24-10A)**, and advanced again to contact the bone. After pulling the needle back 1 to 2 mm off the bone, an additional 2 mL of local anesthetic is injected. A similar procedure is repeated with a medial redirection of the needle **(Fig. 24-10B)**.

▶ Mentally visualize the plane of the needle insertion for the deep peroneal and posterior tibial nerves. Do not move the palpating finger during the injection to ensure proper needle reinsertions (30° laterally and medially) and keep the tip of the needle underneath the skin during redirections.

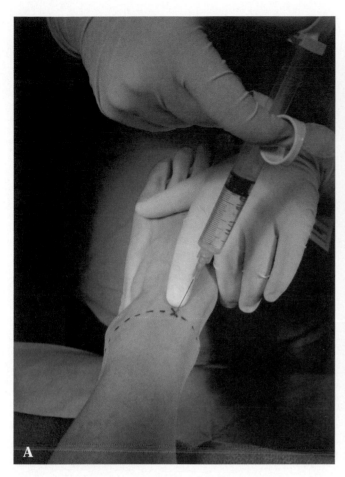

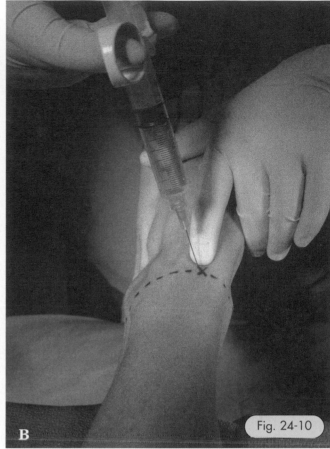

A

B

Fig. 24-10

Posterior Tibial Block

The posterior tibial nerve is anesthetized by injecting local anesthetic just behind the medial malleolus **(Fig. 24-11)**. Similar to that of the deep peroneal nerve, its position is deep to the superficial fascia. With the anesthesiologist facing the medial aspect of the foot, the needle is introduced in the groove behind the medial malleolus and advanced until contact with the bone is felt **(Fig. 24-11)**. At this point, the needle is withdrawn back 1 to 2 mm and 2 to 3 mL of local anesthetic is injected.

TIP

▶ Similar to the procedure used for the deep peroneal nerve, a "fan" technique should be used to increase the success rate. The needle is pulled back to the skin, and two additional boluses of 2 mL of local anesthetic are injected after lateral and medial needle reinsertions **(Fig. 24-12A** and **12B)**.

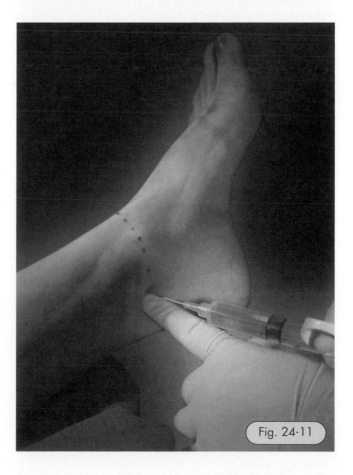

Fig. 24-11

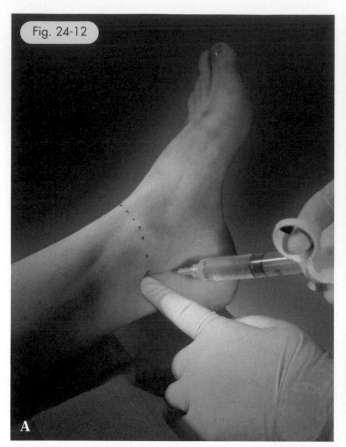

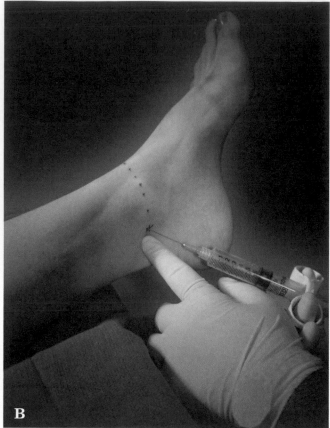

Fig. 24-12

A

B

Block of the Superficial Peroneal, Sural, and Saphenous Nerves

These three nerves are superficial cutaneous extensions of the sciatic and femoral
nerves. Because they are positioned superficially to the deep fascia, an injection of
local anesthetic in the territory through
which they descend to the distal foot is
adequate to achieve their blockade. A
blockade of all three nerves is accomplished using a simple circumferential
injection of local anesthetic subcutaneously **(Figs. 24-12, 24-13, 24-14,** and **24-15)**.

To block the *saphenous nerve*, a $1^{1}/_{2}$-
in, 25-gauge needle is inserted at the level
of the medial malleolus and a "ring" of
local anesthetic is raised from the point of
needle entry to the Achilles tendon and
anteriorly to the tibial ridge **(Fig. 24-13)**.
This can be usually accomplished with
one or two needle insertions. Six (6) milliliters of local anesthetic suffices.

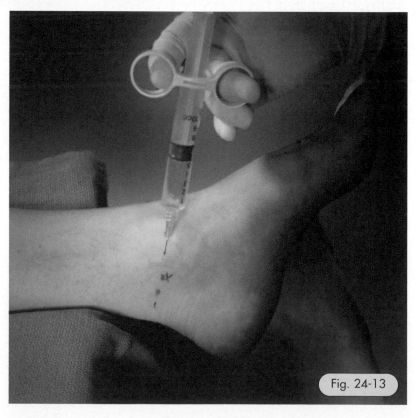

Fig. 24-13

To block the *superficial peroneal* nerve, the needle is inserted at the tibial ridge and extended laterally toward the lateral malleolus **(Fig. 24-14)**. It is important to raise a subcutaneous "wheal" during injection, which indicates injection in the proper, superficial plane. Five milliliters of local anesthetic is adequate.

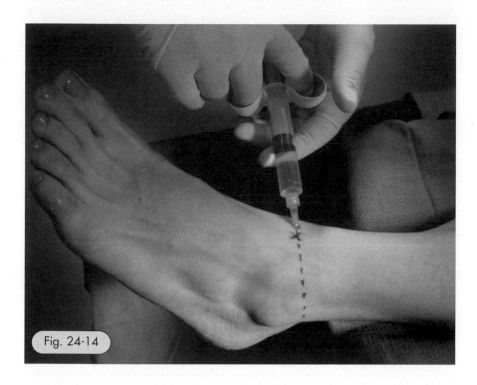

Fig. 24-14

To block the *sural nerve*, the needle is inserted at the level of the lateral malleolus and the local anesthetic is infiltrated toward the Achilles tendon **(Fig. 24-15)**. Six milliliters of local anesthetic is deposited in a circular fashion to raise a skin "wheal."

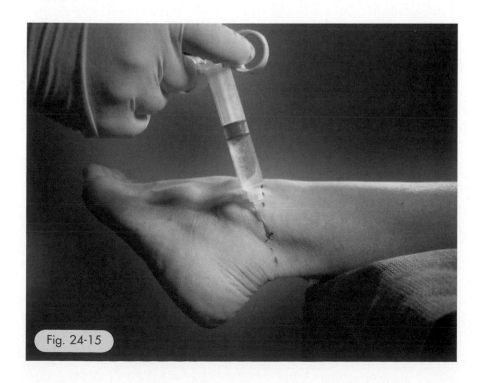

Fig. 24-15

TIP

▶ Remember the subcutaneous position of the superficial nerves and think of their blockade as a "field block." A distinct subcutaneous "wheal." should be seen with injection into a proper plane to block the superficial nerves.

Choice of Local Anesthetic

The choice of the type and concentration of local anesthetic for an ankle block is based on the desired duration of the blockade. Because it is almost always beneficial that the analgesia following an ankle block last some time after surgery, a long-acting local anesthetic is most commonly used. **Table 24.1** provides onset times and durations for some commonly used local anesthetic mixtures.

TABLE 24.1
Choice of Local Anesthetic For Ankle Block

ANESTHETIC	ONSET (min)	DURATION OF ANESTHESIA (h)	DURATION OF ANALGESIA (h)
1.5% Mepivacaine (+ HCO_3)*	15–20	2–3	3–5
2% Lidocaine (+ HCO_3)*	10–20	2–5	3–8
0.5% Ropivacaine*	15–30	4–8	5–12
0.75% Ropivacaine*	10–15	5–10	6–24
0.5% Bupivacaine (or levobupivacaine)*	15–30	5–15	6–30

* The use of epinephrine-containing solutions for ankle block is not recommended.

Block Dynamics and Perioperative Management

Although an ankle block is considered a "superficial block" procedure, it is one of the most uncomfortable block procedures for patients. The reason is that it involves five separate needle insertions, and subcutaneous injections to block the cutaneous nerves result in pressure distension of the skin and nerve endings. Additionally, the foot is supplied by an abundance of nerve endings and is exquisitely sensitive to needle injections. For that reason, this block requires significant premedication to make it acceptable to patients. We routinely use a combination of midazolam (2 to 4 mg intravenously) and a narcotic (500 to 750 μg alfentanil) to ensure the patient's comfort during the procedure.

A typical onset time for this block is 10 to 25 minutes, depending primarily on the concentration and volume of local anesthetic used. Sensory anesthesia of the skin with this block develops faster than the motor block. Placement of an Esmarch bandage or a tourniquet at the level of the ankle is well-tolerated and typically does not require additional blockade in sedated patients.

Complications and How to Avoid Them

Complications following an ankle block are typically limited to residual paresthesias due to inadvertent intraneuronal injection. Systemic toxicity is rare because of the distal location of the blockade. **Table 24.2** provides more specific instructions on possible complications and corrective measures.

TABLE 24.2
Complications of Ankle Block and Preventive Techniques

Infection	• Rare with the use of an aseptic technique.
Hematoma	• Avoid multiple needle insertions. • Most superficial blocks can be accomplished with one or two needle insertions. • Use a small gauge needle and avoid puncturing superficial veins.
Vascular puncture	• Avoid puncturing the greater saphenous vein at the medial malleolus. • Intermittent aspiration should be performed to avoid intravascular injection.
Nerve injury	• Do not inject when the patient complains of pain or high pressures are met on injection. • Do not reinject deep tibial and peroneal nerves.
Other	• Instruct the patient on care of the insensate extremity.

SUGGESTED READINGS

- Delgado-Martinez AD, Marchal-Escalona JM. Supramalleolar ankle block anesthesia and ankle tourniquet for foot surgery. *Foot Ankle Int* 2001;22:836–838.
- Hadžić A, Vloka JD, Kuroda MM. The use of peripheral nerve blocks in anesthesia practice: a national survey. *Reg Anesth Pain Med* 1998;23:241–246.
- Mineo R, Sharrock NE. Venous levels of lidocaine and bupivacaine after midtarsal ankle block. *Reg Anesth* 1992;17:47–49.
- Myerson MS, Ruland CM, Allon SM. Regional anesthesia for foot and ankle surgery. *Foot Ankle Int* 1992;13:282–288.
- Needoff M, Radford P, Costigan P. Local anesthesia for postoperative pain relief after foot surgery: a prospective clinical trial. *Foot Ankle Int* 1999;16:11–13.
- Noorpuri BS, Shahane SA, Getty CJ. Acute compartment syndrome following revisional arthroplasty of the forefoot: the dangers of ankle-block. *Foot Ankle Int* 2000;21:680–682.
- Reilley TE, Gerhardt MA. Anesthesia for foot and ankle surgery: *Clin Podiatr Med Surg* 2002;19:125–147.
- Schurman DJ. Ankle-block anesthesia for foot surgery. *Anesthesiology* 1976;44:348–352.
- Sharrock NE, Waller JF, Fierro LE. Midtarsal block for surgery of the forefoot. *Br J Anaesth* 1986;58:37–40

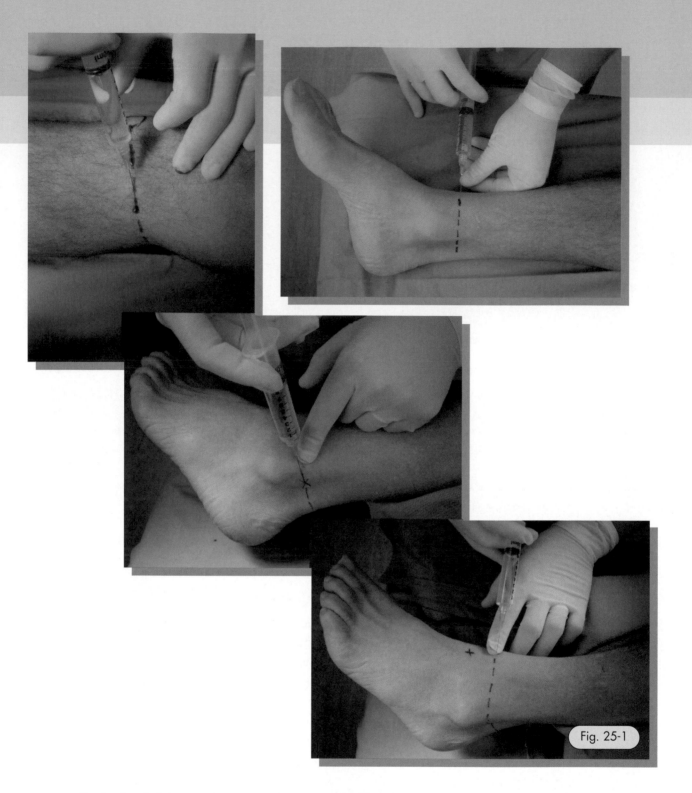

Fig. 25-1

BLOCK AT A GLANCE

- Indications: mostly as a supplement to major blocks of the lower extremity

- Local anesthetic: 5 to 10 mL

- Complexity level: basic

25

CUTANEOUS
NERVE BLOCKS OF THE
LOWER EXTREMITY

GENERAL CONSIDERATIONS

Blocks of the lateral femoral cutaneous, posterior femoral cutaneous, saphenous, sural, and superficial peroneal nerves are useful anesthetic techniques for a variety of superficial surgical procedures. These blocks are simple to learn and perform, they are essentially devoid of complications, and they can nicely complement major conduction blocks of the lower extremity. The combination of their applicability and simplicity should mandate that these blocks be in the armamentarium of every practicing anesthesiologist.

Regional Anesthesia Anatomy

The cutaneous nerves of the lower extremities are blocked by injection of local anesthetic into the subcutaneous layers above the muscle fascia. The subcutaneous tissue contains a variable amount of fat, superficial nerves, and vessels. Deep in this area is a tough membranous layer—the deep fascia of the lower extremity enclosing muscles of the leg. Deep fascia is penetrated by numerous superficial nerves and vessels.

Cutaneous innervation of the lower extremity is accomplished by nerves that are part of the lumbar and sciatic plexuses **(Fig. 25-2** and **25-3)**. The largest cutaneous nerves are the lateral femoral cutaneous, posterior femoral cutaneous, saphenous, sural, and superficial peroneal. A more detailed review of the relevant anatomy is provided with the descriptions of the individual block procedures and in the chapter on anatomy.

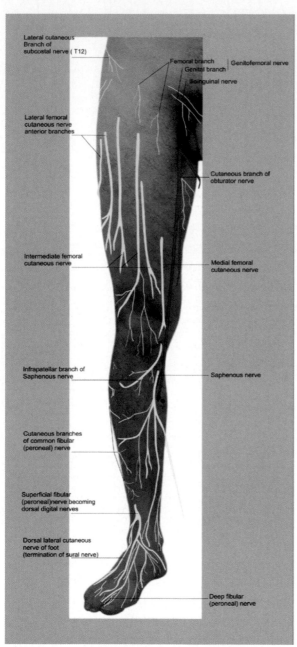

Cutaneous innervation of the lower extremity: Front.

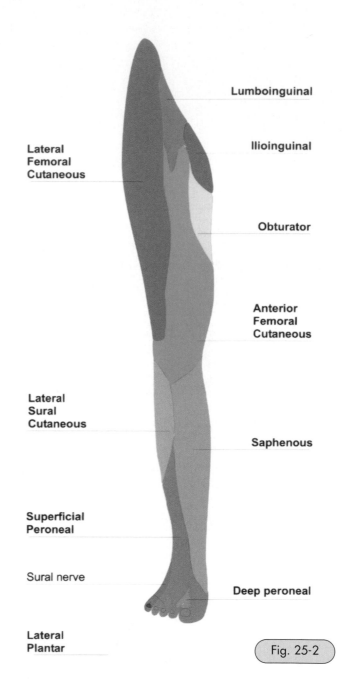

Lumboinguinal

Ilioinguinal

Obturator

Lateral Femoral Cutaneous

Anterior Femoral Cutaneous

Lateral Sural Cutaneous

Saphenous

Superficial Peroneal

Sural nerve

Deep peroneal

Lateral Plantar

Fig. 25-2

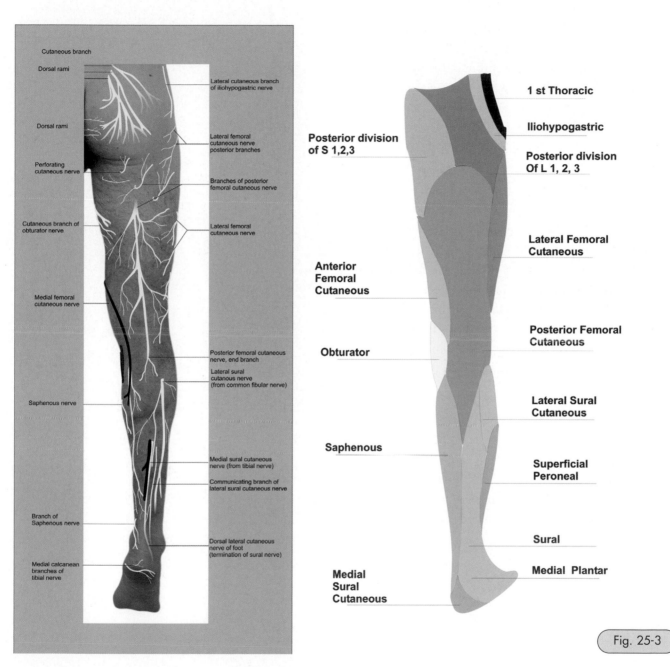

Cutaneous innervation of the lower extremity: Back.

Fig. 25-3

LATERAL FEMORAL CUTANEOUS NERVE

Anatomy

The lateral femoral cutaneous nerve emerges from the lateral border of the psoas major muscle and crosses the iliacus muscle obliquely toward the anterior superior iliac spine, where it supplies the parietal peritoneum of the iliac fossa **(Fig. 25-4)**. The nerve then passes into the thigh behind or through the inguinal ligament, variably medially to the anterior iliac spine (typically about 1 cm) or through the sartorius muscle, dividing into anterior and posterior branches.

The anterior branch becomes superficial about 10 cm distal to the anterior superior iliac spine, innervating the skin of the anterior and lateral thigh as far as the knee. It connects terminally with the cutaneous branches of the anterior division of the femoral nerve and the infrapatellar branch of the saphenous nerve, forming the patellar plexus. The posterior branch pierces the fascia lata higher than the anterior, dividing to supply the skin on the lateral surface from the greater trochanter to about the middle of the thigh and occasionally also supplying the gluteal skin **(Figs. 25-2 and 25-3)**.

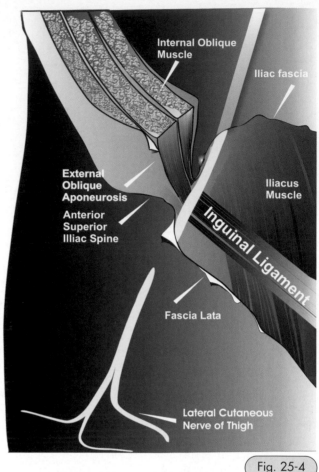

Fig. 25-4

Indications

Lateral femoral cutaneous nerve blockade can be used to provide complete anesthesia in patients undergoing small skin grafts on the lateral aspect of the thigh or can be combined with a femoral block to complement the femoral nerve block for surgery on the knee joint. It also has been reportedly used as a diagnostic tool for myalgia paresthetica, neuralgia of the lateral femoral cutaneous nerve of the thigh.

Technique

The patient is in the supine position with the anesthesiologist at the patient's side to be operated on. The anterior superior iliac spine is palpated and marked **(Fig. 25-5)**. A 4-cm, 22-gauge needle is inserted 2 cm medial and 2 cm caudal to the anterior superior iliac spine **(Fig. 25-6)**. The needle is advanced until a loss of resistance is felt as it passes through the fascia lata. A short-bevel needle is suggested to exaggerate the loss of resistance as it passes through the fascia. Because this fascia "give" is not consistent and its perception may vary among performers, local anesthetic is injected in a fanwise fashion both above and below the fascia lata, from medial to lateral. A volume of 10 mL of local anesthetic is injected for this block. This volume is injected in a "fan" wise fashion to increase the success rate **(Fig. 25-6)**. Although this is a sensory nerve, relatively higher concentrations of long-acting local anesthetic are useful to increase the success rate (0.5% ropivacaine or 0.5% bupivacaine). When used to provide anesthesia for a skin graft harvest site on the lateral thigh, the peripheral innervation of the lateral femoral cutaneous nerve in specific patients is outlined before the procedure is begun.

Because there are no larger vascular structures or other organs nearby, blockade of the lateral femoral cutaneous nerve carries minimal risk of systemic toxicity due to inadvertent intravascular injection. Care should be exercised to avoid forceful injections and use of high pressures. Such injections may result in dysesthesia or hypoesthesia in case of an intraneuronal injection.

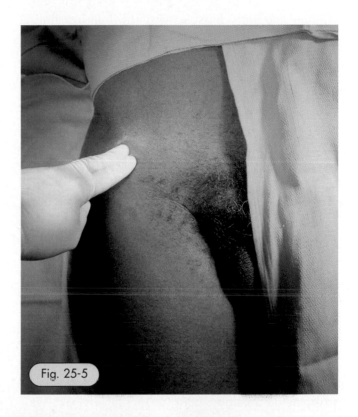

Fig. 25-5

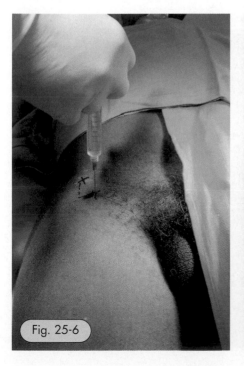

Fig. 25-6

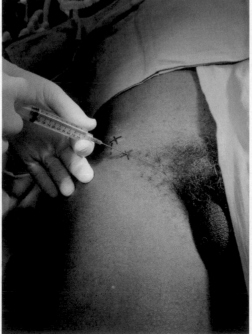

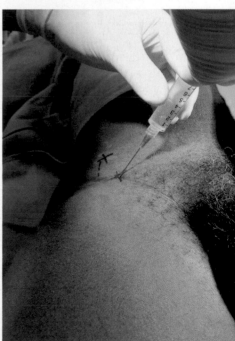

POSTERIOR CUTANEOUS NERVE OF THE THIGH

Anatomy

The posterior femoral cutaneous nerve originates from the dorsal branches of the first and second and from the ventral branches of the second and third sacral rami. It runs through the greater sciatic foramen below the piriformis and descends under the gluteus maximus muscle with the inferior gluteal vessels, posteriorly or medially to the sciatic nerve. The nerve then descends in the back of the thigh, deep to the fascia lata. Its branches are all cutaneous and are distributed to the gluteal region, perineum, and flexor aspect of the thigh and leg **(Fig. 25-3)**.

Indications

This nerve block has been used in burn patients, with donor skin for grafting taken from the posterior thigh in conjunction witho a popliteal or posterior femoral cutaneous nerve block in short saphenous vein stripping.

Technique

The patient can be positioned prone, in the lateral decubitus position, or supine with the leg elevated 90°. The gluteal fold is identified, and 10 mL of local anesthetic is injected subcutaneously to raise a skin "wheal" **(Fig. 25-7)**. In addition, at the midpoint of the gluteal crease, 5 ml of local anesthetic is injected at a deeper level, using a "fan" technique to reach the nerve which has not emerged through the deep fascia.

To block the posterior cutaneous nerve of the thigh above the knee level, such as for short saphenous vein stripping (as a complement to a popliteal block), with the patient in the prone position, 10 mL of local anesthetic is injected subcutaneously along a line 5 cm above and parallel to the popliteal crease **(Fig. 25-8)**.

> **TIP**
>
> ►It should be noted that the posterior cutaneous nerve of the thigh is usually anesthetized with the posterior approach to a sciatic nerve block; therefore, it is not necessary to block it in addition to the sciatic block.

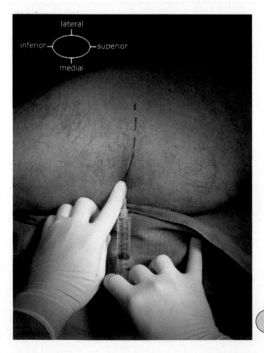

Fig. 25-7

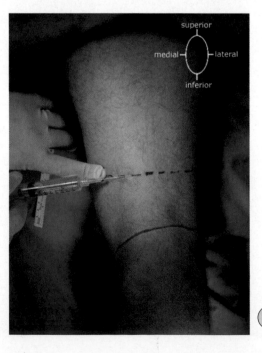

Fig. 25-8

SAPHENOUS NERVE

Anatomy

The saphenous nerve is the largest cutaneous branch of the femoral nerve. It descends laterally to the femoral artery into the adductor canal, where it crosses anteriorly to become medial to the artery. It proceeds vertically along the medial side of the knee behind the sartorius, pierces the fascia lata between the tendons of the sartorius and gracilis, and becomes subcutaneous **(Fig. 25-9)**. From there it descends, with the long saphenous vein, on the medial side of the leg along the medial tibial border. It innervates the skin over the medial, anteromedial, and posteromedial aspects of the lower leg from above the knee (part of the patellar plexus) to as low as the first metatarsophalangeal joint in some instances **(Figs. 25-2 and 25-3)**. The saphenous nerve branches into numerous small branches as it enters the subcutaneous space, and therefore, it is often difficult to achieve blockade of the entire extensive saphenous nerve network. For this reason, it is always preferable to block the saphenous nerve as distally as possible. For instance, to achieve anesthesia of the foot, the saphenous nerve is best approached at the level of the ankle, identically to the technique for performing an ankle block.

Indications

A saphenous nerve block is most commonly used in combination with a sciatic nerve block or a popliteal block to complement anesthesia of the lower leg for various vascular, orthopedic, and podiatric procedures.

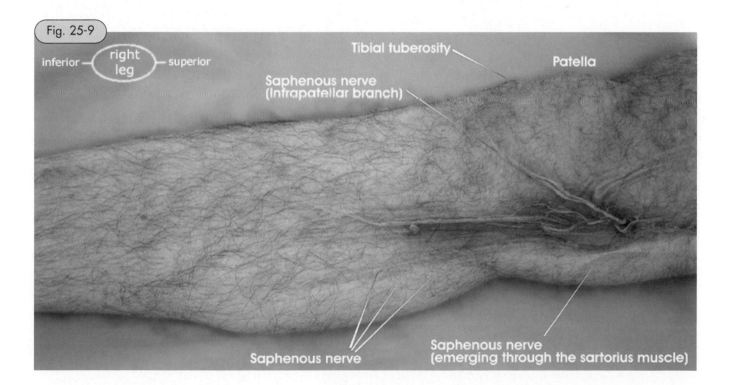

Fig. 25-9

inferior — right leg — superior

Tibial tuberosity
Patella
Saphenous nerve (Infrapatellar branch)
Saphenous nerve
Saphenous nerve (emerging through the sartorius muscle)

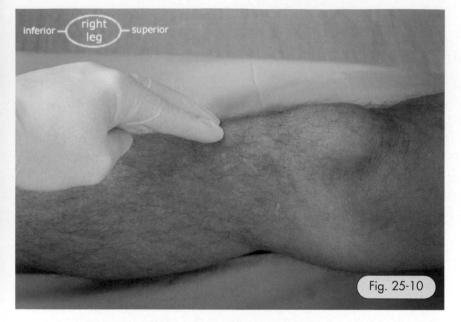

Fig. 25-10

Technique

The main landmark for this block is the tibial tuberosity, an easily recognizable and felt bony prominence on the anterior aspect of the tibia a few centimeters distal to the patella **(Fig. 25-10)**. Several techniques of saphenous nerve blockade have been described; however, in this chapter, we focus primarily on the one we routinely use in our practice. With the patient in the supine position, 5 to 10 mL of local anesthetic is injected subcutaneously as a ring starting at the medial surface of the tibial condyle and ending at the dorsomedial aspect of the upper calf **(Fig. 25-11)**.

TIPS

▶ A paravenous technique has also been described, which is based on the close relationship between the saphenous vein and nerve, to achieve a higher success rate. The technique involves the injection of 5 mL of local anesthetic in a fanlike fashion around the vein on the medial side of the leg just distal to the patella.

▶ In the transsartorial approach, with the patient in the supine position, a skin wheal is raised over the sartorius muscle belly. The sartorius muscle can be palpated just above the knee with the leg extended and actively elevated. A Tuohy needle is inserted at one finger width above the patella, slightly posteriorly to the coronal plane and slightly caudal, through the muscle belly of the sartorius until a loss of resistance identifies the subsartorial adipose tissue. The depth of insertion is typically between 1.5 and 3 cm. After obtaining negative results from an aspiration test for blood, 10 mL of local anesthetic is injected.

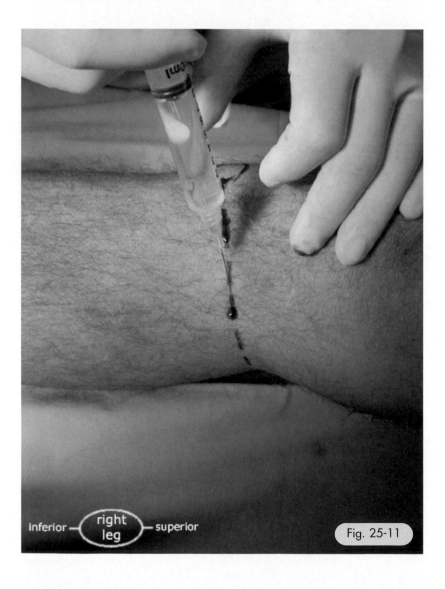

Fig. 25-11

For surgery on the foot, the saphenous nerve is best blocked just above the medial malleolus as in the ankle block technique **(Fig. 25-12)**. With a $1^1/_2$-in needle, 6 to 8 mL of local anesthetic is injected subcutaneously immediately above the medial malleolus in a ringlike fashion. The most commonly reported complication associated with this block is a painless hematoma, resulting from oozing of the punctured caphenous vein at the injection site.

TIP

▶ The most effective method of blocking the saphenous nerve is a low-volume femoral nerve block. The injection of just 10 ml of local anesthetic after obtaining twitches of the patella or vastus medialis muscle results in a nearly 100% success rate.

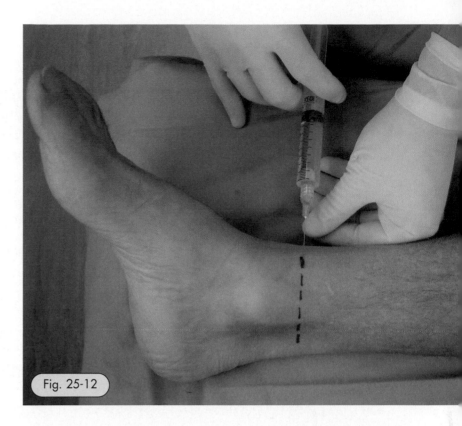
Fig. 25-12

SURAL NERVE

Anatomy

The sural nerve, a branch of the tibial nerve, pierces the deep fascia proximally in the leg and is joined by a branch of the common peroneal nerve. It descends near the lesser saphenous vein and between the lateral malleolus and the calcaneus **(Fig. 25-13)**. It innervates the posterior and lateral skin of the distal third of the leg along the lateral side of the foot and little toe **(Figs. 25-2 and 25-3)**.

Indications

Sural nerve blockade is used for superficial surgery on the lateral aspect of the ankle and foot and in conjunction with an ankle block for foot and toe surgery.

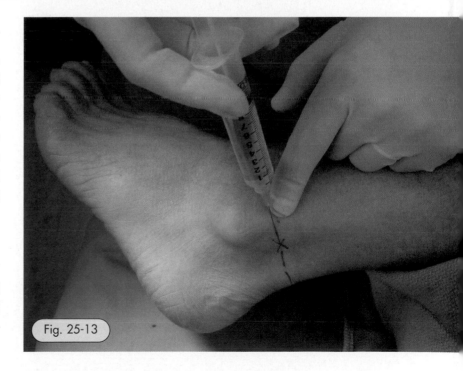
Fig. 25-13

Technique

For the block procedure, the patient can be positioned prone or supine with the ankle supported by a footrest **(Fig. 25-13)**. With a $1^1/_2$-in, 25-gauge needle, a skin wheal is raised lateral to the Achilles tendon and just above the lateral malleolus. The needle is then inserted through the wheal and advanced toward the fibula while injecting 6 to 8 mL of local anesthetic.

SUPERFICIAL PERONEAL NERVE

Anatomy

The superficial peroneal nerve begins at the common peroneal bifurcation. It pierces the deep fascia in the distal third of the leg and descends down the leg adjacent to the extensor digitorum longus muscle where it divides into terminal branches above the ankle. The superficial peroneal branches innervate the dorsal skin of all the toes except that of the lateral side of the fifth and the adjoining sides of the first and second **(Figs. 25-2** and **25-3)**.

Indication

A superficial peroneal block is used alone or in combination with other blocks for foot surgery or ascending venography.

Technique

The superficial peroneal nerve is blocked immediately above and medial to the lateral malleolus by injecting a subcutaneous wheal of 5 to 10 mL of local anesthetic from the site of insertion of the needle for the deep peroneal nerve to the anterior surface of the lateral malleolus **(Fig. 25-14)**.

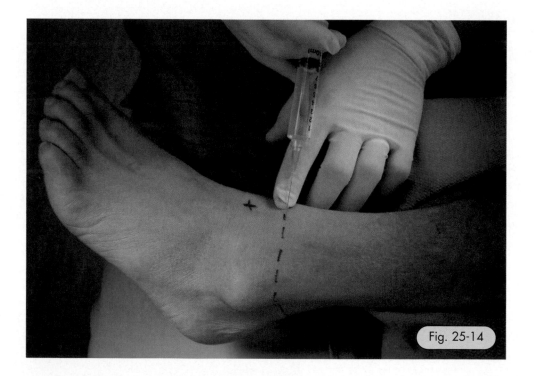

Fig. 25-14

Choice of Local Anesthetic

Any local anesthetic can be used for cutaneous blocks of the lower extremity. The choice of local anesthetic is based primarily on the desired duration of the blockade. Because these blocks do not result in a motor blockade, longer-acting local anesthetics are most commonly chosen (e.g., 0.2 to 0.5% ropivacaine or 0.25% bupivacaine or L-bupivacaine).

Complications and How to Avoid Them

Complications of cutaneous nerve blocks are few; they are listed in **Table 25.1**.

TABLE 25.1
Complications of Cutaneous Blocks of the Lower Extremity and Preventive Techniques

Systemic toxicity of local anesthetic	• The risk is small and may be of concern only when higher volumes local anesthetic are used in conjunction with other high-volume major conduction blocks.
Hematoma	• Avoid multiple needle insertions and insertion of the needle through superficial veins.
Nerve injury	• Usually manifested as transient paresthesias or dysesthesias; injuries result from inadvertent intraneuronal injection. • Injections should not be made when high pressures are felt on injection or when the patient reports pain in the distribution of the nerve.

SUGGESTED READINGS

- Bouaziz H, Benhamou D, Narchi P. A new approach for saphenous nerve block. *Reg Anesth* 1996;21:5.
- Brown DL. *Atlas of Regional Anesthesia*. 2nd ed. Philadelphia, Pa: WB Saunders; 1999.
- Brown TCK, Dickens DRV. A new approach to lateral cutaneous nerve of thigh block. *Anaesth Intensive Care* 1986;14:126–127.
- Cousins MJ, Bridenbaugh PO. Techniques of neural blockade. *Neural Blockade*, 3rd ed. Philadelphia, Lippincott-Raven, 1998.
- Henry G. Anatomy: Descriptive and surgical. In: Pick PT and Howden R (eds.). Portland House, New York, 1977.
- Hughes PJ, Brown TCK. An approach to posterior femoral cutaneous nerve block. *Anaesth Intensive Care* 1986;14:350–351.
- Kim V, Comfort F, Lang SA, Yip RW. Saphenous nerve anaesthesia—a nerve stimulator technique. *Can J Anaesth* 1996;43:852–857.
- Lieberman RP, Kaplan PA. Superficial peroneal nerve block for leg venography, *Radiology* 1987;165:578–579.
- Mansour NY. Sub-sartorial saphenous nerve block with the aid of nerve stimulator. *Reg Anesth* 1993;18:266–268.
- McNicol LR. Lower limb block for children. Anesthesia 1986;41:27–31.
- Mey JC, Deruyck LJ, Cammu G, De Baerdemaeker LE, Mortier EP. A paravenous approach for the saphenous nerve block. *Reg Anesth Pain Med* 2001;26:504–506.
- van der Wal M, Lang SA, Yip RW. Transsartorial approach for saphenous nerve block. *Can J Anaesth* 1993;40:542–546.
- Mussurakis S. Combined superficial peroneal and and saphenous nerve block for ascending venography. *Eur J Radiol* 1992:14:56–59.
- Vloka JD, Hadžić A, Mulcare R, Lesser JB, Koorn R, Thys DM. Combined popliteal and posterior cutaneous nerve of the thigh block for short saphenous vein stripping in outpatients: an alternative to spinal anesthesia. *J Clin Anesth* 1997;9:618–622.
- Wardrop PJ, Nishikawa H. Lateral cutaneous nerve of the thigh blockade as primary anaesthesia for harvesting skin grafts. *Br J Plast Surg* 1995;48:597–600

NOTE: Page numbers followed by f indicate figures; those followed by t indicate tables.

C

G

H

M